Reviewers

GALE CARLI, RN, BSN, MSN, MHED
Assistant Professor
Ohlone College
Fremont, California

JANICE HOFFMAN, RN, BSN, MSN, CCRN
Doctoral Candidate
University of Maryland–Baltimore School of Nursing
Baltimore, Maryland

SUSAN JUNAID, BSN, MSN
Assistant Professor of Nursing
Allen College
Waterloo, Iowa

To my parents
Bill and Jerry Becker
who always encouraged me
to reach for the stars.

To Royal Eaton, MD
who taught me to
listen
to my patients
and
never forget the basics.

Pamela Becker Weilitz

Preface

Health assessment is the process of gathering, verifying, analyzing, and communicating data about a client. The purpose of the initial assessment is to establish a database about the client's level of wellness, health practices, past illnesses, related experiences, and health care goals. The database is derived from a health history, physical examination, and laboratory and diagnostic test results. The information contained in the database is the basis for a client's individualized plan of care.

The *Pocket Guide to Health Assessment*, fifth edition, is a useful guide for performing physical examinations and health assessments in any type of clinical setting. The organization of the guide provides you with a quick reference when assessment focuses on a specific body system or when you conduct a complete physical examination.

Our intent is to make this book a valuable resource to the novice and the experienced examiner. The step-by-step assessment sections takes you through the skill, explaining the Normal and Abnormal Findings. As you become more competent in physical assessment, you will find the new Unexpected Findings section in each clinical chapter helpful. This section includes the finding, significance of the finding, and the next steps you need to take.

Features of the fifth edition guide include:
- The role of critical thinking and the nursing process in the health history and physical examination. A unique, three-column table in each chapter helps the nurse apply knowledge, experience, and standards as they assess clients.
- Summary of preparation for an examination.
- Step-by-step approach to body system assessment.
- Review of Normal and Abnormal Findings of the adult.
- Special insights to assessment methods.
- Nurse Alerts are highlighted in color for easy identification.
- Standard Precaution Alerts advise when to use protective garments.
- Delegation Considerations address the appropriate role of assistive personnel in health assessment.
- Special Gerontologic and Pediatric Considerations.

- Teaching Considerations.
- Cultural Variations alert the nurse to individual clients' preferences and pertinent assessment findings.
- Broadside, three-column format that lists the Area Assessed, Normal Findings, and Variations.
- Tables for Abnormal Findings, Significance, and Next Steps.

New features added in this edition:

- Three column critical thinking table in each clinical chapter to help the nurse apply knowledge, experience, and standards as they assess clients.
- History section stresses the importance of listening to the client during the interview process.
- Key steps bolded in text for quick reference and review.
- Unexpected Assessment Findings section in each chapter presents Abnormal Findings, Significance, and Next Step to alert nurse of dangers/warning signs and needed action.

With the addition of these features, this trusted resource is made even more practical and more user-friendly.

Patricia A. Potter

Pamela Becker Weilitz

Contents

Part II BODY SYSTEM ASSESSMENT

PRELIMINARY SKILLS

1

Critical Thinking and Nursing Judgment

Critical thinking is a complex cognitive process and the foundation of nursing practice. As a nurse, you use a scientific knowledge base, experience, clinical competencies, attitudes, and standards of care to analyze physical assessment data, draw a conclusion, and decide on a plan of nursing care. Clinical decision making is central to nursing practice and requires you to analyze and apply scientific medical and nursing knowledge (Boychuk Duchscher, 1999). Performing health assessment competently ensures that you will make accurate clinical decisions.

Components of Critical Thinking

- *Scientific Knowledge Base*—A knowledge base in nursing, the sciences, and humanities is necessary to think about nursing problems. A nurse caring for a client with low back pain will draw on knowledge from pain physiology, pathophysiology of neuromuscular skeletal injuries, pain relief, cultural considerations, and principles of psychology to accurately interpret the significance pain has for the client. This information will be used to determine the measures that will likely bring pain relief for the client.

- *Experience*—When you encounter a client, information is learned from observing, collecting data, collaborating and consulting with other providers, applying solutions, and evaluating the results. You reflect on the experience, developing a personal database of experiences. The expert nurse uses experience to understand the context of a clinical situation, recognize cues, and interpret them as relevant or irrelevant.

- *Competencies*—Competencies include 1) data collection, 2) hypothesis formation, 3) problem solving, 4) diagnostic reasoning, 5) clinical inferences, 6) clinical decision making, and 7) application of the nursing process. The nursing process gives you a systematic way of thinking through client problems. The nursing process requires you to use critical thinking throughout the assessment, nursing diagnosis, planning, implementation and evaluation. Skills you will develop include the ability to interpret, analyze, infer, and evaluate data.

- *Attitudes*—Central values of attitudes include confidence, independence, fairness, responsibility, risk taking, discipline, perseverance, creativity, curiosity, integrity, and humility. You cannot achieve the best results with a client without being fair in weighing the views of other practitioners, taking risks to generate new solutions to chronic problems, and demonstrating humility when knowledge about a problem is limited. Application of these attitudes ensures client assessment is well thought out and comprehensive.

- *Standards*—Intellectual and professional standards are applied to assist in arriving at the appropriate conclusions (Box 1-1). Intellectual standards are important in critical thinking because they provide a measure of how information is gathered, processed, and presented. Professional standards provide a framework for evaluation, ethical considerations, and your professional responsibilities. Standards are critical elements used to evaluate the client's care and outcomes.

For example, when assessing a client's pain, you obtain precise information from the client and clarify anything the client does not understand. Assess all characteristics of pain for a broad understanding. Assess the degree of pain using a pain scale 0-10, range of motion, and tenderness to palpation. Questions triggered by assessment findings are asked throughout the examination. Professional standards

BOX 1-1 Components of Critical Thinking in Nursing

I. Specific knowledge base in nursing
II. Experience in nursing
III. Critical thinking competencies
  A. General critical thinking competencies
  B. Specific critical thinking competencies
    in clinical situations
  C. Specific critical thinking competency in nursing
IV. Attitudes for critical thinking
  A. Confidence   G. Perseverance
  B. Independence H. Creativity
  C. Fairness   I. Curiosity
  D. Responsibility J. Integrity
  E. Risk taking   K. Humility
  F. Discipline

V. Standards for critical thinking
  A. Intellectual standards
    1. Clear   8. Logical
    2. Precise   9. Deep
    3. Specific   10. Broad
    4. Accurate 11. Complete
    5. Relevant 12. Significant
    6. Plausible 13. Adequate (for purpose)
    7. Consistent 14. Fair
  B. Professional standards
    1. Ethical criteria for nursing judgment
    2. Criteria for evaluation
    3. Professional responsibility

Modified from Kataoka-Yahiro M, Saylor C: A critical thinking model for nursing judgment, *J Nurs Educ* 33(8):351, 1994.
Data from Paul R: The art of redesigning instruction. In Willsen J, Blinker AJA, editors: *Critical thinking: how to prepare students for a rapidly changing world*, Santa Rosa, Calif, 1993, Foundation for Critical Thinking.

such as ethical criteria, clinical practice standards, and guidelines provide a framework for the assessment process and decision making with the use of critical thinking skills.

Application of Critical Thinking to Health Assessment

Critical thinking skills help in guiding health assessment and physical examination (Table 1-1). As a nurse, you must be responsible for conducting a detailed, well-focused exam. You perform the assessment by drawing on your scientific knowledge base, acknowledging the obvious and anticipating possible findings.

For example, when assessing the client with low back pain, you will require knowledge about potential pathophysiological causes of low back pain (ICSI, 1999). This knowledge will alert you to assess not only the character of the pain but also potential musculoskeletal and neurological changes. Your experience will be needed to help recognize physical findings, determine if they are normal or abnormal, and understand the common patterns of symptomatology. You will also recognize that each client is an individual, and each client experiences back pain in a unique way. You will need to apply critical thinking attitudes, such as curiosity and perseverance, when a client's clinical signs are subtle.

All physical measurements should be specific and precise (intellectual standard). Assess if the low back pain is localized or referred down one or both legs. Does movement aggravate the pain? If so, what type of movement? You will learn that a comprehensive pain assessment includes assessment of the client's functional abilities. You will integrate critical thinking competencies from a clinical perspective as well as from the nursing process approach. As a critical thinker, you will use diagnostic reasoning in making any ongoing assessments on the basis of a client's medical problem. The client's low back pain, if related to a herniated disk, will result in clinical signs, such as neurological findings of numbness, tingling, and reduction in muscle strength. In applying the nursing process, you consider how the client's response to pain affects lifestyle, occupation, and daily living activities. A thorough health assessment and physical examination will allow you to identify client problems appropriately and to select those nursing therapies designed to meet desired outcomes.

Table 1-1	Application of the Critical Thinking Model to Health Assessment and Physical Examination
Components of Critical Thinking	Health Assessment and Physical Examination Skills
Specific knowledge base	Understanding normal findings for each body system Understanding normal anatomy and physiology Recognition of variations in findings resulting from aging Knowledge of select pathologies and their related symptomatology
Experience	Familiarity with skills of physical examination (inspection, palpation, percussion, and auscultation) Recognition of client symptoms seen previously Ability to organize examination over time
Competencies	Collecting thorough nursing history Using general and appropriately focused examination techniques Forming accurate nursing diagnoses Evaluation of nursing care through reassessment of findings
Attitudes	Validating findings with another nurse when uncertain Using discipline in being sure examination is systematic and thorough
Standards Intellectual Professional	Applying criteria for symptom analysis Knowing "classic" signs and symptoms of abnormalities Identifying all characteristics of a symptom Telling the client results of the examination

Clinical Judgment in Nursing

Accurate clinical judgment requires a complete and thorough assessment, accurate diagnosis identification, and selection of appropriate therapies. A thorough health assessment and physical examination will include objective and subjective data from which recognizable patterns are formed. You will review and analyze the client's physical, developmental, intellectual, emotional, social, cultural, and spiritual health dimensions.

The subtle and overt signs and symptoms collected from a health history and physical examination provide cues or defining characteristics that lead to formulation of nursing diagnoses (Appendix A). Nursing diagnoses provide a language that enables all nurses to understand the client's health care alterations. A nursing diagnosis is a clinical judgment about individual, family, or community responses to actual and potential health problems and life processes (Gordon, 2000). A nursing diagnosis gives clear direction for you to select, along with the client, the outcomes and associated therapies for which you are accountable and licensed and

competent to implement. A nursing diagnosis has three essential components: the problem, the "related to" component or etiology, and defining characteristics or symptomatology (Gordon, 2000).

Problem: This is the health problem or status of an individual, family, or community. Problems such as pain, body image disturbance, or anxiety are short, clear, precise statements. Actual problems or problems for which the client may be at risk may be diagnosed.

Related to: Related or etiologic factors contribute to the existence or maintenance of a client's health problems. For example, pain may be related to reluctance to take pain medications or failure to follow activity restriction. Related factors may be either external or internal to the client. Identification of a related factor helps a nurse focus on the appropriate interventions for eventual elimination or management of the client's response to health problems. The diagnosis of pain suggests a variety of therapies. However, if a therapy is not selected on the basis of a client's diagnostic-related factor, it is less likely the client will gain pain relief.

Defining characteristics: The defining characteristics or objective and subjective findings validate the presence of a nursing diagnosis. It is a combination of signs and symptoms that reveal a client's health problems (Table 1-2). You use clinical reasoning to cluster the data and form the most appropriate nursing diagnoses.

Collaborative Problems

After you complete an assessment of a client, you may determine that other health care problems exist that are outside your independent scope of practice and that nursing therapies alone will not resolve. Health problems that require collaborative care are certain physiologic complications that a nurse

Table 1-2 Sample Nursing Diagnosis Statements

P Problem	E Etiologic Factors	S Symptomatology (Defining Characteristics)
Impaired skin integrity	Shearing force from positioning and immobilization	Disruption of skin surface Erythema of surrounding skin
Ineffective breathing pattern	Reduced lung expansion from postoperative pain	Shortness of breath Splinting with reduced excursion Tachypnea
Anticipatory grieving	Perceived loss of spouse from terminal illness	Expression of denial Alterations in sleep Expression of sorrow Loss of appetite

monitors to detect onset or changes in status and manages by implementing both physician-prescribed and nurse-prescribed interventions to minimize complications of the events. For example, a client with the medical diagnosis of coronary artery disease may have a collaborative problem such as "Potential complication: cardiac dysrhythmias." This diagnosis will require your ongoing monitoring, as well as actions to reduce any risk factors that might increase the incidence of the dysrhythmia. For example, you will avoid having the client undergo exertional care activities that might increase frequency of dysrhythmias. The same client may also have related nursing diagnoses such as "knowledge deficit regarding disease process related to newly diagnosed status" and "activity intolerance related to oxygen imbalance." There are independent measures you can implement for each nursing diagnosis. If you are able to prevent the onset of a complication, such as the development of a pressure ulcer, or provide primary treatment, such as exercises for an ineffective cough, then the diagnosis is not a collaborative problem. Table 1-3 outlines collaborative problems in comparison with nursing diagnoses.

You do not care for clients by yourself. A significant part of your practice is consultation and collaboration with other health care professionals such as physicians, dietitians, social workers, case managers, and physical therapists. Many times these professionals are comfortable with the nursing language and can collaborate on problems labeled as nursing diagnoses. Other times, professionals may wish to use language with which they are most familiar and to which you as the nurse can easily relate. For example, a problem familiar to the nurse as "activity intolerance" may be stated as "reduced cardiac reserve" by a physical therapist.

You will often serve as the leader of the health care team because of the independent nursing care that must be delivered and the nursing implications related to collaborative problems. Success in helping a client regain function or maintain existing function is best ensured when critical thinking and clinical judgment go hand in hand.

Table 1-3 Collaborative Problems and Nursing Diagnoses

Collaborative Problems	Nursing Diagnoses
Clinical scenario: A client is admitted through the emergency room with a diagnosis of closed head injury and cerebral contusion. At this time the client is unresponsive to verbal stimuli, the right pupil is dilated and slow to react to light, and the client withdraws the left side in response to pain. Glasgow coma scale is 10.	
Potential complication: increased intracranial pressure	Impaired physical mobility
	Tissue perfusion, altered cerebral
	Risk for impaired skin integrity
Clinical scenario: A client enters an acute care medical division with a medical diagnosis of acute lymphocytic leukemia. The client has a fever, pallor, fatigue, and anorexia with a recent 5-lb weight loss. Laboratory data reveal a reduced white blood cell count (neutropenia), reduced platelets (thrombocytopenia), and anemia.	
Potential complication: bleeding	Risk for infection
Potential complication: infection	Risk for activity intolerance
	Altered nutrition: less than body requirements
	Fatigue

Continued

Table 1-3   Collaborative Problems and Nursing Diagnoses—cont'd

Collaborative Problems	Nursing Diagnoses
Clinical scenario: A client comes to a community clinic with a 10-year history of rheumatoid arthritis. In the past 12 months the client's condition has worsened, with symptoms of increasing fatigue, weight loss, and increased pain and stiffness of the hands. Joint range of motion of hands and fingers is making performance of activities of daily living more difficult. The client is placed on steroid therapy for 4 weeks, along with methotrexate.	
Potential complication: systemic inflammation	Pain
Potential complication: joint deformity	Impaired physical mobility
	Fatigue
	Altered nutrition: less than body requirements
	Self-care deficit

2

Nursing Health History and Interview Process

From the moment you first meet a client, you learn to exhibit a sense of caring and respect that wins trust from the client. When successful, the relationship that forms between you and the client enables you to discover information about the client's health status, collaborate with the client on a health care plan, and initiate therapies that maintain and/or improve the client's health.

Health History

In today's complex health care environment, nurses must be able to solve problems accurately, thoroughly, and quickly.

This means that you must be able to review a tremendous amount of information to critically think and make the correct judgments (Potter and Perry, 2001). Your nursing assessment includes collection of data from a primary source (the client) and secondary sources (family member, domestic partner, significant other, and friends) initially in the form of a nursing history. The nursing health history is a client's subjective account of current and past health status and alerts you to key areas that the physical examination must later cover.

The nursing health history can take many forms. Health care settings will design health history and assessment tools to facilitate the collection of histories quickly and easily. The forms usually are designed on the basis of a particular model or framework, which helps to conceptualize the health setting's standards for practice. A form that uses a nursing model helps to conceptualize the scope of nursing practice. Regardless of the model, the history form requires you to collect information thought to be most important in assessing a client's needs. A nursing history form serves as a guideline only. You decide what and how much information needs to be collected.

The nursing assessment must include data that either supports existence of a problem or demonstrates absence of a problem. In other words, data must be relevant. Therefore, you must know what to assess in terms of subjective and objective data. You will use a series of routine questions for each client. You must then have the ability to critically think and know what direction assessment must take based on the client's presenting history, physical signs, culture, and known physiologic or psychological problems.

Clinical situations offer you the opportunity to either conduct a focused overview of a client's condition or collect a comprehensive database about the client's health. When you first meet a client, an overview includes a brief series of questions aimed toward the client or family member and the mea-

surement of specific physical findings. This overview will usually be based on the client's immediate presenting symptoms or the treatment situation. For example, an emergency room nurse uses the A-B-C (airway-breathing-circulation) approach; a psychiatric nurse may focus on the delirious client's reality, anxiety level, and violence potential; and a nurse in a primary care clinic may focus on the client's health maintenance. Once you conclude the focused interview, use cues to direct an intense focused assessment. You will interpret the cues to determine how indepth the assessment should be.

A comprehensive database can provide a more complete view of a client's health status. Data are collected for a client within a variety of established categories. A structured comprehensive database moves from the general to the specific. A comprehensive assessment covers all potential health problem areas. As data begins to reveal a problem or strength in a particular area, you can then choose to expand the assessment to analyze the client's situation thoroughly.

The problem-oriented approach focuses on the client's current situation. The problem-oriented approach to assessment begins with problematic areas, such as pain, and spreads out to relevant areas of the client's life. The pain assessment will begin with a review of the nature of the pain itself and then broaden to include data such as the effect of pain on mobility, lifestyle, and family relationships. Once completed, the problem of pain will be thoroughly analyzed to develop a plan of care to manage the client's pain.

Models for a Health History

Most medical models used in obtaining a health history include a comprehensive interview for an initial encounter. Although this model is referred to as a medical model, the nurse will find the data valuable. Many health care settings develop health history forms that are a combination of nursing and medical models.

Nursing models for a health history may be based on a framework of nursing theory or nursing diagnoses. One common model used for data collection is Gordon's Functional Health Patterns (Gordon, 1994). Health care organizations that use Gordon's model develop their nursing history forms based on functional health patterns. Models provide a framework for organizing the nursing history. The nursing assessment form may also be organized by body system, nursing diagnoses, or defined wellness patterns that are useful to the facility and nurses. The nursing health history usually includes physiologic, psychologic, psychosocial, cultural, and environmental factors affecting the client's health. The history often includes the family and com-

munity as well. Many nursing health histories are designed to complement the medical health history to reduce duplication and lessen the burden of data gathering on the client.

Adult Health History

Table 2-1 summarizes the major areas of an adult health history. The rationale explains the importance that information in each category plays in developing a clear picture of a client's health status. The assessment tips include tips on technique and offer examples of assessment questions. As the nurse, you must decide how indepth to question the client based on their responses.

You will collect historical information directly from the client, family member, domestic partner, or significant other. If available, a previous medical record may be useful to complete the database. Special considerations for obtaining the health history are found in Box 2-1.

Interview

The collection of an appropriate and thorough health history requires you to gather subjective information through a pattern of communication initiated for a specific purpose and focused

Text continued on p. 24

Table 2-1 Adult Health History

Data	Rationale	Assessment Tips
Biographic Information		
• Name, age, date of birth, sex.	• Provides a quick reference for information.	• What is your name?
• Race, ethnic origin.	• Allows a health care provider to identify the client.	• When were you born?
• Living arrangements, marital status.	• Allows health care provider to make contact with the client and appropriate caregivers.	• Do you live with your spouse, domestic partner, significant other, extended family, alone?
• Address, home and work telephone number.	• Information will influence how you interpret physical examination findings collected later.	• Is your address and telephone number correct?
• Employment status, occupation.		• Are you currently working? If so, tell me a little bit about what you do.
• Person to notify in an emergency and telephone numbers.		• Whom do you want notified about illness/hospitalization?
• Religious preference.		• Do you have a religious preference?

Reason for Seeking Health Care (Chief Complaint)

- In the client's own words, describe the reason for the visit.
- Identify client expectations.

- Often can be very useful in focusing and directing the nursing history and physical examination.
- Caution must be used if the client is a poor historian.

- What brings you in today? What do you want to see the doctor about today?
- What do you expect to happen today?
- What do you want to discuss today?

Present Health History (History of Present Illness)

- Overview of reason client is seeking health care.
- Chronologic signs and symptoms, beginning with onset of problem and end with present day.

- Starting point to begin H & P.
- Gives a complete view of principal symptoms and complaint.
- Symptoms may represent potential problems in specific or functional areas.

- Describe your symptoms. When did they start?
- Include severity, onset, duration, frequency, setting, and/or situation when symptoms occur.
- What makes your symptoms better?
- What makes your symptoms worse?
- Perform a focused assessment on the area of concern.

Continued

Nursing Health History and Interview Process **17**

Table 2-1 Adult Health History—cont'd

Data	Rationale	Assessment Tips
Past Health History • Overview of any past medical history or surgeries, any known drug or food allergies. • Current medications. • Immunizations. • Recent visits to other health care providers.	• Information from the past health history often can immediately explain the related cause for the client's symptoms. • Put together information, referring to past experiences. • A list of current medications can provide an indication of current and past medical conditions, especially if the client is a poor historian. • Information is useful in assessing the client's health promotion activities. • Provides information about the client's history and how client cares for self.	• Do you have any chronic illnesses (e.g., heart disease, lung disease, cancer, diabetes, Tuberculosis (TB)? • Have you ever had surgery? What type? When? • Have you had any accidents or injuries? • Can you remember your childhood illnesses (measles, mumps, rubella, chickenpox, whooping cough [pertussis], strep throat, rheumatic fever, scarlet fever, poliomyelitis)? • Are you allergic to any medications or foods? What kind of reaction do you have? • What are your current medications? • Are you taking any over-the-counter medications, herbal therapies, or vitamins? • Do you use cocaine, marijuana, street drugs, or overuse prescription medications? (See Box 2-2.) • Do you have your childhood immunizations record?

- When was your last influenza or pneumococcal vaccine, tetanus immunization, and TB skin test?
- Have you had Hepatitis A or B series vaccine?
- When did you last see your primary care physician, dentist, and optometrist/ophthalmologist?

Nutritional Assessment

- 24-hour diet recall.

- Provides a snapshot of dietary habits.

- What did you eat yesterday?
- Was yesterday a typical day?
- What dietary supplements do you take?
- Do you take any appetite suppressants or stimulants?

Woman's Health History

Overview of obstetrics and gynecological history. Includes:
- Pregnancies.
- Births.
- Menstrual history.
- Well woman maintenance.

- Information gives complete woman's health status.
- Provides opportunity to discuss safe sex, contraception, and sexual problems.

- At what age did your menarche (onset of menstruation) begin?
- How frequently do your menstrual periods occur?
- When was your last menstrual period?
- Have you had any excessive bleeding, cramps, or irregularity during your menstrual cycle?
- Have you had a hysterectomy? Why? When?

Continued

Table 2-1 Adult Health History—cont'd

Data	Rationale	Assessment Tips
Woman's Health History—cont'd • Mammograms. • Breast self-examination.	• Provides opportunity to teach women's health promotion, maintenance, and prevention.	• How many times have you been pregnant? Any miscarriages or abortions? • How many deliveries occurred in which the fetus reached viability (after 20 weeks)? • What is your current method of contraception? • What is your current plan for safe sexual practice? • When was your last PAP smear? Have you ever had an abnormal PAP? When? Results? • Do you perform monthly breast self-examination? Are you currently concerned about any lumps? • When was your last mammogram? • Did your mother use DES or any other medication while pregnant? • Do you have any history of sexually transmitted diseases? • Do you have any history of chronic vaginal infections? • Do you practice safe sex? What percentage of the time?

Man's Health History

Overview of health maintenance and promotion. Includes:
- Testicular self-examination.
- Prostate-specific antigen (PSA) testing.
- Sexually transmitted diseases.

- Provides baseline for ongoing evaluation.
- Information gives complete man's health status.
- Provides opportunity to discuss safe sex, contraception, and sexual problems.
- Provides opportunity to teach health promotion, maintenance, and prevention.

- Do you perform testicular self-examination?
- Have you had a PSA test? What was the PSA level? When was your last level drawn?
- Have you ever had a sexually transmitted disease?
- Do you practice safe sex? What percentage of the time?

Family History

Includes:
- Health status of the immediate family and living blood relatives.
- Cause of death of blood relatives.

- Can reveal risk factors for major illnesses such as alcoholism, arthritis, cancer, heart disease, diabetes mellitus, hypertension, sickle cell disease, and mental disorders.

- Have any of your family members had heart disease, cancer, stroke, high blood pressure, diabetes, sickle cell disease, TB, or kidney disease?
- If so, who?
- Do any family members have illnesses similar to the client's illness?

Continued

Table 2-1 Adult Health History—cont'd

Data	Rationale	Assessment Tips
	• The client's presenting signs and symptoms could be the first sign of a serious illness.	• Has any family member suffered from a mental illness? • What was the cause of death of each of your parents? • How old were they at the time of their deaths? • If there is a hereditary disease, assess both sides of the client's family for at least two generations.
Environmental History Review environment where client lives and works. Determine whether client: • Lives or works around pollutants or hazardous wastes and chemicals. • Is exposed to noise or physical safety risks.	• Can be at risk for a variety of chronic diseases as a result of exposure to pollutants and hazardous materials. • Chronic exposure to loud noise can cause hearing problems. • Failure to use safety equipment during work and recreation will reveal additional risks.	• Are you exposed to any sources of pollution or hazardous wastes where you live? At the workplace? • When you participate in sports or hobbies, do you wear protective equipment (e.g., helmet and safety glasses)? • Are you exposed to extremely loud noise at home or work? Do you wear earplugs?

BOX 2-1 Special Considerations for Collecting a Nursing History

- Assessment data sources include the client, family or significant other, health team members, and the client's health record.
- Do not allow interruptions to occur during the interview. Data collected on the nursing history tool are subjective; do not challenge this information but explore it with the client to clarify any vagueness.
- When the client is critically ill, disoriented, confused, mentally handicapped, or very young, the family, domestic partner, significant other, or previously recorded health histories are necessary sources of information for the nursing history.
- Clients with physical or emotional handicaps require an assessment approach that adapts to their needs.

- The client must be involved even if mental or physical limitations prevent full discussion and participation.
- Family members, domestic partner, significant other, and friends can be useful resources, but do not allow them to make decisions for the client when the client is capable of doing so independently.
- Family members may know tips on how to make the client comfortable or how to communicate more effectively with the client.
- Deaf clients often read, write, or read lips. Blind clients can usually hear; talking louder is unnecessary.
- Review previous medical records to help with clarification or prior medical and nursing problems.

on a specific content area. During a health history you use therapeutic communication skills to learn not only about the client's level of wellness but also about issues that can often be of a sensitive nature (Table 2-2, Box 2-3). You also help the client to understand changes that are occurring or will occur in life based on the client's illness or potential health problem.

All information shared by the client must be kept confidential. Careful word choice, professional behavior, direct eye contact, and a nonjudgmental attitude will help put the client at ease and make the client feel comfortable sharing important but sometimes embarrassing information. You need to be able to show an understanding of the client's intellectual and emotional needs before the client is willing to discuss important issues about his or her health.

You prepare for the health history interview by reviewing available information about the client in the medical record before meeting with the client. This may include demographic data and a client-completed health assessment. If you have seen the client previously or are familiar with the client's situation, review the literature related to the client's health problem before the interview. Conduct the interview in a comfortable, quiet, private setting when possible. In the outpa-

---

BOX 2-2   Red Flags for Suspicion of Substance Abuse

Frequently missed appointments
Frequent requests for work excuses
Frequent requests for controlled substances
Vague complaints of pain, insomnia, anxiety, "nerves"
Lost prescriptions for controlled substances
Frequent emergency room visits
Use of multiple pharmacies
Frequent changes of doctors
Calls made after office hours to get controlled substances from on-call physician
Client wears long-sleeved shirt and long pants in hot weather
Family history of addiction

Table 2-2 Interviewing Techniques

Technique	Description	Examples
Problem solving	• Focuses on gathering indepth data on specific problems identified by the client or obvious to the nurse.	• It looks like you are having trouble walking. • What activities are associated with your chest pain?
Direct questions	• Ask for specific information. • Often clarify previous information or offer additional data. • Do not encourage more information than requested. • Can be answered with short answers or *Yes* or *No*. • Useful in gathering biographic information or in dealing with a rambling historian.	• How long have you been diagnosed with hypertension? • Do you have pain every day? • When did you start on lipid-lowering medications?
Open-ended questions	• Aimed at obtaining a response of more than one or two words. • Lead to clients actively describing their health status.	• Tell me about the pain you are having. • Describe how you have been feeling.

tient setting, the client remains in street clothes until the health history is completed to enhance client comfort and put you and the client on a similar social level.

One additional step in preparation is to know oneself (Seidel et al, 1999). You should understand what you bring to an interaction. Do you have any preexisting biases about the client or the client's diagnosis? Are you angry over reasons that are unrelated to the client but are difficult to control? Are you overzealous in wanting to be liked by the client? Are you afraid of doing harm? Are you worried about "catching something?" You need to be aware of past experiences and personal emotions and thoughts. Displacement of anger or nonverbal expressions of disapproval can destroy a client relationship.

Begin the interview by addressing the client formally, such as "Mr. Ruiz," or "Mrs. Chan." Allow clients to tell you how they would like to be addressed. Then introduce yourself in the manner in which you wish to be addressed. Extend your hand for a handshake in the customary greeting of the United States. Be aware of cultural differences, especially where touch is concerned (Table 2-3). Both you and the client should be seated comfortably, within a comfortable distance of one another. Take cues from the client. If you are seated too close, the client may lean backward or shift position in the chair frequently.

BOX 2-3   Approaching Sensitive Issues

Topics such as death, sexual practices or preferences, drug or alcohol use, and history of abuse can be uncomfortable for the client and you. Seidel et al (1999) recommend the following tips:

- Privacy is essential.
- Do not waffle; be direct and firm.
- Do not apologize for asking a question.
- Do not pass judgment.
- Be patient.
- Give the client time to respond to your questions.
- Do not push too hard.
- If the client is defensive, proceed slowly.
- Show respect for the client's feelings, beliefs, and practices.
- Avoid "Why" questions.

Table 2-3 Cross-Cultural Variations in Clients' Response to Touch	
Nation of Origin	Space
Asian	Noncontact people (however, Japanese require less personal space)
China	
Hawaii	
Philippines	
Korea	
Japan	
Southeast Asia	
African	Close personal space
West coast (as slaves)	
African countries	
West Indian Islands	
Dominican Republic	
Haiti	
Jamaica	

Continued

Table 2-3 Cross-Cultural Variations in Clients' Response to Touch—cont'd

Nation of Origin	Space
European	
Germany	Noncontact people: aloof; distant
England	Southern countries: closer contact and touch
Italy	
Ireland	
Other European countries	
Native American	Space very important and has no boundaries
170 Native-American tribes	
Aleuts	
Eskimos	
Hispanic countries	Tactile relationships: touch; handshakes; embracing
Spain	
Cuba	Value physical presence
Mexico	
Central and South America	
Arabic countries	Require less personal space; common to touch persons of same sex

Modified from Giger JN, Davidhizar RE: *Transcultural nursing: assessment and intervention*, ed 3, St Louis, 1999, Mosby.

Explain to the client the purpose of the visit, the history and physical examination process, and the approximate length of time the interview and physical examination will last. Assure the client regarding confidentiality of information. Your professional approach evokes the client's trust. This is particularly important if you are to learn about a client's motivations, strengths, and resources. You help the client resolve any anxiety, feelings of helplessness, and concerns about the personal nature of information to be shared.

Focus the interview on the client's health dimensions, using a model that forms a database for eventual nursing diagnosis identification. Use interviewing skills to clarify and validate information so that appropriate clinical problem solving takes place. Health history information is later confirmed by findings from the physical examination. Work closely with the client to identify problems and select goals of care.

Close the interview by summarizing information collected. Validate problems, nursing diagnoses, and goals of care with the client. Explain how additional contact will be made with the client, including preparation for the physical assessment. Give a client an idea of when the interview will end; for example, "We will finish in about 5 minutes." Thus the client can maintain attention without wondering when the interview will end.

Basic Communication Strategies

- *Silence*—Communicates to the client that he or she has time to organize thoughts and present complete information without interruption. During this time, observe any nonverbal behavior, positioning, physical deformities, or limitations.

- *Attentive Listening*—Shows your interest and concern and helps ensure that accurate data are collected. Notice client's posturing, body movement, and voice tone while you listen to what client says.

- *Conveying Acceptance*—Communicates a willingness to listen nonjudgmentally. EXAMPLES: Sitting at eye level with the client, assuming a comfortable and open posture, and using good eye contact.

- *Related Questions*—Focuses the interview on particular health issues or body systems to prevent rambling. For example, the client might report, "I have had this pain in my stomach for so long, it just never seems to go away." A related question might be, "Tell me specifically what you were doing when the pain began."

- *Paraphrasing*—Restates what you have heard the client communicate. Paraphrasing validates in more specific terms what the client has said and lets the client know if you understand the message. For example, the client might say, "I guess this illness will be a problem for my family. I have been able to live by myself for a long time. I'm worried about what I will be able to do for myself. My daughter has talked about me moving to Arizona with her." You may paraphrase, "Let me see if I understand. You are concerned as to how your illness will limit your ability to live alone. You feel your family may want you to live with them?"

- *Clarifying*—Ask the client to restate information in more specific or different terms when the client's word choice is confusing. Clarifying helps you understand the client's intended message better. Having the client give examples to clarify meaning is very helpful. For example, the client might report, "I seem to notice a twinge in my back whenever I try to sleep on my side or I notice it when I dress in the morning." Your clarifying remark might be, "Now tell me what part of your back is affected. Are you saying your back hurts whenever you turn or rotate your body?"

- *Focusing*—Helps eliminate vagueness in communication by asking follow-up questions, requesting the client to be more complete with data. Point to inconsistencies in

statements. For example, you might say, "Now you told me that you have difficulty sleeping at night. Let's be specific; are you having difficulty falling asleep, reawakening, or both?"

- *Stating Observations*—Gives client feedback and encourages the client to offer additional pertinent information. EXAMPLE: "You seem to be holding your right arm still when you move in that direction."

- *Confronting*—A constructive approach informing a client what you think or feel about a behavior, feeling, or statement that the client has communicated during the interaction. You may describe the client's visible behavior, using responses aimed at understanding and using constructive feedback. This skill focuses on your perception of a client's overt or subtle behavior. For example, "You look nervous; would you like to talk about it?" or "You said your knee does not hurt, but when I palpated it you winced."

- *Giving Feedback*—Gives client information about what you observe or deduce. Effective feedback focuses on:

  Behavior rather than on the client
  Observations rather than inferences
  Description rather than judgment

Exploration of alternatives rather than answers or solutions

Its value to the client rather than catharsis it provides the nurse

What is said rather than why it is said

EXAMPLE: "As I watch you now, you are able to prepare the medication much more quickly in the syringe. Plus, you did not contaminate the needle."

- *Offering Information*—Information offered should not be mistaken for advice. Similarly, if you share personal information, the interaction may no longer be therapeutic. EXAMPLE: "When you have a cataract, it is normal to have a reduction in depth perception. It can be difficult to make out the edges of stairs, for example."

- *Summarizing*—Highlights the main ideas of any interview or discussion. Summarizing validates data from the client and signals the end of one part of the interview before continuing with the next part. EXAMPLE: "Let me quickly review what you have shared. You want to start an exercise plan to help manage the stress you have been feeling at work and to help you better control your weight. You prefer swimming and walking. Your husband wants to exercise with you as well.

Setting up a daily schedule would help you plan time for exercise."

 Cultural Phenomena Influencing Health Assessment

A client's cultural heritage presents the need for a unique approach to health assessment and physical examination. Giger and Davidhizer (1999) provide an excellent model for assessing clients from multicultural backgrounds (see Appendix B). Their model includes six important variables to incorporate in any interaction with a client: communication, space, social organization, time, environmental control, and biologic variation. Each factor influences how to approach a physical examination. For example, you must understand the importance of nonverbal communication and use of silence in different cultures. Do not assume they are indicative of a physiologic or psychological abnormality. Touch is an important skill to use during palpation and may not be well received by clients from a variety of cultures (Table 2-3). A client's comfort with you will be influenced by the space you maintain with the client. If you make biased assumptions about a client's social organization and the type of familial support that should be present, the nursing history may be inaccurate.

 Pediatric Considerations

- Routine examinations of children have a focus on illness prevention, particularly for care of well children with competent parenting and no serious health problems (Wong, 1999). The focus is on growth and development, sensory screening, dental examination, and behavioral assessment.

- Children who are chronically ill, disabled, foster children, or foreign-born adopted may require additional examination visits.

- When obtaining histories for infants and children, gather all or part of the information from the parent or guardian. Institutions that provide health care services for children will have specially adapted assessment forms.

- Parents often think the interviewer is testing them. Offer support and do not pass judgment:

  - Use first names with children and last names with parents (unless parents prefer otherwise).

- If a young child becomes restless or uncooperative, divide the assessment into two sessions. Use of a toy, as well as the presence of parents, may have a calming effect.

- Interviewing children in the presence of parents or guardians allows you to observe parent-child interactions. Children are often unable to express their feelings and tend to act out their problems instead.

- Children who experience a traumatic event, such as loss of a parent, a pet, or close friend, may experience an acute episode of depression.

- Children with psychosocial problems may have difficulty at school.

- Adolescents tend to respond best when treated as adults and individuals. Ask adolescents how they prefer to be addressed (for example, "Billy" or "Mr. Smith").

- Parents' reliability in providing a health history can vary. Concrete facts such as birth weight and birth date tend to be recalled most accurately; minor illnesses tend to be forgotten more easily than major ones; parents of several children tend to be less accurate in their recall of most items than are parents of single children; and the parents' educational level is directly related to the accuracy of recall for some data, such as immunizations.

Gerontologic Considerations

- In addition to the basic components of a health history, assess the following categories with an older adult: functional, cognitive, affective, and social well-being (Lueckenotte, 2000).
- Older adults often have lengthy and complicated histories. It is important to stay focused and help the client share pertinent information.
- Do not stereotype aging clients. They are able to adapt to change and learn about their health.
- Sensory or physical limitations (especially hearing or visual impairments) can affect how long you can inter-

view and assess an older client. Plan for more than one encounter to complete the examination. Be sensitive to the older client's sense of fatigue (Lueckenotte, 1999).

- Clients may find that giving certain types of health information is stressful; they may not discuss change or problems confirming their fear of illness or old age.
- Data provided depend on what the older adult feels is important at the time.
- Touch is often well accepted by older adults (Lueckenotte, 2000). Use touch with respect and sensitivity.
- Explanations and rationales of what you are doing are very important to the older adult who may not hear or see clearly.

Physical Assessment Skills

3

The four basic skills used during a physical examination are inspection, palpation, percussion, and auscultation. The specific uses of these skills are outlined in the assessment sections for the different body systems. In addition, olfaction is an important skill you will use throughout an examination. You will detect and analyze the nature and source of odors associated with bodily alterations (Table 3-1). The following sections summarize general principles for the use of the basic physical assessment skills.

Technique	Knowledge	Competency
Inspection		
• The process of observation. It is a visual examination of body parts to detect normal characteristics or significant physical variations.	• Know normal physical characteristics of clients of all ages before trying to distinguish abnormal findings. Experience helps you to recognize normal variations among clients.	• Learn to make several observations at once, while becoming perceptive of early warnings of abnormalities.
		• Be thorough and systematic in inspecting every body part. If hurried,

- Variations among clients exist, as well as ranges of normal in an individual.

- Experience is needed to distinguish abnormal findings.

- Learn to make several observations at the same time, while becoming perceptive of early warning of abnormalities.

- you may overlook significant findings or make incorrect conclusions about a client's condition.

- Good lighting and exposure of body parts are essential for careful inspection.

- Inspect each area for size, shape, color, symmetry, position, and the presence of any abnormalities.

- Compare each area with the same area on the opposite side of the body.

- Pay attention to detail.

- Inspection is a visual skill, but you should also include olfaction. The sense of smell can sometimes detect abnormalities that may not be recognized by other means.

- Ask a colleague to confirm findings if you are unsure about an odor.

Technique	Knowledge	Competency
Palpation • Palpation involves use of the sense of touch. The hands can make delicate and sensitive measurements of specific physical signs, including temperature, moisture, texture, mobility, and resilience.	• Use palpation with or after visual inspection. (The only exception to this is after inspection of the abdomen (see Chapter 16.) This allows you to focus on any abnormalities noted during inspection. • Know the normal location of body organs. • Experience will improve your ability to detect subtle differences in qualities such as texture, temperature, and resistance.	• Use different parts of the hand to detect characteristics (e.g., texture, shape, temperature, perception of vibration, or movement and consistency) (Fig. 3-1). • Be sure client is relaxed and positioned comfortably to avoid muscle tension that may distort palpation findings. • Have the client take slow, deep breaths to enhance muscle relaxation. • Palpate any suspected area of tenderness last.

Table 3-1	Assessment of Characteristic Odors	
Odor	Site or Source	Potential Causes
Alcohol	Oral cavity	Ingestion of alcohol; diabetes
Ammonia	Urine	Urinary tract infection
Body odor	Skin, particularly in areas where body parts rub together (e.g., under arms, breasts)	Poor hygiene, excess perspiration (hyperhidrosis), foul-smelling perspiration (bromidrosis)
Feces	Wound site	Wound abscess
	Vomitus	Bowel obstruction
	Rectal area	Fecal incontinence
Foul-smelling stools in infant	Stool	Malabsorption syndrome
Halitosis	Oral cavity	Poor dental and oral hygiene, gum disease
Sweet, fruity ketones	Oral cavity	Diabetic acidosis
Stale urine		Uremic acidosis
Sweet, heavy, thick odor	Skin	*Pseudomonas* (bacterial) infection
	Draining wound	
Musty odor	Casted body part	Infection inside cast
Fetid, sweet odor	Tracheostomy or mucous secretions	Infection of bronchial tree (*Pseudomonas* bacteria)

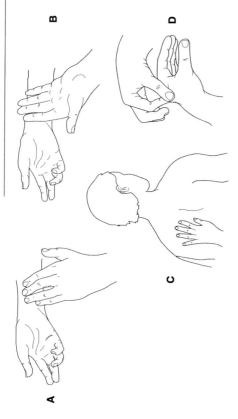

Fig. 3-1
A, Fingertips are the most sensitive parts of the hand; used to assess texture, shape, size, and consistency. **B**, Dorsum or back of hand used to assess temperature. **C**, Palm of hand used to assess vibration. **D**, Grasp the skin with fingertips to assess turgor.

Technique	Knowledge	Competency
		• Have the client point out more sensitive areas and note any nonverbal signs of discomfort.
		• Keep fingernails short, warm hands before touching client, and use a gentle approach.
		• Always use light palpation before deep palpation.
		• Apply tactile pressure in a slow, gentle, deliberate manner.
		• The sensation of touch is best preserved with light, intermittent pressure.
		• Any tender areas should be examined further, because tenderness may reveal a serious abnormality.
		• Methods of palpation include the following (Fig. 3-2):

Technique	Knowledge	Competency
		• *Light palpation*—used to examine superficial abnormalities. Fingers are gently applied over the skin surface; fingers depress the skin about 1 cm (1/2 inch).

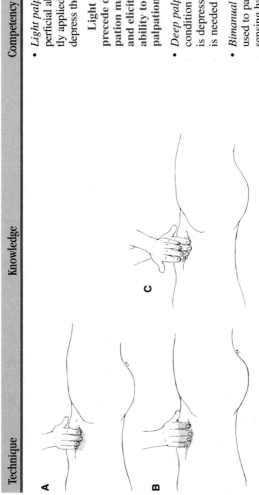

Fig. 3-2
Three techniques of palpation. **A,** Light palpation.
B, Deep palpation. **C,** Bimanual palpation.

Light palpation should always precede deep palpation. Deep palpation may disrupt fluid or tissue and elicit tenderness, limiting your ability to gather data with light palpation (Seidel et al, 1999).

• *Deep palpation*—used to examine the condition of organs and masses; skin is depressed 2.5 cm (1 inch). Caution is needed to prevent internal injury.

• *Bimanual palpation*—both hands are used to palpate deeply; one hand (the sensing hand) is relaxed and placed lightly on the client's skin. The active hand applies pressure to the sensing hand. The lower sensing hand remains sensitive to detect organ characteristics.

- Palpation techniques depend on the body area being examined and the client's condition. For example, when there is risk of a fractured rib, palpate with extreme care; when palpating an artery, avoid applying pressure that may obstruct the blood flow.

- Characteristics measured by palpation in major body areas are found in Box 3-1.

- Table 3-2 describes the five basic percussion sounds, the sites at which they are normally heard, and the sound characteristics to assess.

- *Direct method of percussion:* The body surface is struck directly with one or two fingertips.

Percussion

- Percussion involves tapping the body with the fingertips to evaluate the size, borders, and consistency of organs and to discover fluid in body cavities. Percussion determines the location, size, and density of underlying structures to verify abnormalities assessed by palpation and auscultation.

- Know the location of body organs in relation to typical anatomic landmarks such as the costal margin, umbilical area, and costovertebral angle.

- Much experience is needed to become competent at percussion.

BOX 3-1   Exercises to Increase Familiarity With Stethoscope

1. Place earpieces in both ears with tips of earpieces turned toward the face. *Lightly* blow into the stethoscope's diaphragm. Again place earpieces in both ears, this time with ends turned toward the back of the head. *Lightly* blow into the stethoscope's diaphragm. The earpiece should follow the contour of the ear canal. After learning the right fit for the loudest sound, wear the stethoscope the same way each time.

2. Put the stethoscope on and *lightly blow* into the diaphragm. If sound is barely audible, *lightly* blow into the bell. Sound is carried through only one part of the chestpiece at a time. If sound is greatly amplified through the diaphragm, the diaphragm is in position for use. If sound is barely audible through the diaphragm, the bell is in position for use.

3. Listen while moving the diaphragm lightly over the hair on your arm. The bristling sound created by rubbing of hair against the diaphragm mimics a sound heard in the lungs. Also, always be sure to keep the diaphragm stationary and firm to reduce extraneous sounds.

4. Place the stethoscope on and gently tap tubing. The sound can distract from being able to hear sounds created by body organs. Always avoid stretching or moving the tubing; it should hang freely.

Table 3-2 Sounds Produced by Percussion

Sound	Intensity	Pitch	Duration	Quality	Common Location
Tympany	Loud	High	Moderate	Drumlike	Enclosed, air-containing space; gastric air bubble, puffed-out cheek
Resonance	Moderate to loud	Low	Long	Hollow	Normal lung
Hyperresonance	Very loud	Very low	Longer than resonance	Booming	Emphysematous lung
Dullness	Soft to moderate	High	Moderate	Thudlike	Liver
Flatness	Soft	High	Short	Flat	Muscle

Technique	Knowledge	Competency
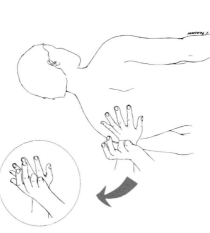		• *Indirect method of percussion:* The middle finger of the nondominant hand (pleximeter) is placed firmly against the body surface (Fig. 3-3). With palm and fingers staying off the skin, the tip of the middle finger of the dominant hand (plexor) strikes the base of the distal joint of the pleximeter. Use a quick, sharp stroke with the plexor finger, keeping the forearm stationary. Keep the wrist relaxed. Once the finger has struck, the wrist snaps back. A light, quick blow produces the clearest sounds. • Apply the same force at each area of the body to make an accurate comparison of sounds produced by percussion.

Fig. 3-3
Technique for performing indirect percussion.

- If the blow is not sharp, if the pleximeter hand is held loosely, or if the palm rests on the body surface, the sound is dampened or softened, preventing detection of underlying structures.

Auscultation

- Auscultation is listening to sounds produced by the body. Some sounds can be heard with the unaided ear, although most sounds are heard only through the stethoscope.

- Know normal sounds created by the body (e.g., passage of blood through an artery, bowel sounds, heart sounds).

- Be aware of the location in which sounds can be most easily heard.

- Experience will help you learn what areas normally do not emit sounds.

- Listen in a quiet environment.

- Listen for the presence of sound, as well as its characteristics.

- Be sure the earpieces of the stethoscope fit snugly and comfortably, with the binaurals angled and the earpieces following the contour of the ear canal (usually the earpieces are pointed toward the face).

- Rubber or plastic tubing of the stethoscope should be flexible and only 30 to 40 cm (12 to 18 inches) in length for best sound transmission.

Technique	Knowledge	Competency
		• If you have a hearing disorder, use a stethoscope with greater amplification or ask colleagues to validate findings.
		• Always place either the diaphragm or bell of the stethoscope on bare skin, because clothing obscures sound.
		• Use the stethoscope bell for low-pitched sounds such as abnormal heart and vascular sounds.
		• Use the diaphragm for high-pitched sounds such as bowel, lung, and normal heart sounds.
		• To assess deviations from normal, you should consider the origin and cause of the sound, the exact site at which the sound is heard best, and the expected normal qualities of the sound.
		• Through auscultation note four characteristics of sound (Table 3-3) (Box 3-1).

Table 3-3 Characteristics of Sound

Characteristic	Description
Frequency	Number of sound wave cycles generated per second by a vibrating object. The higher the frequency, the higher the pitch of a sound and vice versa.
Loudness	Amplitude of a sound wave. Auscultated sounds are described as *loud* or *soft*.
Quality	Sounds of similar frequency and loudness from different sources. Terms such as *blowing* or *gurgling* describe quality of sound.
Duration	Length of time sound vibrations last. Duration of sound is *short*, *medium*, or *long*.

Preparation for the Examination

Proper preparation of the environment, equipment, and client ensures a smooth physical examination with few interruptions. A disorganized approach when preparing for a physical examination can cause errors and incomplete findings.

Preparing for the Examination

Environment	Equipment	Physical Preparation of Client
• Ensure privacy for the client.	• Wash hands thoroughly before preparing equipment for the examination.	• Ensure the client's physical comfort before starting the examination.

Environment	Equipment	Physical Preparation of Client
• Conduct the examination in a well-equipped room if possible. If you are examining the client in a semiprivate hospital room, close the room curtains or dividers. In the home use the client's bedroom.	• Have all equipment readily available. Be sure all equipment is functioning properly. Have spare batteries and light bulbs available for the otoscope and ophthalmoscope.	• Ask the client to empty bladder or bowel if needed, and collect urine and fecal specimens at this time.
• Be sure lighting is adequate, without distortion from shadows.	• Arrange equipment in order of use before the examination begins.	• Provide privacy while the client changes into a gown and give the client time to undress, assisting if necessary.
• A sound-proofed room is ideal; minimize any outside noise.	• Be sure any equipment that touches the client's skin is warmed (e.g., run warm water over speculum blades; rub diaphragm of stethoscope briskly between the hands).	• Focused examinations (e.g., head and neck) may not require the client to completely undress.
• Do not allow interruptions from other health care workers during the examination.	• Be familiar with all equipment before beginning the examination.	• Be sure client is dressed and draped properly. Hospitalized clients usually wear a simple patient gown. Outpatients can change into a linen or disposable gown.
• Raise the head of the table about 30 degrees when the client is supine.		• Provide a drape for over the lap or lower trunk.
• Have examination bed or table at examiner's waist level.		

- Make sure the room is sufficiently warm to maintain comfort.

- Provide adequate space for an examination, particularly for older adults who use mobility aids.

- Eliminate drafts, control room temperature, and provide warm blankets.

- Periodically ask whether the client is comfortable.

- Seriously ill or older clients are more likely to become chilled.

- Help the client move onto and off the table.

- Offer a drink of water, tissue, or pillow to help the client relax.

- Help the client assume proper positions (Table 4-1) during the examination so that body parts are accessible and the client stays comfortable. Some clients have limited strength and need assistance.

Table 4-1 Positions for Examinations

Position	Areas Assessed	Rationale	Limitations
Sitting	Head and neck, back, posterior thorax and lungs, anterior thorax and lungs, breasts, axillae, heart, vital signs, and upper extremities	Sitting upright provides full expansion of lungs and provides better visualization of symmetry of upper body parts.	Physically weakened client may be unable to sit. Examiner should use supine position with head of bed elevated instead.
Supine	Head and neck, anterior thorax and lungs, breasts, axillae, heart, abdomen, extremities, pulses	This is most normally relaxed position. It provides easy access to pulse sites.	If client becomes short of breath easily, examiner may need to raise head of bed.
Dorsal recumbent	Head and neck, anterior thorax and lungs, breasts, axillae, heart, abdomen	Position is used for abdominal assessment because it promotes relaxation of abdominal muscles.	Clients with painful disorders are more comfortable with knees flexed.
Lithotomy*	Female genitalia and genital tract	This position provides maximal exposure of genitalia and facilitates insertion of vaginal speculum.	Lithotomy position is embarrassing and uncomfortable, so examiner minimizes time that client spends in it. Client is kept well draped.

Position	System/Area		Notes
Sims'	Rectum and vagina	Flexion of hip and knee improves exposure of rectal area.	Joint deformities may hinder client's ability to bend hip and knee.
Prone	Musculoskeletal system	This position is used only to assess extension of hip joint.	This position is poorly tolerated in clients with respiratory difficulties.
Lateral recumbent	Heart	This position aids in detecting murmurs.	This position is poorly tolerated in clients with respiratory difficulties.
Knee-chest*	Rectum	This position provides maximal exposure of rectal area.	This position is embarrassing and uncomfortable.

*Clients with arthritis or other joint deformities may be unable to assume this position.

Environment	Equipment	Physical Preparation of Client
		• Adjust draping during positioning to be sure the body part being examined is not unnecessarily exposed. Keep other areas covered.
		• Some positions are uncomfortable and/or embarrassing; keep the client in a position no longer than is necessary.
		• When alternative positions can be used for a particular examination, choose the position best suited for weakened clients.

- Position older adults to avoid having them look into the source of light, which can cause discomfort from the light's glare.

- For disabled clients, special body positions may be used (see Chapter 19).

- Sequence an examination to keep position changes to a minimum.

- Be efficient throughout the examination to limit client movement.

- Do not leave confused, combative, or uncooperative clients unattended on the examination table.

BOX 4-1 Equipment and Supplies for Physical Examination

- Cotton applicators
- Cytobrush
- Disposable pad
- Drapes
- Eye chart (e.g., Snellen chart)
- Flashlight and spotlight
- Forms (e.g., physical, laboratory)
- Gloves (sterile or clean)
- Goniometer
- Gown for client
- Water-soluble lubricant
- Ophthalmoscope
- Otoscope
- Glass microscope slides and slip covers
- Paper towels
- Percussion hammer
- Ruler
- Safety pin
- Scale with height measurement rod
- Specimen containers and microscope slides
- Sphygmomanometer and cuff
- Stethoscope
- Swabs or sponge forceps
- Tape measure
- Thermometer
- Tissues
- Tongue depressor
- Tuning fork
- Vaginal speculum
- Wristwatch with second hand or digital display

The equipment and supplies typically needed by examiners for physical assessment are listed in Box 4-1 and displayed in Figure 4-1. Special equipment for special procedures is listed in later chapters.

Psychological Preparation of the Client

Begin the assessment by explaining in general terms the purpose of the examination, how it will be performed, what the client should expect to feel, and how the client can cooperate.

Tell the client to feel free to ask any questions and to describe any discomfort felt during the examination. Provide an opportunity for those questions.

EXAMPLE: "Mrs. Smith, I am now going to perform a physical examination so I can have a good idea of whether you have any health problems. As we go along I will explain to you exactly what I will be doing. Please feel free to ask any questions. If you become uncomfortable, please tell me. We will start with an examination of the head and neck area."

As you examine each body system, explain the procedure in greater detail. Use simple terms when describing steps of the examination. EXAMPLE: "As I examine your breasts, I want you to relax lying down. First I will look at the color, size, and

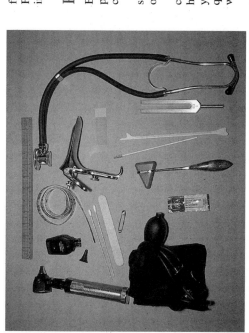

Fig. 4-1
Equipment used during a physical examination.

shape of your breasts. Then I'll gently use my hands to feel the breast tissue itself." If a client speaks a foreign language, determine if a family member, significant other, domestic partner, or friend can interpret. Ask the client if that caregiver can be present during the examination.

■ Put the client at ease.
■ Convey an open, receptive, and professional approach.
■ Use a relaxed tone of voice and facial expression when making explanations.
■ Maintain good eye contact.
■ Perform each physical examination maneuver smoothly and confidently (take your time).
■ If a client seems highly anxious, back away and re-explain your intent. Then begin again.
■ Have a third person (of the client's gender) in the examination room during the examination of the genitalia. Having a third person in the room should make the client feel more comfortable and reduce any fears the client may have. The additional person also protects the examiner and the client because there is a witness to the examination.
■ Monitor the client's emotional responses throughout the examination. Observe fear or concern in facial expressions.
■ Observe for body movements such as tensing when touched or clutching the drape around the body.
■ If the client is overly afraid, anxious, or uncomfortable, postpone the examination until a time when relaxation and cooperation can lead to greater accuracy in the assessment.
■ Never force a client to continue.
■ Pace or time the examination process according to the client's physical and emotional tolerance. Older adults in particular take more time to assume necessary body positions.

Respect the client's cultural differences. A client's health beliefs, use of alternative therapies, nutritional habits, relationships with family, and comfort with close physical contact during an examination must be considered.

5

Organizing and Completing the History and Physical Examination

Organization of the Examination

Always obtain a nursing history and general survey before the initial physical examination. Information from the history and survey provides a useful road map for you to follow when making detailed physical measurements. Historical information, survey findings, and vital signs help to localize physical signs later during the examination. The client's health status, the health care setting, and your experience may require different approaches for organizing an examination. For example, a client in acute distress may require a focused physical examination before any historical information can be gathered.

When a client is admitted to a hospital or is a first-time visitor to a clinic, a complete examination is usually performed. An experienced nurse often learns to incorporate history taking with an examination, especially if time with the client is limited. Again, critical thinking is important in deciding what information to gather from the client and how extensive an examination should be.

Once a complete examination is done, you will perform ongoing assessments of a client's condition. The nature and extent of these focused examinations depend on the client's clinical status and needs. In hospital settings, you will typically perform a focused examination at the beginning of each shift to gain a good sense of the client's status. The shift-to-shift assessment provides a comparison with previous assessments and gives you a reference point from which to evaluate the client's progress during the remainder of the shift.

In the ambulatory setting, the client may be acutely ill or initiating care with a new primary care provider. You will adjust your examination based on the needs of the client. If the client is acutely ill, a focused assessment may be completed to meet the needs of the client. A complete history and physical can be conducted when the client improves. A complete health history and physical will be appropriate for the client who is initiating care and has no acute illness.

The physical examination follows certain priorities when a client is ill or has specific symptoms. Body systems most at risk for being abnormal should be examined first; less critical parts of the examination can be deferred until the client can tolerate a more thorough examination. For example, a client who has shortness of breath usually first undergoes a complete thoracic (see Chapter 13) and cardiac (see Chapter 14) assessment. A more comprehensive examination can wait until the client's fatigue is relieved.

GENERAL TIPS FOR ORGANIZING AN EXAMINATION

- Follow a head-to-toe approach, using each of the four examination skills, to ensure that all body systems are reviewed.
- Always inspect, palpate, percuss, and then auscultate *except during the abdominal examination.* Auscultate and percuss before palpating the abdomen, to avoid causing alterations in bowel sounds.
- Assess the structure and function of each body part and organ, such as the appearance of external eye structures, as well as visual function.
- Compare both sides of the body for symmetry. A degree of asymmetry is normal. (For example, the biceps muscle of the dominant arm may be more developed than the same muscle in the nondominant arm.)
- Integrate client education throughout the examination. Demonstrations can often be given during an examination, such as for breast self-examination.
- Perform painful assessment procedures near the end of the examination.

- If a client becomes fatigued, offer rest periods between assessments.
- Record quick notes during the examination to avoid keeping the client waiting.
- Complete all documentation after the examination. Use the institution's nursing history and physical examination form.
- Record findings in specific anatomic and scientific terms so that any professional can interpret the findings.
- Use common and accepted medical abbreviations to keep notes brief and concise.

Critical Thinking

Knowledge

Throughout the examination, concentrate on one step at a time. Ask yourself the following questions: "What are the skills appropriate for this part of an examination? What are my findings? What should the findings normally be? Is my technique causing the findings, or is there evidence of a true abnormality?"

Experience

Use your experience. If you have ever cared for a client with similar abnormal findings, consider in what way(s) the two clients are the same or different. Prior experience with a similar finding may help you in determining the nature of any abnormalities. In addition, recall what approaches to examination were most effective with previous clients.

Standards

Always apply appropriate standards for data gathering. For example, to assess any symptom, such as nausea or pain, always follow the standard of assessing location, onset, severity, frequency, aggravating and relieving factors, and concomitant symptoms. There are many standards available in the literature.

Delegation Considerations

The general survey requires critical thinking and knowledge application unique to a professional nurse. Assistive personnel may conduct follow-up monitoring (for example, measure height and weight, take vital signs, record intake and output [I&O] and report a client's subjective signs and symptoms. Assistive personnel are capable of data collection, including gathering the information provided by monitoring equipment and measuring vital signs. Assistive personnel must report all monitoring data to you for assessment considerations. Delegation of assessment to assistive personnel is inappropriate. Assessment requires grouping and organizing the data obtained to interpret the meaning. Grouping and organizing the data requires critical thinking skills in order for you to make correct clinical decisions.

COMPLETING THE EXAMINATION

Recording and Reporting the Physical Assessment Findings

When recording information gathered in a physical assessment, you must condense and organize information into a meaningful written summary. Standardized forms are usually available in hospitals and other health care institutions. The standardized forms allow all health professionals to review the client's status. The summary of the assessment is a legal document, and the information must be presented by incorporating the following characteristics: accuracy, conciseness, thoroughness, currentness, organization, confidentiality, and legible penmanship.

During the examination, take brief notes about findings and the client's concern. Measurements such as vital signs, extent of edema, and the size of an organ should be written down as they are obtained. Do not try to record all data during the examination, because you may become detracted away from the client.

Conduct the examination in an efficient sequence. Be sure to follow the same pattern every time to decrease the risk of missing an assessment parameter and to increase your competency. You may find that combining assessments of body systems is indicated. Record your results by the categories on the assessment form used by your institution. Review entries made during the examination for accuracy and thoroughness. Communicate significant findings to appropriate medical and nursing personnel depending on the seriousness and urgency of the need for intervention. Record the findings communicated to other health care providers. The process of conducting the examination is the same in the ambulatory care setting.

Guidelines for Description of Findings

The report of a client's physical assessment should leave no questions in the minds of readers as to the client's current physical and psychological condition (Box 5-1). Data should be concise and accurate so subsequent examiners can compare their data with the baseline database. Helpful guidelines for recording details of the client's examination include the following:

- A client's presenting problem or illness helps you to anticipate what an assessment will reveal. Use the client's own words to foster consistency.
- Record both expected and unexpected findings with integration of subjective and objective data.
- One way to record expected findings is to indicate the absence of symptoms. For example, "No cough, shortness of breath, dyspnea."
- Record unexpected findings, such as pain, by the quality or character.
- Relate physical findings to the processes of inspection, palpation, percussion, and auscultation.
- Refer to topographic or anatomic landmarks when describing findings. The location of the apical pulse, a breast mass, the site of abdominal pain, or the liver span measurement must be documented to provide a comparison for future assessments. For example, "The apical impulse is 4 cm from the midsternal line at the fifth intercostal space."
- Assessment findings are sometimes reported as variations by degree. Extent of edema, pulse amplitude, and heart murmur intensity are examples of findings reported on incremental scales.
- Organs, masses, and lesions are consistently recorded on the basis of seven characteristics: texture, size, shape, mobility, tenderness, color, and location. In addition, characteristics such as heat, induration, scarring, or discharge may be noted. Record how long the client has had the abnormality or when the abnormality was first discovered.
- Describe discharge from any site by color, consistency, odor, and amount.
- Drawings or illustrations may prove helpful in describing the location of findings. A picture of the abdomen divided into quadrants may be useful in drawing the location of a lesion or mass. Similarly, a stick figure can be used to compare findings in extremities, such as pulse amplitude or reflexes.

Recording Conclusions

After organizing and recording all information from the examination, review findings and consider the client's signs and symptoms, both overt and subtle. A repeat assessment or having a colleague confirm a finding may be necessary. Do not be afraid to rely on previous experience in examining clients. The more you perform assessments, the more proficient you will become. You will increase your competency with consistent, organized assessment and reporting of findings. You will analyze the findings to reach a conclusion and select an accurate nursing diagnosis.

You will become more expert at selecting the nursing diagnoses after examination of hundreds of clients. Your intuition, coupled with scientific knowledge of a client's presenting condition, helps to ensure that all possible questions have been asked and assessment data gathered.

Review all available assessment data and consider the patterns that emerge from the physical findings. Your selection of accurate nursing diagnoses is critical to ensure that an appropriate plan of care is developed for the client (Appendix A).

BOX 5-1	Sample Documentation for Complete Physical Examination

VITAL SIGNS:	Weight 150	Temp 99.2	Pulse 90	Blood Pressure 120/78
HEAD:	Normocephalic.			
EARS:	Tympanic membranes and canals are clear bilaterally. Good light reflex.			
EYES:	PERRLA, EOMI, sclera anicteric, conjunctiva normal, fundi benign.			
NOSE:	Clear. No polyps.			
THROAT:	Clear without exudate or drainage. Tonsils 1+.			
NECK:	Supple, without lymphadenopathy or thyromegaly.			

HEART:	PMI nondisplaced. RRR, S1 and S2 WNL. No murmurs, rubs or gallops. No carotid bruits.
LUNGS:	Clear to auscultation and percussion.
BREAST:	Symmetrical in size and shape. No nodules, lesions, or masses palpable. No nipple discharge. No axillary lymphadenopathy.
ABDOMEN:	Nondistended, BS present. Soft, nontender without hepatosplenomegaly or mass.
GU:	Male: Normal circumcised male genitalia with normal distribution of pubic hair. No testicular masses of nodules are palpable. No penile lesions or discharge. Female: Normal external genitalia with normal distribution of pubic hair. Labia are without masses, nodules, or lesions. Vagina pink and moist with thin, clear vaginal secretions. Multiparous os. No lesions observed. Bimanual: No cervical motion tenderness or adnexa fullness. Ovaries and uterus WNL.
RECTAL:	No external lesions, hemorrhoids, masses, or tenderness. Normal anal sphincter tone. No masses or nodules. (Male: prostate smooth, firm, sulcus palpated.) Stool is brown and heme negative.
EXTREMITIES:	Without clubbing, cyanosis or edema. No scoliosis or kyphosis. Flexibility WNL. ROM WNL. Pedal pulses 2+ bilaterally.
NEUROLOGICAL:	Cranial nerves II through XII intact. Sensation intact to pin and position. Muscle strength 5/5. Rhomberg negative without pronator drift. DTR's 2+, toes downgoing and symmetrical. Finger to nose and heel to shin normal. Gait normal including tandem, heel, and toe.

BODY SYSTEM
ASSESSMENT

General Survey

The assessment process begins with a history of the client's present illness or the reason for seeking health care. Complete a general survey of the client while obtaining the history. An experienced nurse can do this simultaneously. Initially you may need to focus on the history, then complete the general survey. You will need to practice the skills of observation and history taking to gain experience and develop competency.

The general survey begins a review of the client's primary health problems. The assessment includes the client's mental status, general appearance and behavior, vital signs, height, and weight. The survey can effectively point out problems early by providing information about characteristics of an illness, a client's hygiene and body image, emotional state, recent weight changes, and developmental status. If you find abnormalities or signs of problems, direct attention to specific body systems later during the examination. The survey can also reveal important information about the client's behavior that can influence how you communicate instructions to the client and conduct portions of the examination.

Critical Thinking Application—General Survey and Vital Signs

Knowledge	Experience	Standards
• Be familiar with the normal and variations for vital signs of adults and children.	• There are variations in body temperature that are associated with the time of day.	Apply the following standards when performing the general survey and health history.
• Be familiar with factors that can affect vital signs.	• Blood pressure may vary from one arm to the other.	• Always apply the appropriate standards for data gathering.
• Knowledge of effective interviewing skills such as questioning, reflection, encouragement, and paraphrasing will increase your success in obtaining needed history.	• History-taking skills will improve with practice.	• Always follow the standard of assessing location, onset, severity, frequency, aggravating and relieving factors, and concomitant symptoms for complaints such as pain.
• General knowledge of anatomy will be needed to perform the general survey.	• Maintaining a consistent structure and order will result in efficient and precise interviewing skills.	• Always proceed in the same order in completing the physical examination.

Equipment

The equipment necessary for the general survey and physical examination is found in Chapter 4, Box 4-1, p. 50.

General Survey and Vital Signs Assessment

Delegation Considerations

Evaluation of vital sign data requires critical thinking and knowledge application and is not appropriate to delegate to assistive personnel. Assistive personnel are trained to obtain vital signs and report them to you. Be sure to clearly define the vital signs that should be reported to you immediately. Assistive personnel can be very helpful in collecting vital sign data and documenting the findings.

Client Preparation

- Conduct the general survey with the client sitting or standing.
- Be sure the client is as fully awake as possible before conducting the mental status examination.

- The client may sit or lie comfortably during vital signs.
- Ask the client to remove shoes and any heavy outer clothing before you measure height and weight.
- When weighing a hospitalized client, always weigh at the same time of day, with the same scale, and with the client wearing the same clothing.

History

The nursing health history and interview are presented in Chapter 2. The following points are specific for the general survey:

- Data may be collected initially during the nursing history or as the nurse performs physical measurements.
- Ask the client's reason for seeking health care and expectations for this encounter.
- Review nursing history for the client's primary health problems.
- Review nursing history for medications that the client is currently taking.

- Note if client is in any acute distress (e.g., difficulty breathing, pain, anxiety). If present, focus on the client's chief complaint and obtain vital signs. A focused history would be appropriate because it relates to the client's signs and symptoms.

- Ask the client for current height and weight. Asking for this information is helpful in determining the client's body image perception. Compare the actual height and weight with the client's response.

- Ask whether the client has had a recent change in weight, the amount, and over what period of time the change occurred.

- Ask if client has recently been dieting or following an exercise program.

- Determine type of client's diet and fluid intake. Ask the client to recall intake over the past 24 hours if the client is diabetic, has nutritional problems, is elderly, or is immunocompromised.

- Before measuring body temperature, ask if client is experiencing headaches, myalgia, chills, nausea, or weakness. Inspect condition of oral mucosa for coating, lesions, and decreased salivation.

- Identify the client's normal baseline heart rate and blood pressure.

- Ask if client has noticed recent change in pulse or heart rate.

Consider any factors that might influence vital signs (Table 6-1).

Table 6-1 Factors That Influence Vital Signs

Factor	Vital Sign	Effect
Exercise	Pulse	Short term—increases rate
		Long term—strengthens heart muscle, causing lower-than-normal rate at rest and quicker return to resting rate after exercise
	Respiration	Increases rate and depth
	Blood pressure	Increases cardiac output and mean arterial pressure
	Temperature	Strenuous exercise may raise temperature
Fever, heat	Pulse	Increases rate
	Respirations	Increases rate
Acute pain, anxiety	Pulse	Sympathetic stimulation—increases rate
	Respirations	Increases rate and depth; alters rhythm
	Blood pressure	Increases pressure
Unrelieved severe chronic pain	Pulse	Parasympathetic stimulation—slows rate
Medications		
Atropine	Pulse	Increases rate
Digitalis	Pulse	Slows rate

Modified from Hazinski MF: Children are different. In Hazinski MF, ed: *Nursing care of the critically ill child*, ed 2, St Louis, 1991, Mosby; Kinney MR et al: *AACN's clinical reference for critical care nursing*, ed 4, St Louis, 1998, Mosby; and USDHHS National High Blood Pressure Education Program; National Heart, Lung, and Blood Institute, National Institutes of Health: *The sixth report of the Joint National Committee on Prevention, Detection, Evaluation, and Treatment of High Blood Pressure*, Bethesda, Md, January 1997, NIH.

Continued

Table 6-1	Factors That Influence Vital Signs—cont'd	
Factor	Vital Sign	Effect
Medications—cont'd		
Beta blocker	Pulse	Slows rate
	Blood pressure	Lowers pressure
Antidysrhythmic	Pulse	Slows rate
Diuretics	Blood pressure	Lower pressure
Adrenergic inhibitors	Blood pressure	Lower pressure
Ace inhibitors	Blood pressure	Lower pressure
Narcotic analgesics	Respirations	Decrease rate and depth or affect rhythm
	Blood pressure	Lower pressure
General anesthetics	Respirations	Lower rate and depth
	Blood pressure	Lower pressure
Amphetamines and cocaine	Respirations	Increase rate and depth
Age	Respirations	From infancy to adulthood, lung vital capacity increases
		With old age, depth of respiration decreases
	Pulse	Infant 120 to 160 beats/min
		Toddler 90 to 140 beats/min
		Preschooler 80 to 110 beats/min
		School-age 75 to 100 beats/min
		Adolescent 60 to 90 beats/min
		Adult 60 to 100 beats/min

	Respirations	Newborn 35 to 40 breaths/min
		Infant 30 to 50 breaths/min
		Toddler 25 to 32 breaths/min
		Child 20 to 30 breaths/min
		Adolescent 16 to 19 breaths/min
		Adult 12 to 20 breaths/min
	Blood pressure	1 Month 85/54
		1 Year 95/65
		6 Years 105/65
		10 to 13 Years 110/65
		14 to 17 Years 120/75
		Middle adult 120/80
		Older adult 140/90
Body position	Pulse	Lying prone decreases rate
		Standing or sitting increases rate
	Respirations	Straight posture—full chest expansion
		Slumped posture—reduced rate and volume
	Blood pressure	Standing suddenly—may lower pressure

Modified from Hazinski MF: Children are different. In Hazinski MF, ed: *Nursing care of the critically ill child*, ed 2, St Louis, 1991, Mosby; Kinney MR et al: *AACN's clinical reference for critical care nursing*, ed 4, St Louis, 1998, Mosby; and USDHHS National High Blood Pressure Education Program; National Heart, Lung, and Blood Institute, National Institutes of Health: *The sixth report of the Joint National Committee on Prevention, Detection, Evaluation, and Treatment of High Blood Pressure*, Bethesda, Md, January 1997, NIH.

ASSESSMENT TECHNIQUES—GENERAL SURVEY AND VITAL SIGNS

Assessment	Normal Findings	Deviations From Normal
General Survey **Mental Status** For clients who are alert and responsive to conversation, conduct a mental status examination, using a mental status questionnaire such as the MSQ or MMSE Sample Items (Box 6-1).	Test should only take 5 to 10 minutes to administer. Concentrates on cognitive function. The maximum score on the test is 30; average score is 27.	Scores below 20 may indicate dementia and delirium (see Chapter 20).
If client's alertness is questioned, assess client's level of consciousness (see Chapter 20 for neurological examination).	Client is alert, oriented, and responds appropriately to all questions.	Client is confused, at times difficult to arouse by verbal stimulus. Client not consistently oriented to person, place, event, or time.

BOX 6-1   MMSE Sample Items

Orientation to Time

"What is the date?"

Registration

"Listen carefully, I am going to say three words. You say them back after I stop. Ready? Here they are. . ."
HOUSE (pause), CAR (pause), LAKE (pause). Now repeat those words back to me."
(Repeat up to 5 times, but score only the first trial.)

Naming

"What is this?" (Point to a pencil or pen.)

Reading

"Please read this and do what it says." (Show examinee the words on the stimulus form.)
CLOSE YOUR EYES

Assessment	Normal Findings	Deviations From Normal
General Appearance		
Observe for signs of distress (e.g., shortness of breath, client's subjective complaint of chest pain or difficulty breathing). These signs help to establish priorities about what to examine first. For any acute sign or symptom, determine onset, duration, severity, predisposing and aggravating factors, and conditions that bring relief.	None	Perform a focused examination if the client is in distress. Implement appropriate nursing interventions to attempt to relieve the distress. Observe and report to the physician if the client's condition worsens.
If no signs of distress are observed, proceed with the general survey and physical examination.		
Assess client's gender and race while observing client's physical features.	Ask the client "What is your race?" Normal physical characteristics vary according to age and race.	
Note if client appears to be stated age.	Ability to participate in examination may be affected by client's age.	Client appears much older or younger than stated age.

Observe client's dress.

A person's culture, lifestyle, socioeconomic level, and personal preference affect the type of clothes that the person wears.

| Type of clothing worn is appropriate for occasion, temperature, and weather conditions. Appears clean and fits the body. Older adults may wear extra clothing because of their sensitivity to cold. Be aware of cultural variations for dress, such as head coverings and long pants in warm weather. | Clothing is dirty or unkempt. Depressed or mentally ill persons may be unable to choose proper clothing. |

Hygiene and grooming

Note the client's level of cleanliness; observe the appearance of the hair, skin, and fingernails. The client's degree of illness or type of activity performed before the examination may affect grooming.

| Dressed for occasion. Hair is neatly groomed or brushed. Appears clean and groomed appropriately for age, culture, or socioeconomic group. | Appearance is unkempt and disheveled. Hair is not groomed. Fingernails and hands may appear soiled. |

Note the amount and type of cosmetics used.

| Makeup is appropriate for age and culture. | Note excessive, nontraditional application of cosmetics. |

Assessment	Normal Findings	Deviations From Normal
Note the presence of any body odor. An unpleasant body odor may simply be the result of physical exercise or may be caused by poor hygiene. Observe for dressings, ostomy devices, or open wounds.	No body odor is noted. Be aware of cultural norms for bathing. European and middle eastern countries do not bathe as often as Americans because of availability of water.	Foul body odors, fetid breath, fruity odor. Note that the odor of alcohol does not always mean alcoholism. Foul odor can be localized to a draining wound or ostomy.
Body Structure and Mobility Observe the following:		
Body type	Client appears fit, trim, and muscular. Body type reflects level of health, age, and lifestyle.	Client appears obese or extremely thin.
Posture	Normal standing posture is an upright comfortable stance with parallel alignment of hips and shoulders. Normal sitting involves some rounding of the shoulders.	Posture is slumped or bent. May reflect mood or presence of pain. Kyphosis, lordosis, or scoliosis may be detected.

Gait

Observe the client walk into the room or along the bedside (if ambulatory). Note whether movements are coordinated or uncoordinated.

Walks with the arms swinging freely at the sides and with head and face leading the body.

Walks hesitantly or tends to list. May fall one way, backward, forward, consistent direction (see Chapter 19).

Body movements

Observe purposeful body movements (e.g., shaking of examiner's hand, grasping hold of an object).

Able to perform movement smoothly, without hesitation.

Tremors present, involving the extremities. Body part is limited in motion or is immobile.

Behavior

Facial expression

Note client's eye contact. (Be aware of cultural norms.) Are expressions appropriate to the situation?

Maintains good eye contact during discussions. Smiles and shows thoughtful reflections to questions.

Facial expression does not match verbal message or other nonverbal signs. Be aware that some cultures do not make eye contact and may feel threatened. Makes no eye contact, has motionless face and fixed stare. Hides mouth behind hand when speaking.

Assessment	Normal Findings	Deviations From Normal
Mood and affect Affect is a person's feelings as they appear to others. A person's mood or emotional state is expressed verbally and nonverbally. Observe whether the client's verbal expressions match nonverbal behavior and note whether the client's mood is appropriate for the situation.	Client is comfortable and cooperative with examiner; answers questions freely and appropriately.	Client appears unusually happy or withdrawn. Hesitates to answer questions; is quick to anger.
Speech Note client's ability to articulate words and pace sentences. Does client speak in a normal tone of voice? Is speech pattern congruent with age?	Follows simple instructions and answers questions. Normal speech is understandable, moderately paced, and shows an association with the person's thoughts. Voice tone is moderate and changes appropriately with context of discussion.	Has difficulty responding to questions or instructions. Talks rapidly or slowly. An abnormal pace may be caused by emotions or neurological impairment. Speaks loudly or very softly.

Suspected Abuse

If abuse is suspected, interview further in private (Table 6-2).

The abuse of children, women, and older adults is a growing health problem. Assess for the following:

• Client has suffered obvious physical injury or neglect (e.g., evidence of malnutrition or presence of bruising on extremities or trunk).

• Client is fearful of spouse or partner, caregiver, parent, or adult child.

• Partner/caregiver has history of violence, alcoholism, or drug abuse.

• Caregiver is unemployed, ill, or frustrated in caring for client.

• Client denies history or shows no physical sign of injury.

• Presence of clinical indicators of abuse should be reported to a social service center (consult agency policy).

Table 6-2   Clinical Indicators of Abuse

Physical Findings	Behavioral Findings
Child Sexual Abuse	
Vaginal or penile discharge	Problem in sleeping or eating
Blood on underclothing	Fear of certain people or places
Pain or itching in genital area	Play activities recreate the abuse situation
Genital injuries	Regressed behavior
Difficulty sitting or walking	Sexual acting out
Pain while urinating	Knowledge of explicit sexual matters
Foreign bodies in rectum, urethra, or vagina	Preoccupation with other's or own genitals
Venereal disease	

Domestic Abuse

Injuries and trauma are inconsistent with reported cause
Multiple injuries involving head, face, neck, breasts, abdomen, and genitalia (black eyes, orbital fractures, broken nose, fractured skull, lip lacerations, broken teeth, strangulation marks)
X-rays show old and new fractures in different stages of healing
Burns
Human bites

Attempted suicide
Eating or sleeping disorders
Anxiety
Panic attacks
Pattern of substance abuse (follows physical abuse)
Low self-esteem
Depression
Sense of helplessness
Guilt
Increased forgetfulness

Continued

Modified from Haviland S, O'Brien J: *Orthop Nurs* 8(4):11, 1989; Stanley SR: *Orthop Nurs* 8(1):33, 1989; and Moss VA; Taylor WK: *AORN J* 53(5):1158, 1991.

Table 6-2   Clinical Indicators of Abuse—cont'd

Physical Findings	Behavioral Findings
Older Adult Abuse	
Injuries and trauma are inconsistent with reported cause (cigarette burn, scratch, bruise, or bite)	Dependent on caregiver
	Physically and/or cognitively impaired
Hematomas	Combative
Bruises at various stages of resolution	Wandering
Bruises, chafing, excoriation on wrist or legs (restraints)	Verbally belligerent
Burns	Minimal social support
Fractures inconsistent with cause described	
Dried blood	
Prolonged interval between injury and medical treatment	

Modified from Haviland S, O'Brien J: *Orthop Nurs* 8(4):11, 1989; Stanley SR: *Orthop Nurs* 8(1):33, 1989; and Moss VA, Taylor WK: *AORN J* 53(5):1158, 1991.

Assessment	Normal Findings	Deviations From Normal

Vital Signs

Temperature Measurement

Body temperature is usually measured by the oral route. Axillary and tympanic membrane measurements are also common. Have client assume a comfortable sitting or supine position. Box 6-2 shows how to convert Fahrenheit to Centigrade and Centigrade to Fahrenheit.

Wait 20 to 30 minutes after client ingests any hot or cold foods or liquids, after smoking, or after strenuous exercise.

Wash hands and apply disposable glove to dominant hand for measuring oral and rectal temperatures.

BOX 6-2 Temperature Conversion Chart

Convert Fahrenheit to Centigrade

Subtract 32 from the Fahrenheit reading and multiply the result by $\frac{5}{9}$.

$C = (F - 32°) \times \frac{5}{9}$

Example:　$40° C = (104° F - 32° F) \times \frac{5}{9}$

Convert Centigrade to Fahrenheit

Multiply the Centigrade reading by $\frac{9}{5}$ and add 32 to the product.

$F = (\frac{9}{5} \times C) + 32°$

Example:　$104° F = (\frac{9}{5} \times 40° C) + 32°$

Assessment	Normal Findings	Deviations From Normal
Oral Temperature Place clean, covered electronic thermometer probe under client's tongue in sublingual pocket, lateral to center of lower jaw, until audible signal is heard (about 30 seconds).	Normal adult body temperature is 36° C (96.8° F) to 38° C (100.4° F).	A single temperature reading does not indicate a fever. A persistent elevation above normal warrants therapy. Monitor for trends over time, noting the time of day and any pattern.
Rectal Temperature With client in Sims' position and upper leg flexed, separate buttocks and gently insert lubricated probe into anus in direction of umbilicus. Insert 3.5 cm (1½ inches) for adult. *Do not force thermometer.* Hold in place until audible signal occurs on electronic digital display.	Adult: Rectal temperatures are usually 0.5° C (0.9° F) higher than oral temperatures.	A persistent elevation above normal warrants therapy.

Assessment	Normal Findings	Deviations From Normal
Axillary Temperature	Adult: Axillary temperatures are usually 0.5° C (0.9° F) lower than oral temperatures.	A persistent elevation above normal warrants therapy.
Move clothing or gown from client's shoulder and arm. Insert thermometer into center of axilla, lower arm over thermometer, and place arm across client's chest. Leave in place until audible signal is heard.		
Tympanic Membrane Temperature		
Insert tympanic probe into client's ear canal, directed toward the nose. Apply a gentle but firm pressure (Fig. 6-1). *Do not force the thermometer into the ear.* Initiate starter and leave in place until audible or visual signal indicates temperature reading. **Presence of impacted cerumen can cause a false low reading.**		

Pulse Measurement

Wait 5 to 10 minutes before assessing pulse if client has been active or exercising.

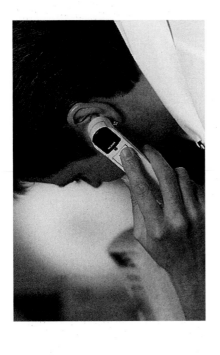

Fig. 6-1
Tympanic thermometer inserted into auditory canal.

Assessment	Normal Findings	Deviations From Normal
Radial Pulse		
Position the client supine with a forearm across the lower abdomen or chest or at the side of the body. If the client is seated, bend the elbow 90 degrees and support the lower arm on the chair or on your arm. Slightly extend the wrist with palm facing down.		
Place tips of first two fingers of hand over groove along radial or thumb side of client's inner wrist.		
Lightly compress against radius, obliterate pulse initially, and then relax pressure so that pulse becomes easily palpable.		
Count rate for 30 seconds if regular and multiply by 2.		
Count rate for 60 seconds if irregular.		

Assess client's pulse for the following:

Rate   See Table 6-1 for normal findings.

Rate >100 beats/minute is tachycardia (abnormally elevated rate). Rate <60 beats/minute is bradycardia (abnormally low rate; *exception: highly conditioned athletes*).

Rhythm   Normally a regular interval occurs between each pulse or heartbeat.

A dysrhythmia is indicated by an interval interrupted by an early or late beat or a missed beat. The pulse will feel irregular.

Strength   Pulse strength or amplitude remains equally strong bilaterally.

Pulse strength may be graded:

0 Absent, not palpable

1+ Pulse diminished, barely palpable, easy to obliterate

2+ Easily palpable, normal

3+ Full, increased

4+ Strong, bounding, cannot be obliterated

Assessment	Normal Findings	Deviations From Normal
Equality	Both radial pulses are symmetric.	One pulse is unequal in strength or absent.
Apical Pulse		
• Expose client's sternum and left side of chest. Locate fifth intercostal space at left midclavicular line.		
• Place diaphragm of stethoscope over apical impulse and auscultate until you hear normal S_1 and S_2 heart sounds (Fig. 6-2).		
• Count rate for 1 full minute.		
Rate	Adult: Normal rate is 60 to 100 beats/minute.	Rate >100 beats/minute is tachycardia; rate <60 beats/minute is bradycardia.
Rhythm	Regular interval occurs between S_1 and S_2 and between S_2 and next S_1.	A dysrhythmia involves interruption in successive heart sounds.

Respiration Assessment

To assess respirations, have the client assume a comfortable position sitting or laying supine with the head of the bed or examination table elevated 45 to 60 degrees.

Wait 5 to 10 minutes if client has been active or exercising.

Be sure client's chest is visible. Observe a complete respiratory cycle, then count rate for 30 seconds if regular and multiply by 2. If rhythm is irregular or rate is less than 12 or more than 20, count for 1 full minute.

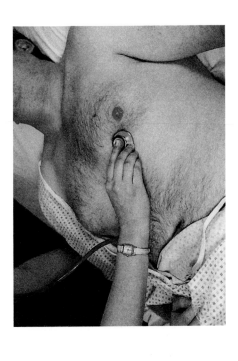

Fig. 6-2
Auscultation of apical pulse.

Assessment	Normal Findings	Deviations From Normal
Assess the following:		
Rate	See Table 6-1 for normal findings.	Rate <12 breaths/minute is brady-pnea; rate >20 breaths/minute is tachypnea.
Rhythm	A regular interval occurs after each respiratory cycle.	Intervals occur irregularly between respiratory cycles.
Depth	Excursion or movement of chest wall is full and equal bilaterally.	Excursion is shallow or excessively deep. One side of chest may expand more than the other, indicating pain, positioning restriction, or possible pathology.

Blood Pressure

Determine the best site for obtaining blood pressure measurement. Do not apply the blood pressure cuff above an IV line where intravenous fluids are infusing or an arteriovenous shunt, on the same side where breast or axillary surgery has been performed, when the arm or hand has been traumatized or diseased, or client has lower arm cast or bulky bandage.

Have client avoid caffeine intake and smoking for 30 minutes before assessment (USDHHS, 1997).

Table 6-3 outlines common mistakes in measuring blood pressure.

Table 6-3 Common Mistakes in Blood Pressure Measurement

Error	Effect
Bladder or cuff too wide	False low reading
Bladder or cuff too narrow	False high reading
Cuff wrapped too loosely	False high reading
Deflating cuff too slowly	False high diastolic reading
Deflating cuff too quickly	False low systolic and false high diastolic reading
Stethoscope that fits poorly or impairment of the examiner's hearing, causing sounds to be muffled	False low systolic and false high diastolic reading
Inaccurate inflation level	False low systolic reading
Multiple examiners using different Korotkoff sounds for diastolic readings	Inaccurate interpretation of systolic and diastolic readings

Assessment	Normal Findings	Deviations From Normal

Be sure restrictive clothing has been removed from client's arm. Palpate brachial artery and position cuff 2.5 cm (1 inch) above site of brachial pulsation. Center bladder of cuff above artery and wrap cuff evenly and snugly around upper arm. With manometer positioned vertically at eye level, palpate brachial or radial artery while inflating cuff rapidly to a pressure 30 mm Hg above point at which pulse disappears. Slowly deflate cuff. Point at which pulse reappears is approximate systolic pressure.

Wait 30 seconds. Then place diaphragm of stethoscope over brachial artery. Inflate cuff to 30 mm Hg above palpated systolic pressure. Slowly release the valve and allow mercury to fall at rate of 2 to 3 mm Hg per second. Note point on manometer when first clear sound is heard. Continue deflation, noting point when the sound disappears (diastolic pressure in adult).

See Table 6-1 for normal blood pressure findings.

The severity of hypertension is classified by stages (Table 6-4). Hypotension is present when the systolic blood pressure falls to 90 mm Hg or below. A high reading of 150/90 mm Hg warrants another checkup within 2 months (Table 6-5) for hypertension.

Table 6-4   Classification of Blood Pressure For Adults Age 18 Years and Older*

Category	Systolic (mm Hg)	Diastolic (mm Hg)
Optimal[†]	<120	<80
Normal*	<130	<85
High normal	130-139	85-89
Hypertension[‡]		
Stage 1 (mild)	140-159	90-99
Stage 2 (moderate)	160-179	100-109
Stage 3 (severe)	180-209	110-119
Stage 4 (very severe)	≥210	≥120

Modified from USDHHS Sixth Report of Joint National Committee on Prevention, Detection, Evaluation, and Treatment of High Blood Pressure: National Heart, Lung and Blood Institute; National Institutes of Health: *Sixth report of the Joint National Committee on Detection, Prevention, Evaluation, and Treatment of High Blood Pressure,* Bethesda, Md, January 1997, NIH.

*Not taking antihypertensive drugs and not acutely ill. When systolic and diastolic pressures fall into different categories, the higher category should be selected to classify the individual's blood pressure status. For instance, 160/92 mm Hg should be classified as Stage 2, and 180/120 mm Hg should be classified as Stage 4. Isolated systolic hypertension (ISH) is defined as SBP ≥140 mm Hg and DBP <90 mm Hg and staged appropriately (e.g., 170/85 mm Hg is defined as Stage 2 ISH).

[†]Unusually low readings should be evaluated for clinical significance.

[‡]Based on the average of two or more readings taken at each of two or more visits following an initial screening.

NOTE: In addition to classifying stages of hypertension based on average blood pressure levels, the clinician should specify presence or absence of target-organ disease and additional risk factors. For example, a patient with diabetes and a blood pressure of 142/94 mm Hg plus left ventricular hypertrophy should be classified as "Stage 1 hypertension with target-organ disease (left ventricular hypertrophy) and with another major risk factor (diabetes)." The specificity is important for risk classification and management.

Table 6-5	Recommendations For Follow-Up Based on Initial Set of Blood Pressure Measurements For Adults Age 18 and Older

Initial Screening Blood Pressure (mm Hg)*		Follow-Up Recommended[†]
Systolic	Diastolic	
<130	<85	Recheck in 2 years
130-139	85-89	Recheck in 1 year[‡]
140-159	90-99	Confirm within 2 months
160-179	100-109	Evaluate or refer to source of care within 1 month
≥180	≥110	Evaluate or refer to source of care immediately or within 1 week

From USDHHS Sixth Report of Joint National Committee on Prevention, Detection, Evaluation, and Treatment of High Blood Pressure; National High Blood Pressure Education Program; National Heart, Lung and Blood Institute; National Institutes of Health: *Sixth report of the Joint National Committee on Detection, Prevention, Evaluation, and Treatment of High Blood Pressure.* Bethesda, Md, January 1997, NIH.

*If the systolic and diastolic categories are different, follow recommendations for the shorter time follow-up (e.g., 160/85 mm Hg should be evaluated or referred to source of care within 1 month).

[†]The scheduling of follow-up should be modified by reliable information about past blood pressure measurements, other cardiovascular risk factors, or target-organ disease.

[‡]Consider providing advice about lifestyle modifications.

Assessment	Normal Findings	Deviations From Normal
Height and Weight		
Weigh clients capable of bearing weight on a standing scale. Use a stretcher scale for clients who are unable to bear weight.		A weight gain of up to 5 lbs (2.3 kg) in a day may indicate a fluid retention problem.
Calibrate the scale by setting weight at *zero*; note whether the balance beam registers in the middle of the mark. Scales with a digital display should read *zero* before use.		
Be sure client is wearing light clothing and no shoes. Have client stand on scale platform and remain still. Adjust scale weight on the balance beam until the tip of the beam registers in the middle of the mark. Weight is measured in pounds or kilograms (2.2 lb /1 kg). Digital scales display results immediately.		

With the client standing erect on a scale, raise the metal rod attached to the scale up and over the client's head. The rod should be placed level horizontally at a 90-degree angle to the measuring stick. Height is measured in inches or centimeters.

Infants and Children

Height and Weight

Using a table scale for infants, weigh the infant unclothed and protected from falling from the scale basket.

See Appendix C for standardized height and weight tables. The body mass index (BMI) is calculated by dividing the client's weight (in kg) by the height (in meters squared) (BMI × Wt [kg]/ht [m²]). A BMI between 20 and 25 in men and 19 and 24 in women is expected (see Appendix D).

Healthy term newborns vary in weight between 2500 and 4000 g (5 lb 8 oz to 8 lb 13 oz). In general they double their birth weight by 4 to 5 months of age and triple their birth weight by 12 months of age (Seidel et al, 1999).

A BMI above 27 corresponds with being at least 20% overweight. A BMI of 30 and above indicates obesity. See Appendix C.

Assessment	Normal Findings	Deviations From Normal
Portable devices are available to measure infant length. Place the infant on the firm surface and have a parent or assistant hold the infant's head against the headboard. With the infant's legs straight at the knees, place the footboard against the bottom of the infant's feet. Record length in the nearest 0.5 cm or ⅕ inch.	See Appendix E for physical growth curves for children.	
Head Circumference With the child supine, place the measuring tape snugly around the child's head at the occipital protuberance and supraorbital prominence (Fig. 6-3). Measure to the nearest 0.5 cm or ⅕ inch.	Head circumference for term newborns ranges from 12.5 to 14.8 inches (31.5 to 37 cm).	A head circumference increasing rapidly and rising above percentile curves suggests increased intracranial pressure. A head circumference growing slowly to fall off percentile curves suggests microcephaly.

Chest Circumference

Wrap the measuring tape around the infant's chest at the nipple line, firmly but not tight enough to cause an indentation of the skin. Take the measure midway between inspiration and expiration to the nearest 0.5 cm or ⅕ inch.

The newborn's head circumference may equal or exceed the chest circumference by 2 cm (⅘ inch) for the first 5 months of age (Seidel et al, 1999). Between 5 and 24 months of age, the infant's chest circumference should closely approximate the head circumference. After 24 months, the chest circumference exceeds the head circumference.

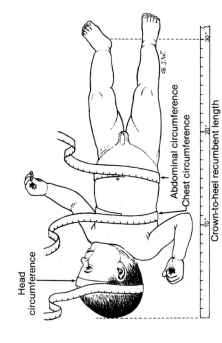

Fig. 6-3
Measuring infant's head, chest, and abdominal circumferences.

Pediatric Considerations

- When weighing an infant in a basket scale, remove the infant's clothing and diaper. Be sure the room is warm. Place the infant in the basket and hold a hand lightly above to prevent an accidental fall.
- When a child is below minimum height on the standing scale, position the child against a wall. Place a book on top of the child's head perpendicular to the wall and mark the wall at the point of contact. Measure the distance between the floor and the mark on the wall to determine the child's height.
- Count respirations in an infant or a young child for a full minute. Infant respirations are primarily diaphragmatic and are observed by abdominal movement.
- Apnea monitors may be made available in the home for premature infants or newborns who are at risk for respiratory compromise or arrest.
- Wait at least 15 minutes after any activity or anxiety before measuring a child's blood pressure. To determine the diastolic pressure in a child, deflate the cuff, noting the point when sound becomes muffled.
- Insert a rectal thermometer 1.2 cm (½ inch) for an infant.

Gerontologic Considerations

- Many older adults assume a stooped, forward-bent posture, with hips and knees somewhat flexed and arms bent at the elbows, raising the level of the arms.
- Aging causes ossification of costal cartilage and downward slant of the ribs with an increase in the intercostal spaces, causing a more rigid rib cage and reduction in chest wall expansion.
- Older adults may have a decrease in height as a result of osteoporosis and kyphosis.
- Body weight changes because of a decline in lean body mass and a loss of body water. From age 25 to age 75, the fat content of the body increases by 16% (Ebersole and Hess, 1998).
- Older adults have a diminished immune response to pyrogens, and therefore body temperature might not rise as high in the presence of a fever.

Client Teaching

- The general survey can be a time to instruct the client about the importance of regular health examinations.
- Encourage parents to keep postnatal care follow-up visits to assess child's ongoing growth pattern.
- All clients should know how to measure body temperature. Measuring body temperature is particularly important to teach clients with febrile illnesses or conditions that increase the risk of infection. Instruct the client on the parameters to report to the physician or to treat at home. Review over-the-counter treatment options with the client.
- Teach clients with preexisting respiratory disease preventive measures for avoiding respiratory infections, such as routinely having flu shots or pneumonia vaccines. Special breathing and coughing exercises may be necessary for clients with chronic lung disease.
- Educate clients about hypertension risk factors: family history, obesity (>30% overweight), cigarette smoking, excessive alcohol consumption, elevated blood cholesterol

Cultural Considerations

- Italian, Jewish, African-American, and Spanish-speaking persons smile readily and use many facial expressions and gestures to communicate happiness, pain, or displeasure. Irish, English, and Northern European persons tend to have less facial expression (Giger, 1999).
- Orientals and some Native Americans often find eye contact to be impolite and an invasion of privacy. Persons of certain cultures avoid eye contact with persons of a higher or lower socioeconomic status, such as Indian and Vietnamese cultures.
- African-American infants generally weigh 181 to 240 g less than white infants at birth. Oriental, Filipino, Hawaiian, and Puerto Rican babies generally also weigh less than white infants (Seidel et al, 1999).
- Mexican-American children tend to have greater weight-for-height values than the average white child (Seidel et al, 1999).
- African-Americans are less responsive to beta blockers for hypertension (USDHHS, 1997).

levels (total cholesterol >200 mg/dl or LDL cholesterol
>130 mg/dl), and continued exposure to stress.

- Educate clients with hypertension about long-term follow-up care, medication schedules, and the importance of a consistently followed treatment plan.

Integument

The integument, consisting of the skin, hair, and nails, provides external protection for the body, helps regulate body temperature, and is a sensory organ for pain, temperature, and touch. Inspect all integumentary structures, making mental or written notes as needed. As you become more comfortable and confident with the assessment skills, begin to incorporate integumentary assessment when other body systems are examined. You will use the skills of inspection, palpation, and olfaction.

Anatomy and Physiology
The Skin

The skin has three primary layers: epidermis, dermis, and subcutaneous tissue (Fig. 7-1). The epidermis, the outer layer, is composed of several thin layers undergoing different stages of maturation. The outer layer shields underlying tissue against water loss and mechanical and chemical injury, and prevents the entry of disease-producing microorganisms. The innermost layer of the epidermis generates new cells that migrate toward the skin's surface to replace dead cells that are continuously shed from the skin's outer surface. The innermost epidermis also resurfaces wounds and restores skin integrity. Special cells called *melanocytes* can be found in the epidermis. Melanocytes produce melanin, the dark pigment of the skin. Darker-skinned clients have more active melanocytes.

The dermis is a thicker skin layer containing bundles of collagen and elastic fibers that support the epidermis. It is elastic and durable and contains a complex network of nerve endings, sweat glands, sebaceous glands, hair follicles, and blood vessels. The skin insulates the body against extremes of cold and facilitates heat loss. When the body's temperature rises, the skin acts as a radiator. Therefore the skin promotes the radiation of heat from the skin's surface by way of vasodilation and by providing a surface for the evaporation of sweat.

The third layer, subcutaneous tissue, contains blood vessels, nerves, lymph nodes, and loose connective tissue filled with fat cells. The fatty tissue serves as a heat insulator and provides support for upper skin layers.

The skin exchanges oxygen, nutrients, and fluid with underlying blood vessels; synthesizes new cells; and eliminates dead, nonfunctioning cells. The cells require adequate nutri-

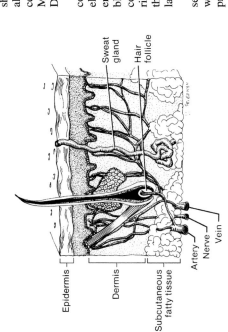

Fig. 7-1
A cross-section of the skin.

Epidermis

Dermis

Subcutaneous
fatty tissue

Sweat
gland

Hair
follicle

Artery

Nerve

Vein

to become secondary lesions that require more extensive nursing care.

The Nails

The most visible portion of the nails is the nail plate, the transparent layer of epithelial cells covering the nail bed (Fig. 7-2). The vascularity of the nail bed creates the nail's underlying color. The semilunar, whitish area at the base of the nail bed from which the nail plate develops is called the *lunula*.

The Hair

Two types of hair cover the body: terminal hair (long, coarse, thick hair easily visible on the scalp, axillae, pubic areas, and in the beards of males) and vellus hair (small, soft, tiny hairs covering the whole body except for palms and soles). Assessment of the hair occurs during all portions of the examination.

The condition of the nails and hair can reflect a person's general health, state of nutrition, occupation, and level of self-care. Even a person's psychological state may be revealed by evidence of conditions such as nail biting.

tion and hydration to resist injury and disease. Adequate circulation is needed for cell life. The skin reflects changes in a person's physical condition by alterations in color, thickness, texture, turgor, temperature, and hydration.

The skin provides a window to detect a variety of conditions, including changes in oxygenation, circulation, nutrition, local tissue damage, and hydration. In a hospital setting the majority of clients are older adults, debilitated clients, or young but seriously ill clients. Older adults are at risk for skin lesions resulting from trauma during administration of care, from exposure to pressure of immobilization, or from reaction to medications used in treatment. Clients most at risk for integumentary injury are the neurologically impaired; diabetic; chronically ill; orthopedic clients; and clients with diminished mental status, poor tissue oxygenation, low cardiac output, and inadequate nutrition. In nursing homes and extended care facilities, clients may be at risk for many of the same problems depending on their level of mobility and presence of chronic illness. You must routinely assess the skin for primary or initial lesions that may develop. Without proper care, primary lesions can quickly deteriorate

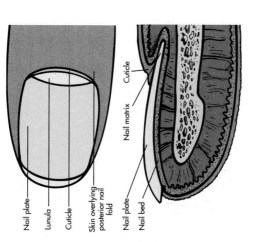

Fig. 7-2
Components of the nail unit. (From Thompson SM et al: *Mosby's manual of clinical nursing*, ed 2, St Louis, 1989, Mosby.)

Nail plate

Lunula

Cuticle

Skin overlying posterior nail fold

Nail matrix

Cuticle

Nail plate

Nail bed

Critical Thinking Application—Integument

Knowledge	Experience	Standards
Use basic knowledge of structure and function of the skin.	Reflect on different clients you have cared for and the cultural variations in the hair, skin and nails.	Apply the following principles when examining the integument:
• Recall knowledge of risk of infection posed by any break or disruption of the skin.	• Wide variations exist in the condition of clients' integument.	• Begin with a brief but careful overall visual sweep of the entire body.
• Become familiar with cultural variations of skin color.	• Recall previous clients who presented with lesions or changes in the condition of the skin.	• Do not ignore "hard-to-see" locations such as under the female client's breasts, under the arms, or in the pubic area.
• Be familiar with common pathologic conditions that may be reflected by changes in the integument. Examples: generalized pallor (anemia), marked localized pallor (arterial insufficiency), jaundice (liver disease), orange-green or gray color in light-skinned clients (renal failure), hyperemia as seen with inflammation or fever.	• Locate sites where problems commonly develop (e.g., basal cell cancers occurring over sun-exposed areas, plantar warts on the soles of the feet).	• Skin temperature changes can reflect alterations in blood flow and may require attention to vascular assessment (see Chapter 14).
		• Use the client as a resource. He or she will be best informed as to whether skin lesions are newly developed or old.

- Measure skin lesions accurately, using a centimeter ruler. Carefully note the location of any lesions.

Equipment

- Adequate lighting
- Disposable gloves (for broken skin, moist or draining lesions, and lice or scabies)
- Centimeter ruler

Delegation Considerations

The physical examination of the hair, skin and nail requires critical thinking and knowledge application unique to a professional nurse and should not be delegated to assistive personnel. Instruct assistive personnel to alert you to changes in the client's hair, skin or nails when administering client's care.

Client Preparation

- To view all skin surfaces and intertriginous areas (tissue-to-tissue), the client will need to assume multiple positions.
- The area to be examined must be fully exposed with both direct and tangential lighting.
- If an area is not clean or is covered with cosmetics, it may be necessary to cleanse the skin for adequate inspection.
- Assessment occurs throughout the examination.
- Explain the need to separate parts of hair to detect obvious problems. Clients may be sensitive to having hair examined.

History
Skin

Ask the client about:

- History of changes in the skin, such as dryness, pruritus, sores, rashes, lumps, color, texture, odor, and lesions that do not heal. Consider if heat, cold, stress, exposure to toxic material or skin care products, or travel to exotic places cause alterations.
- Identify risk factors for skin cancer (Box 7-1).
- Determine if client works or spends excessive time outside. If so, ask whether a sunscreen is worn and the level of protection.
- Question client about frequency of bathing and type of soap used. Excessive bathing or harsh soaps can dry the skin.
- Ask if client has had recent trauma to the skin.
- Does client have a history of allergies? If so, what skin changes, if any, normally occur?
- Ask if client uses topical medications or home remedies on the skin.

BOX 7-1 Skin Cancer Risk Factors

Age >50 years
Male
Light-colored hair or eyes
Fair, freckled or ruddy complexion
Tendency to sunburn easily
Family history of skin cancer
Repeated trauma or irritation to skin, such as:
   Excessive overexposure to frost, wind, or ultraviolet
   B radiation from the sun
   Exposure to arsenic, creosote, coal tar, and/or petro-
   leum products
   Overexposure to radium, radioisotopes, x-rays
   Living near the equator or at high altitudes
Precancerous dermatoses

Adapted from Seidel HM et al: *Mosby's guide to physical examination*, ed 4, Mosby, 1999, St. Louis.

- Ask if client goes to tanning parlors, uses sun lamps, or takes tanning pills.
- Does client have family history of serious skin disorders such as skin cancer or psoriasis?

Nails

- Does client work with creosote, coal tar, and/or petroleum products?
- Ask whether the client has experienced recent trauma or changes to the nails (e.g., splitting, breaking, discoloration, thickening).
- Determine the client's nail care practices and occupation.
- Has the client had other symptoms of pain, swelling, presence of systemic disease with fever, psychological or physical stress?
- Ask the parents whether a pediatric client bites the nails.
- Determine if client has risks for nail or foot problems (for example, diabetes, older adulthood, obesity).

Hair and Scalp

- Ask whether the client is wearing a wig or hairpiece and request that it be removed.
- Determine whether the client has noted a change in growth or loss of hair or lesions of the scalp.
- Identify type of shampoo, other hair care products, and curling irons used for grooming. Does client use a rinse or dye in hair?
- Has client had recent trauma to the scalp?
- Determine if client has recently taken chemotherapy if hair loss is noted, or vasodilators (minoxidil) if growth is noted.
- To rule out risk of ticks, ask if client recently spent time outdoors (for example, camping).

Ask if client has noted changes in diet or appetite (see Chapter 7).

ASSESSMENT TECHNIQUES—INTEGUMENT

Assessment	Normal Findings	Deviations From Normal
⊙ **Standard Precautions Alert** *If client has moist or open lesions, wash hands and apply gloves.*		
SKIN		
Inspection		
• Inspect the skin for color and pigmentation.	• Skin color is usually uniform over the body. Normal pigmentation ranges in tone from ivory to light pink to ruddy pink in light-skinned persons and light to deep brown or olive in dark-skinned persons. Be aware of cultural diversity.	• Pallor can be seen in the face, buccal mucosa, conjunctivae, and nail beds.
• Inspect for abnormalities on skin surfaces with the least amount of pigmentation. For example, inspect color of volar aspect of forearms, palms of hands, soles of feet, buccal (mouth) mucosa, abdomen, nail beds, and conjunctivae.	• Dark-skinned clients have lighter-colored palms, soles, lips, and nail beds than the rest of their skin.	• Cyanosis is best observed in the lips, nail beds, and palms.
		• Jaundice usually appears first in the sclera.
• Compare color on both sides of the body.	• Areas exposed to the sun, such as the face, arms, knees, and elbows will be darker.	• Increased vascularity of the face (see Table 7-1 for skin color abnormalities).
		• Basal cell carcinomas.

Color	Condition	Causes	Assessment Locations
Bluish (cyanosis)	Increased amount of deoxygenated hemoglobin (associated with hypoxia)	Heart or lung disease, cold environment	Nail beds, lips, mouth, skin (severe cases)
Pallor (decrease in color)	Reduced amount of oxyhemoglobin	Anemia	Face, conjunctivae, nail beds, palms of hands
	Reduced visibility of oxyhemoglobin resulting from decreased blood flow	Shock	Skin, nail beds, conjunctivae, lips
Loss of pigmentation	Vitiligo	Congenital or autoimmune condition causing lack of pigment	Patchy areas on skin over face, hands, arms
Yellow-orange (jaundice)	Increased deposit of bilirubin in tissues	Liver disease, destruction of red blood cells	Sclera, mucous membranes, skin
Red (erythema)	Increased visibility of oxyhemoglobin caused by dilation or increased blood flow	Fever, direct trauma, blushing, alcohol intake	Face, area of trauma, sacrum, shoulders, other common sites for pressure ulcers
Tan-brown	Increased amount of melanin	Suntan, pregnancy	Areas exposed to sun: face, arms; areolae, nipples

Table 7-1 Skin Color Variations

Assessment	Normal Findings	Deviations From Normal
• Inspect hard-to-see areas such as those around casts, traction, splints, or dressings.	• Skin is intact, with absence of inflammation.	• Skin will become reddened from pressure and excoriated from friction.
• Note any patches or areas of skin with color variations.	• Variations are absent.	• Localized skin changes, such as pallor or erythema.
		• Petechiae: tiny, pinpoint-size red or purple spots.
		• Localized changes such as rash, inflammation, or swelling.
• Pay close attention along arms and legs where major veins are distributed, looking for presence of injection sites.	• Skin overlying major veins is intact and clear.	• Reddened, edematous, and warm areas along the arms and legs.
		• Hyperpigmented and shiny areas.

- Inspect condition of skin over regions exposed to pressure.

  Never massage reddened areas. Massage increases breaks in capillaries in underlying tissues and increases risk of pressure ulcer.

- Normal reactive hyperemia (redness) is a visible effect of localized vasodilation, the body's normal response to lack of blood flow to underlying tissue. Normal hyperemia over pressure area lasts less than 1 hour after client repositions.

- Pallor and mottling.

- Absence of superficial skin layers. (Box 7-2).

BOX 7-2   Staging for Pressure Ulcers

Stage I: Skin is reddened and not broken
Stage II: Epidermis and dermis layers are damaged
Stage III: Damage is through to the subcutaneous tissue
Stage IV: Involvement of muscle and possible bone.

Adapted from Seidel HM et al: *Mosby's guide to physical examination*, ed 4, Mosby, 1999, St Louis.

Assessment	Normal Findings	Deviations From Normal
Palpation		
• Assess additional areas of potential pressure: skin of nares around nasogastric tubes, intravenous sites, drainage tube sites, and sites where Foley catheters exit the meatus.	• Skin and mucosa are intact, with minimal redness.	• Redness and excoriation.
• Using ungloved fingertips, palpate skin surfaces to feel the skin's moisture.	• Skin is normally smooth and dry, with minimal perspiration or oiliness (Seidel et al, 1999). Skin folds, such as the axillae, are normally moist.	• Flaking (appearance of dandrufflike flakes when the skin is rubbed) and scaling (fishlike scales easily rubbed off the skin) are indicators of abnormally dry skin.
• Observe mucous membranes (see Chapter 12) for dullness, dryness, and flaking.	• Increased perspiration may be associated with activity, warm environment, obesity, anxiety, or excitement.	• Lack of perspiration.
• Palpate skin temperature with the dorsum or the back of the hand. Compare symmetric body parts. Compare upper and lower body parts. Palpate over pressure sites.	• Skin is normally cool or warm to the touch.	• Temperature variation may reveal localized warmth at an infected wound site or coolness resulting from reduced blood flow. Example: A Stage I pressure ulcer will feel warm to the touch.

- Lightly stroke skin with fingertips; gently palpate to determine texture. Be aware of cultural variations.
  - Skin texture is normally smooth, soft, even, and flexible. Texture is not uniform throughout the body. Palms of hands and soles of feet are thicker.

- Note if skin is smooth or rough, thin or thick, tight or supple, and soft or indurated (hardened).
  - Normally the skin is firm, without tenderness or lesions.
  - Localized changes may result from trauma, surgical wounds, or lesions.

- Palpate skin lightly for tenderness, firmness, and depth of surface lesions.

- Palpate areas that appear irregular more deeply.
  - Localized areas of hardness.

- Assess turgor by grasping a skin fold on the back of the forearm or sternal area and releasing (Fig.7-3).
  - Skin moves and snaps back into place easily and quickly.
  - Skin stays pinched (tented ≥5 seconds), indicating dehydration.

- If areas of redness over the skin are noted, place fingertip over area and apply gentle pressure, then release.
  - Normal reactive hyperemia (redness) is the visible effect of localized vasodilation. Affected areas of skin will blanch with fingertip pressure.
  - No blanching.

- Normally the skin snaps back immediately to resting position in a person under 65 years of age.

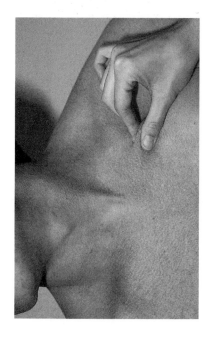

Fig. 7-3

Assessment for skin turgor. (From Seidel HM et al: *Mosby's guide to physical examination*, ed 4, St Louis, 1999, Mosby.)

Assessment	Normal Findings	Deviations From Normal
• Inspect and palpate for edema. • Palpate for mobility, consistency, and tenderness of the edema.	• No edema.	• Skin in dependent areas looks stretched, swollen, and shiny.
• To assess pitting edema, press the area firmly with thumb for 5 seconds and release.	• No pitting edema.	• Pitting edema can be measured by degree of indentation: 1+, 2+, 3+, 4+ (Fig. 7-4). Record depth of pitting in millimeters (Seidel et al, 1999).
• Inspect any lesion for color, location, texture, size, shape, type, grouping (clustered or linear), and distribution (localized or generalized). Observe exudate for color, odor, amount, and consistency.	• Skin should be free of lesions, except common freckles or age-related changes such as skin tags, senile keratosis (thickening of skin), cherry angiomas (ruby red papules), and atrophic warts.	• Lesions are present (see Table 7-2).

Assessment	Normal Findings	Deviations From Normal
• Gently palpate any lesion to determine mobility, contour (flat, raised, or depressed), and consistency (soft or hard). Note if client complains of tenderness during palpation.	• Skin is free of lesions.	• Tumors are elevated and solid. • Scabs, blisters, or pimples are early signs of skin damage from pressure.

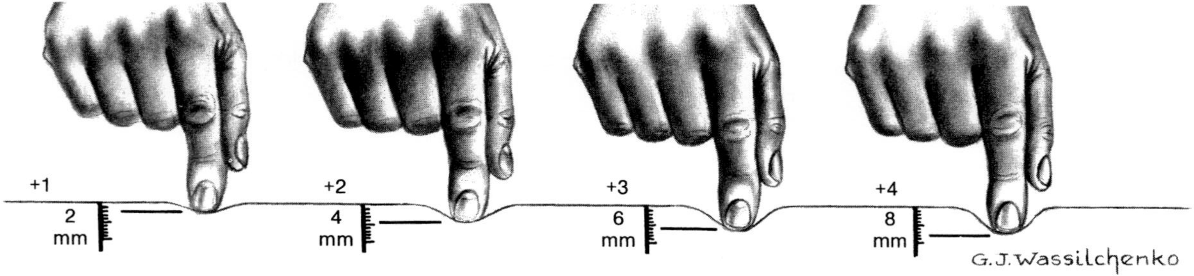

G.J.Wassilchenko

+1   +2   +3   +4
2   4   6   8
mm   mm   mm   mm

Fig. 7-4

Assessing for pitting edema.

(From Seidel HM et al: *Mosby's guide to physical examination*, ed 4, St Louis, 1999, Mosby.)

Table 7-2 Types of Skin Lesions

Primary Skin Lesions

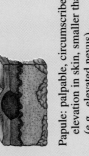

| Macule: flat, nonpalpable change in skin color, smaller than 1 cm (e.g., freckle, petechia) | Papule: palpable, circumscribed, solid elevation in skin, smaller than 0.5 cm (e.g., elevated nevus) | Nodule: elevated solid mass, deeper and firmer than papule, 0.5 to 0.2 cm (e.g., wart) |

Modified from Smoller J, Smoller BR: Skin malignancies in the elderly: diagnosable, treatable, and potentially curable. *J Gerontol Nurs* 18(5):19, 1992. Illustrations from Belcher AE: *Cancer nursing*, St Louis, 1992, Mosby; Habif TP: *Clinical dermatology*, ed 3, St Louis, 1996, Mosby; and Zitelli B, Davis H: *Atlas of pediatric physical diagnosis*, ed 2, St Louis, 1991, Mosby.

Continued

Table 7-2   Types of Skin Lesions—cont'd

Primary Skin Lesions

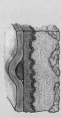

Tumor: solid mass that may extend deep through subcutaneous tissue, larger than 1 to 2 cm (e.g., epithelioma)

Vesicle: circumscribed elevation of skin filled with serous fluid, smaller than 0.5 cm (e.g., herpes simplex, chickenpox)

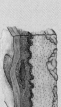

Wheal: irregularly shaped, elevated area or superficial localized edema, varies in size (e.g., hive, mosquito bite)

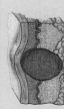

Pustule: circumscribed elevation of skin similar to vesicle but filled with pus, varies in size (e.g., acne, staphylococcal infection)

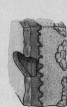

Ulcer: deep loss of skin surface that may extend to dermis and frequently bleeds and scars, varies in size (e.g., venous stasis ulcer)

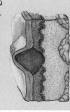

Atrophy: thinning of skin with loss of normal skin furrow with skin appearing shiny and translucent, varies in size (e.g., arterial insufficiency)

Skin Malignancies in the Older Adult

Basal Cell Carcinoma

0.5-cm to 1.0-cm crusted lesion that may be flat or raised
and may have a rolled, somewhat scaly border.
Frequently there are underlying, widely dilated blood
vessels that can be seen clinically within the lesions.

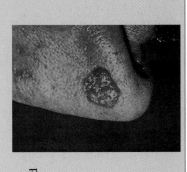

Modified from Smoller J, Smoller BR: Skin malignancies in the elderly: diagnosable, treatable, and potentially curable. *J Gerontol Nurs* 18(5):19, 1992. Illustrations from Belcher AE: *Cancer nursing,* St Louis, 1992, Mosby; Habif TP: *Clinical dermatology,* ed 3, St Louis, 1996, Mosby; and Zitelli B, Davis H: *Atlas of pediatric physical diagnosis,* ed 2, St Louis, 1991, Mosby.

Continued

Table 7-2 Types of Skin Lesions—cont'd

Skin Malignancies in the Older Adult

Squamous Cell Carcinoma

Occurs more often on mucosal surfaces and nonexposed areas of skin, compared to basal cell.
0.5-cm to 1.5-cm scaly lesions, may be ulcerated or
crusted. Frequently appear and grow more rapidly
than basal cell.

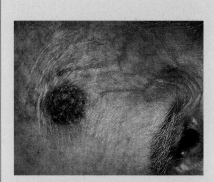

Melanoma

0.5-cm to 1.0-cm brown, flat lesions that may arise on sun-exposed or nonexposed skin. Variegated pigmentation, irregular borders, and indistinct margins. Ulceration, recent growth, or recent change in long-standing mole are ominous signs.

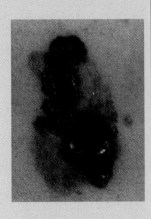

Modified from Smoller J, Smoller BR: Skin malignancies in the elderly: diagnosable, treatable, and potentially curable. *J Gerontol Nurs* 18(5):19, 1992. Illustrations from Belcher AE: *Cancer nursing,* St Louis, 1992, Mosby; Habif TP: *Clinical dermatology,* ed 3, St Louis, 1996, Mosby; and Zitelli B, Davis H: *Atlas of pediatric physical diagnosis,* ed 2, St Louis, 1991, Mosby.

Continued

Table 7-2 Types of Skin Lesions—cont'd

Pressure Ulcers in Stages

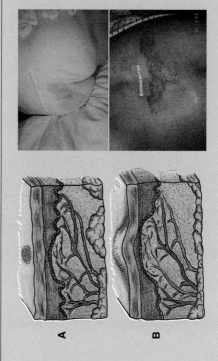

Stage I

A

Stage II

B

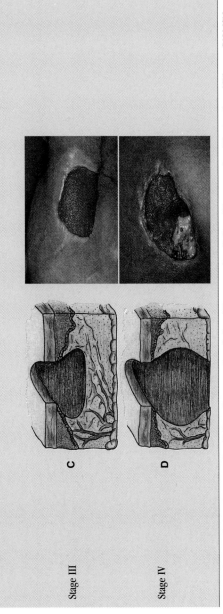

Stage III

Stage IV

Diagram of Stages. **A,** Stage I pressure ulcer. **B,** Stage II pressure ulcer. **C,** Stage III pressure ulcer. **D,** Stage IV pressure ulcer. (Courtesy Laurel Wiersma, RN MSN, Clinical Nurse Specialist, Barnes-Jewish Hospital, St Louis, Mo.)

Assessment	Normal Findings	Deviations From Normal
• Measure size of a lesion using a centimeter ruler. Measure height, width, and depth when possible.		
Nails		
• Inspect the nail bed color, cleanliness, length, thickness and shape of the nail plate, texture of the nail, and condition of tissue around the nail.	• Nails are normally transparent, smooth, well rounded, and convex, with surrounding cuticles smooth, intact, and without inflammation.	• Nails are ragged, dirty, and poorly kept. Erythema around cuticles. • Bluish-black. See Box 7-3 for abnormalities of the nail bed.
• Inspect the angle between the nail and nail bed. Have client place the nail (dorsal) surfaces of the fingertips of corresponding fingers of the right and left hand together. If nails are clubbed, a diamond-shaped window at base of the nails disappears and angles between distal tip increases.	• Normal nail bed angle is 160 degrees.	• Change in angle between nail and nail base larger than 180 degrees.

BOX 7-3 Abnormalities of the Nail Bed

160 degrees

Normal nail: Approximately 160-degree angle between nail plate and nail

180 degrees

Clubbing: Change in angle between nail and nail base (eventually larger than 180 degrees) nail bed softening, with nail flattening; often enlargement of fingertips

Causes: Chronic lack of oxygen: heart or pulmonary disease

180 degrees

Beau's lines: Transverse depressions in nails indicating temporary disturbance of nail growth (nail grows out over several months)
Causes: Systemic illness such as severe infection, nail injury

Continued

BOX 7-3 Abnormalities of the Nail Bed—cont'd

Koilonychia (spoon nail): Concave curves
Causes: Iron-deficiency anemia, syphilis, use of strong detergents

Splinter hemorrhages: Red or brown linear streaks in nail bed
Causes: Minor trauma, subacute bacterial endocarditis, trichinosis

Paronychia: Inflammation of skin at base of nail
Causes: Local infection, trauma

Assessment	Normal Findings	Deviations From Normal
• Inspect the lateral and proximal nail folds around the nail.	• Nail folds are smooth and intact.	• Nail folds are inflamed, rough, and have torn edges.
• Inspect the nail plate. Look for ridges, grooves, depressions, and pitting.	• Nail plate is smooth. Beading and longitudinal ridging are common.	• Splinter hemorrhages (longitudinal red or brown streaks).
		• Beau lines (transverse depression of the nail at the base of the lunula).

- Palpate the nail base for firmness by gently squeezing the nail between your thumb and the pad of your finger. Does nail adhere to nail bed?

- Assess adequacy of circulation and capillary refill by palpation: grasp the client's finger and observe the color of the nail bed. Next, apply gentle, firm pressure with thumb to nail bed. As pressure is applied, the nail bed appears white or blanched. Release pressure quickly for return of pink color.

- Inspect surfaces of sides and bottoms of toes and sides of fingers.

- Nail bed is firm and adherent.

- White color of nail bed under pressure should return to pink within 2 or 3 seconds, or the time it takes to say "capillary refill."

- Skin is smooth and not swollen.

- Softening and flattening of nail caused by clubbing.

- Prolonged capillary refill.

- Calluses and corns are flat and painless, resulting from thickening of epidermis caused by friction. Changes are harmless but may be a source of discomfort from eventual pressure against shoes.

Assessment	Normal Findings	Deviations From Normal
Hair and Scalp		
⊙ *Standard Precautions Alert* *Apply gloves if lice are suspected. After inspecting for lice, discard gloves in appropriate container and wash hands thoroughly before continuing examination.*		
• Inspect the color, distribution, quantity, thickness, texture, and lubrication of body hair. Be aware of cultural variation.	• Hair is normally evenly distributed, is neither excessively dry nor oily, and is pliant. Balding is common in men, occurring from the front of the scalp.	• Hirsutism. • Reduction of hair covering the extremities.
• Separate sections of scalp hair to observe characteristics of color, texture, and coarseness. Be aware of cultural variation.	• Scalp hair may be coarse or fine, curly or straight, and it should be shiny, smooth, and pliant.	• Hair loss. • Excessively oily hair.
	• It is not excessively oily or dry.	• Dry, coarse, or discolored hair.
	• Color varies from very light blond to black to gray and may show alterations from rinses or dyes.	• Brittle hair.

- Inspect the scalp for lesions, which easily go unnoticed in thick hair; separate hair for thorough examination.

- Inspect hair follicles on the scalp and pubic areas for lice or other parasites. Lice attach their eggs to hair. Avoid close contact of your clothing to prevent transmission of lice.

- Scalp is smooth and inelastic, with even coloration. Moles are common.

- No lice, scabies, or crabs are observed.

- Scaliness or dryness of scalp.
- Lumps or bruises.

- Lice are difficult to see. The tiny eggs look like oval particles of dandruff.

- Head and body lice are very small with grayish-white bodies.

- Crab lice have a red appearance. Lice leave bites or pustular eruptions in the hair follicles and in areas where skin surfaces meet (e.g., behind the ears).

UNEXPECTED ASSESSMENT FINDINGS—INTEGUMENT

Abnormal Finding	Significance	Next Step
Changes in Skin Color		
• Pallor.	• Consider anemia.	• Review lab results for low hemoglobin (Hgb)/hematocrit (Hct). Consider bleeding sources. Check BP.
• Cyanosis.	• Client may be cold. Late sign of diminished oxygenation.	• Check for central cyanosis, mucous membranes of mouth. Assess for diminished oxygenation (see Chapter 13).
• Petechiae.	• May indicate blood clotting disorders, drug reactions, or liver disease.	• Review chart for previous documentation of petechiae. If none, notify physician. Assess for other skin changes.
• Increased vascularity of the face.	• May be related to chronic alcohol ingestion or some dermatological condition.	• Review chart for previous documentation of change. Record and report findings.
• Localized changes such as rash, inflammation, or swelling.	• May result from allergic reaction to cosmetics, soap, laundry detergent, or fragrance.	• Review any changes in product use. • Record and report findings.

Finding	Interpretation	Action
Reddened, edematous, warm and hardened areas along the arms and legs.	Suggests recent injections.	Review medical record for medically indicated injections (e.g., insulin, heparin, Vitamin B_{12}).
		Ask client about substance abuse with injectable medications.
Hyperpigmented and shiny areas.	Suggests old injection sites.	Record and report findings.
Absence of superficial skin layers.	Early pressure ulcer formation.	Record and report findings.
		Implement nursing measures to reduce and prevent pressure ulcer formation.
Localized skin changes with irregular findings in texture.	May result from trauma, surgical wounds, or lesions.	Ask client about changes, trauma, and surgery.
		Record and report findings.
Skin of dependent areas look stretched, swollen, and shiny (see Table 7-2).	May indicate poor venous return.	Record and report findings.
	Direct trauma will also cause edema.	Quantify amount of edema by using objective measure of edema from none to 4+ (see Fig. 7-4, p. 124).

Abnormal Finding	Significance	Next Step
• Skin lesions.	• May indicate an acute or chronic infection. • May indicate a fungal infection such as tinea curis (ringworm) or tinea pedis (athletes foot). • May indicate a mole or skin tag.	• Ask client about changes. Is a mole asymmetric? Are borders irregular? Is color uneven or irregular? Has diameter changed? Is the lesion larger than a pencil eraser?
• Impaired nail growth.	• May be caused by direct injury such as nail biting or generalized disease.	• Review history for indication of injury or illness that may result in impaired nail growth. • Record and report findings.
• Bluish-black discoloration.	• Usually indicates hemorrhage under the nail from trauma.	• Review history for indication of injury. • Record and report findings.
• Splinter hemorrhages (longitudinal red or brown streaks).	• Can occur as the result of a minor injury or severe psoriasis of the nail matrix (Seidel et al, 1999).	• Assess for history of injury or psoriasis. • If new findings, notify physician. • Record and report findings.

• Beau lines (transverse depression of the nail at the base of the lunula).	• The result of a temporary interruption of nail formation resulting from systemic illness such as nail infection or nail injury. • The Beau lines are seen on all of the nails (Seidel et al, 1999).	• Review laboratory data for indication of hypercalcemia or other diseases. • Record and report findings, noting when client first observed changes.
• Paronychia (inflamed, swollen nail bed).	• Caused by infection and trauma.	• Record and report findings. • Determine if injury occurred. • Notify physician of findings. Usually prescribe an antibiotic for the infection.
• Clubbing of nails.	• Caused by chronic hypoxemia.	• Record and report finding.
• Changes in shape or curvature of nail body	• Can indicate systemic disease.	• Assess for adequate oxygenation (see Chapter 13).
• A mass or hardening in area just below nail bed in interphalangeal joint.	• Can be from traumatic injury to interphalangeal joint capsule from repetitive striking of finger.	• Assess for history of recent or prior trauma to the hand. • Record and report findings including any change in function of the hand and/or finger.

Abnormal Finding	Significance	Next Step
• Decreased capillary refill.	• Caused be circulatory insufficiency.	• Record and report findings. • If new finding, report to physician.
Abnormalities in hair • Hirsutism in women.	• Hair growth on the upper lip, chin, and cheeks, with vellus (fine) hair becoming coarser over the body.	• Record and report findings. • Physician may order laboratory tests to determine levels of progesterone, estrogen, and testosterone.
• Excessively oily hair.	• May result from androgen hormone stimulation.	• Review laboratory data, if available, for evidence of increased androgen hormone.
• Dry, coarse, or discolored hair.	• May be the result of poor nutrition.	• Review nutritional habits.
• Brittle hair.	• May be caused by excessive use of shampoo or chemical agents.	• Determine client's use of hair care products. • Record and report findings.

Scaliness or dryness of scalp.	• Dandruff or psoriasis.	• Determine client's use of hair care products. • Record and report findings.
Lumps or bruises to scalp.	• May indicate trauma.	• Assess for recent trauma to the head. • Record and report findings.
Reduction of hair covering the extremities.	• May be result of arterial insufficiency. • Do not confuse this with loss of hair from shaven legs or chronic rubbing of calves from men's pants legs.	• Assess peripheral pulses, temperature, and sensation. • Record and report findings, including the level on lower extremity where there is a change in hair distribution or sensation.
Hair loss.	• Can be related to endocrine disorders such as diabetes, thyroiditis, and even menopause.	• Review medical record for disorders. • Review with client when hair loss was first noticed. • Evaluate for genetic predisposition, such as family history of male pattern baldness. • Record and report findings.

Abnormal Finding	Significance	Next Step
• Scabies.	• Result of close contact with a person infested with scabies.	• Notify care provider who may want to isolate scabies for indentification. • Use a piece of transparent tape to secure a single scabie. Unlike lice, they are not attached to a hair follicle, but rather are moving on the skin. • Review with physician, using a microscope.
• Head lice.	• Head lice are acquired by use of a hair brush or comb of infested individuals. Easily transmitted in classrooms among children who readily share personal items.	• Notify care provider who may want to isolate lice for identification. • Select hair follicule with attached nit. Cover with transparent tape and remove single hair. • Review hair follicule with physician, using a microscope.

there are three flexion creases. When the two distal creases are fused to form a single horizontal crease (simian crease), this may indicate Down syndrome.
- Localized loss of hair such as on the back of the head may indicate that the infant lies too frequently in one position and may have unmet stimulation needs.
- Tufts of hair anywhere along the spine, especially over the sacrum, can indicate the site of spina bifida occulta.
- During adolescence a change in the amount and distribution of hair growth occurs.

Be familiar with skin changes common in communicable diseases:

- Chickenpox (varicella)—Rash highly pruritic, begins as macule, rapidly progresses to papule, and then vesicle (surrounded by erythematous base) becomes cloudy, breaks easily, and forms crusts; all three stages (papule, vesicle, crust) are present in varying degrees at one time. Rash is distributed centripetally, spreading to face and proximal extremities but sparse on distal limbs and less on areas not exposed to heat (Wong, 1999).
- Measles (rubeola)—Stages of rash development: appears 3 to 4 days after onset of prodromal stage; begins as

Pediatric Considerations

- When exposing an infant to an examination of the skin, be sure the room is comfortably warm because air conditioning can cause a cold-induced cyanosis, and excessive heat can produce flushing.
- Skin color of light-skinned children varies from a milky-white and rosy color to a more deeply hued pink color. Dark-skinned children, such as Hispanic, African American, Latin, or Mediterranean, have inherited various brown, red, yellow, olive-green, and bluish tones in their skin, which can falsely alter assessment.
- Common changes in texture may indicate cradle cap, eczema, diaper rash, or excessive dryness (xeroderma) (Wong, 1999).
- Skin rashes are common in infants because of food allergies or diaper irritation.
- Periorbital edema may normally be evident in children who have been crying, sleeping, or who have allergies.
- Developmental changes may cause skin changes, such as facial acne in adolescents.
- Assess the dermatoglyphics, or pattern of handprint, in children. Note the flexion creases in the palm of the hand. (They also can be seen in the sole of the foot.) Normally

erythematous maculopapular eruption on face and gradually spreads downward; more severe at earlier sites and less intense at later sites. After 3 to 4 days it assumes a brownish appearance, and fine desquamation occurs over areas of extensive involvement (Wong, 1999).

- German measles (rubella)—Rash first appears on face and rapidly spreads downward to neck, arms, trunk, and legs; after first day body is covered with a discrete, pinkish-red maculopapular exanthema. The rash disappears in same order it began and is gone by third day. Communicable 7 days before to about 5 days after appearance of rash (Wong, 1999).

- Scarlet fever—Rash appears within 12 hours after onset of fever, chills, and abdominal pain. Red, pin-head-size punctate lesions rapidly become generalized but are absent on the face, which becomes flushed with striking circumoral pallor. Rash is more intense in folds of joints, and by end of first week, desquamation begins (fine, sandpaper-like on torso; sloughing on palms and soles). Communicable during incubation period. Clinical illness approximately 10 days and during first 2 weeks of carrier phase (Wong, 1999).

- Exanthema subitum (roseola)—Rash is discrete rose-pink macules or maculopapules appearing first on trunk, then spreading to neck, face, and extremities; nonpruritic, fades on pressure, lasts 1 to 2 days (Wong, 1999).

Gerontologic Considerations

- Older adults may have difficulty reaching all body parts for cleansing. Difficult-to-reach areas may have body odor.
- Pigmentation of the skin increases unevenly, causing discolored skin.
- With increasing age, the skin becomes wrinkled and leathery, with decreased turgor. Overall there is an increase in skin folds and laxness in the skin's ability to return to normal position. Skin turgor is best checked in older adults over the sternum, forehead, or abdomen.
- Skin may be drier because of diminished sebaceous and sweat gland activity.
- A common skin lesion that develops with aging is seborrheic, or senile, keratosis. Keratosis appears as a benign, wartlike growth appearing on the trunk, face, and scalp as

single or multiple lesions. The lesions are superficial, circumscribed, raised areas that thicken and darken over time.

- Actinic keratosis, common in men past middle age, is a lesion that can become cancerous. This type of lesion appears in areas exposed to the sun, such as bald heads, hands, and faces. The lesion is a localized thickening of the skin that begins as a reddish, scaly, superficial area.
- In the older adult, evidence of delayed healing of bruises, lacerations, and excoriations is considered normal.
- Older adults' hair becomes dry, brittle, dull gray, white, or yellow. Hair thins over the scalp, axillae, and pubic areas.
- Older men lose facial hair.
- With aging, the nails of the fingers and toes develop longitudinal striations and grow at a slower rate.
- Because of insufficient calcium, nails may turn yellow in older adults.
- The cuticle also becomes less thick and wide.

Cultural Considerations

- Cultural variations in skin color influence ability to detect abnormalities; in white skin, pallor may be an extreme paleness of the skin, whereas in dark skin there is a loss of red tones. Erythema is noted by palpation of increased warmth in dark-skinned clients. Cyanosis may be easier to detect in the lips and tongue of dark-skinned clients, where cyanosis appears an ashen gray.
- White and African-American adolescents and adults generally have body odor, but Oriental and Native-American adolescents and adults generally do not. The difference is caused by few functioning apocrine glands and a difference in the glands' secretions (Seidel et al, 1999).
- Rashes in dark-skinned clients may need to be palpated, because the rash may not be readily visible to the eye (Giger, 1999). Note induration and warmth of the area.
- African Americans often develop keloids, rope-like scars that occur as a result of an exaggeration of the wound-healing process following trauma or inflammation to the skin.
- When assessing the darkly pigmented client for specific color changes such as pallor or jaundice, inspect the conjunctivae and oral membranes of the buccal mucosa (see Chapter 12).
- Mongolian spots (bluish pigment from fetal migratory melanocytes) found generally in the lumbosacral region are present in 80% of Orientals at birth (Giger, 1999). These spots can be mistaken for bruises.

- In whites, nail beds are pink with translucent white tips. In African Americans, a brown or black pigmentation is normally present in longitudinal streaks.
- Asian and African Americans have less hair over the chest and legs than do whites, and Native Americans have little or no hair on their bodies.
- The hair of African Americans is usually thicker and drier than the hair of whites. Hispanics have hair that is usually dark and may be curly and woolly, straight, or wavy.

Client Teaching

Skin

Instruct client to conduct a complete monthly self-examination of the skin, noting moles, blemishes, and birthmarks. Tell the client to inspect all skin surfaces. Cancerous melanomas start as small, molelike growths that increase in size, change color, become ulcerated, and bleed. Follow the ABCD rule (American Cancer Society, 2000):

A is for Asymmetry

B is for Border irregularity; edges are ragged, notched, or blurred

C is for Color; pigmentation is not uniform

D is for Diameter; greater than 6 mm

- Tell client to report to a physician or care provider any change in skin lesions or a sore that bleeds or does not heal. Especially instruct older adults, who tend to have delayed wound healing.
- Instruct client to reduce risk of skin cancer by avoiding over-exposure to the sun by wearing wide-brimmed hats and long sleeves, using sunscreens with SPF greater than or equal to 15 approximately 20 minutes before going into sun and after swimming or perspiring, avoiding tanning at midday (10 AM to 3 PM); and not using indoor sunlamps, tanning parlors, or tanning pills. Medications such as oral contraceptives and antibiotics can make skin more sensitive to the sun. Children require special protection from the sun. (Keep children clothed and in the shade.)
- To treat "winter itch," client should avoid hot water, harsh soaps, and drying agents such as rubbing alcohol. Use a superfatted soap such as Dove, and pat rather than rub the skin dry.
- Tell the client to apply alcohol-free lotion and moisturizer regularly to the skin to reduce itching and drying.
- Inform the client that baths need not be taken daily.

- Instruct adolescents regarding proper skin cleansing and the importance of a balanced diet and adequate rest.

Nails

- Instruct the client to cut nails only after soaking them at least 10 minutes in warm water. (EXCEPTION: Diabetics should not soak nails.)
- Caution client against use of over-the-counter preparations to treat corns, calluses, or ingrown toenails.
- Tell the client to cut nails straight across and even with tops of fingers and toes. If client has diabetes, tell client to file, not cut, nails.
- Instruct client to shape nails with a file or emery board.
- If your client is a diabetic, client should wash feet daily in warm water. Inspect the feet each day in a place with good lighting, looking for dry places and cracks in the skin. Soften dry feet by applying a cream or lotion such as Nivea, Eucerin, or Alpha Keri. Do not put lotion between the toes. Caution against using sharp objects to poke or dig under the toenail or around the cuticle. Have client see a podiatrist for treatment of ingrown toenails and nails that are thick or tend to split.

Hair and scalp

- Clients may require instruction about basic hygiene measures, including shampooing and combing the hair.
- Instruct clients who have head lice to shampoo thoroughly with a pediculicide (shampoo available at drug stores) in cold water, comb thoroughly with fine-tooth comb, and discard comb. After combing, remove any detectable nits or nit cases with tweezers or between the fingernails. A dilute solution of vinegar and water may help loosen nits.
- Ways to reduce transmission of lice include the following:
  - Do not share personal care items with others.
  - Vacuum all rugs, car seats, pillows, furniture, and flooring thoroughly and discard vacuum bag.
  - Use thorough hand washing.
  - Launder all clothing, linen, and bedding in hot soap and water and dry in hot dryer for at least 20 minutes. Dry-clean nonwashables.
  - Instruct client that his or her partner must be notified if lice were sexually transmitted.

8

Head and Neck

Assessment of the head and neck includes assessing the general appearance of the head and then focusing on neck structures, including neck muscles, lymph nodes, carotid arteries and jugular veins, the trachea, and the thyroid gland. The assessment of the carotid arteries and jugular veins can be deferred until conducting assessment of the vascular system (see Chapter 14).

Anatomy and Physiology

The head provides a protective cover for the brain and special sensory organs. The skull consists of seven bones (two frontal, parietal, and temporal, and one occipital) that are fused together and covered by the scalp. Describe the assessment findings by bone location.

The facial skull contains cavities for the eyes, nose, and mouth. The bony structure of the face is formed from the fused frontal, nasal, zygomatic, ethmoid, lacrimal, sphenoid, and maxillary bones, which serve as additional landmarks (Fig. 8-1).

The structure of the neck is formed by the cervical vertebrae, the ligaments, and sternocleidomastoid and trapezius muscles. The two sets of muscles divide each side of the neck into two triangles (Fig. 8-2). The anterior triangle contains the trachea, thyroid gland, carotid artery, and anterior cervical lymph nodes. The posterior triangle contains the posterior lymph nodes. The lymph nodes collect drainage of lymphatic fluid from the head and neck areas. The immune system protects the body from foreign antigens, removes damaged cells from the circulation, and provides a partial barrier to growth of malignant cells within the body. Fig. 8-3 shows the location of major lymphatic chains in the head and neck.

The thyroid gland lies in the anterior lower neck on both sides of the trachea, with the isthmus of the gland overlying the trachea (Fig. 8-4). The thyroid gland has two lateral lobes, which are butterfly shaped and joined by the isthmus at their lower aspect. The lobes curve posteriorly around the cartilage and are in large part covered by the sternocleidomastoid muscles. The trachea is located midline above the suprasternal notch.

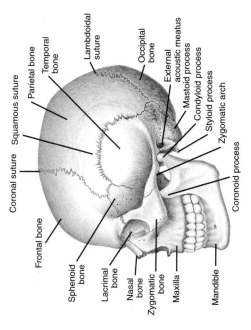

Coronal suture · Squamous suture · Parietal bone · Temporal bone · Lambdoidal suture · Occipital bone · External acoustic meatus · Mastoid process · Condyloid process · Styloid process · Zygomatic arch · Frontal bone · Sphenoid bone · Lacrimal bone · Nasal bone · Zygomatic bone · Maxilla · Mandible · Coronoid process

Fig. 8-1
Bones of the skull.

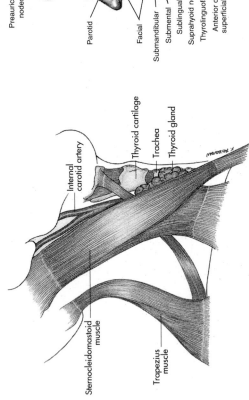

Fig. 8-3

Head and neck lymphatic system.
(From Seidel HM et al: *Mosby's guide to physical examination*, ed 4, St Louis, 1999, Mosby.)

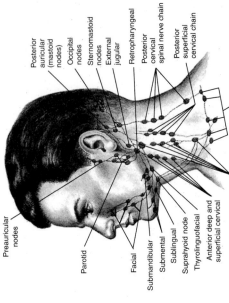

Fig. 8-2

Anatomic position of major neck structures.

You inspect the head to determine presence of any obvious deformities or trauma. Examination of the neck determines the integrity of neck structures and the lymphatic system. The lymphatic system is examined region by region during the assessment of other body systems (for example, breast, genitalia, and extremities). Superficial lymph nodes aid in identifying the presence of infection or malignancy. Examination of the thyroid and trachea can also alert the examiner to potential malignancies.

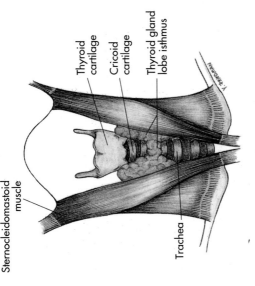

Sternocleidomastoid muscle

Thyroid cartilage

Cricoid cartilage

Thyroid gland lobe isthmus

Trachea

Fig. 8-4
Anatomic position of the thyroid gland.

Critical Thinking Application—Head and Neck

Knowledge	Experience	Standards
• Refer to previous knowledge regarding infectious disease and the immune system. Clients with suspected immunosuppression or compromise may have involvement of the lymphatic system. • Knowledge of neurological function must be applied when examining the head. The presence of trauma poses risk for neurological injury and requires a thorough neurological assessment (see Chapter 20). Be alert for a cervical neck injury, a life-threatening injury requiring immediate immobilization.	• Gaining expertise in palpation of lymph nodes and the thyroid gland takes considerable practice. • Have a more experienced clinician confirm any findings you make. **You will find a certain positioning technique works best for you to palpate structures consistently.**	• Be methodical in examining each lymph node chain on both sides of the neck. • Be consistent and proceed in the same order with each examination (e.g., anterior cervical chain, posterior cervical chain, and thyroid).

Head and Neck Assessment

Equipment

- Stethoscope
- Cup of water

Delegation Considerations

Physical examination of the head and neck requires critical thinking and knowledge application unique to a professional nurse. The examination should not be delegated to unlicensed assistive personnel. Staff should know to report any instances of clients noting reduced range of motion (ROM) in the neck or lumps in the neck.

Client Preparation

Client assumes a sitting position, with head upright and still during examination. Be sure clothing is loosened or removed so neck is fully exposed. Palpate the lymph nodes from the front so you can palpate bilaterally at the same time. Palpate the thyroid gland from either the front of or behind the client.

History

- Determine if client experienced recent trauma to the head. If so, assess state of consciousness after injury (immediately upon return of consciousness, 5 minutes later, and duration of unconsciousness). Also note any predisposing factors (for example, seizure, blackout).
- Ask if client has history of headache; note location, onset, duration, character, pattern, associated symptoms, and precipitating factor.
- If the client has experienced trauma, does client have neck pain? **Immobilization of cervical vertebrae may be necessary.**
- Determine length of time client has experienced neurological symptoms.
- Review client's occupational history for use of safety helmets (if appropriate).
- Ask if the client participates in contact sports, cycling, rollerblading, or skateboarding.
- For infants, assess birth history and shape of head on delivery.
- Has the client had a recent cold or infection? Does the client feel fatigued or weak?

- If an enlarged lymph node exists, consider several factors (for example, infection, malignancy). If client has risk factors for human immunodeficiency virus (HIV) infection, review for history of intravenous (IV) drug use, hemophilia, sexual contact with persons infected with HIV, history of blood transfusion, multiple sexual contacts, or homosexual or bisexual tendencies (if client is male).
- Has the client been exposed to radiation, toxic chemicals, or infection?

- To rule out thyroid problems, ask if client has had change in temperature preference (more or less clothing); swelling in neck; change in hair texture, skin, or nails; or change in emotional stability.
- Does client have history of thyroid disease? Are thyroid medications taken?
- Review medical history for pneumothorax (collapsed lung) or bronchial tumor.

ASSESSMENT TECHNIQUES — HEAD AND NECK

Head

Inspection

Assessment	Normal Findings	Deviations From Normal
• Note position of head in relation to shoulders and trunk.	• Head is normally held upright, still, and midline to trunk.	• Tilting of head to one side. • Horizontal jerking.
• Inspect client's facial features (eyelids, eyebrows, palpebral fissures, nasolabial folds, and mouth) for symmetry at rest, shape, movement, and expression.	• Slight asymmetry is common. Facial characteristics vary with race and sex.	• Facial asymmetry. • A rounded or "moon-shaped" face. • Dull, puffy, yellow skin with peri-orbital edema and temporal loss of eyebrows.
• Inspect the head for size, shape, and contour.	• The skull is generally round, with prominence in the frontal area anteriorly and occipital area posteriorly.	• Local skull deformities. • A large head.

Assessment	Normal Findings	Deviations From Normal
Palpation		
• Palpate the skull for nodules or masses by gently rotating fingertips down the midline of the scalp and then along the sides of the head.	• Skull is symmetric and smooth. Bones are not distinguishable.	• Indentation, depression of skull, tenderness, or swelling.
• Palpate the temporal arteries along the temporal-sphenoid bones; note course, elasticity, and presence of tenderness.	• Pulse palpable; vessel easily distensible.	• Thickening, hardening, and tenderness of temporal artery.
Neck		
Inspection		
• Have client sit facing you. Begin by inspecting the neck in the usual anatomic position, in slight hyperextension.	• Neck is slightly hyperextended, without masses or asymmetry. Trachea is midline. Veins and arteries are flat. Thyroid gland cannot be visualized.	• Edema of neck.
• Observe for symmetry of the neck muscles, alignment of the trachea, and any subtle fullness at base of neck.		• A mass at the base of the neck, visible as the client swallows.

- Note any distention or prominence of jugular veins and carotid arteries. During inspection ask the client to swallow a drink of water.

- Ask the client to flex the neck with the chin to the chest, then hyperextend the neck backward, and rotate the head to each side and sideways so that the ear moves toward the shoulder. This tests the sternocleidomastoid and trapezius muscles.

- Moves freely; full range of motion without discomfort or dizziness:
  - Flexion = 45 degrees
  - Extension = 55 degrees
  - Lateral abduction = 40 degrees

- Limited ROM.

- With the client's chin raised and head tilted slightly back, carefully inspect the area of the neck where lymph nodes are distributed.

- Nodes are not visible and nodal areas are without inflammation.

- Enlarged mass.

- Compare both sides and look for apparent enlargement, erythema, or red streaks.

Assessment	Normal Findings	Deviations From Normal
• To examine lymph nodes, have the client relax with neck flexed slightly forward or toward side of the examiner to relax tissues and muscles. Examine both sides of the neck.		
Palpation		
• Use the pads of the middle three fingers and gently palpate in a rotary motion for superficial and deep lymph nodes (see Fig. 8-3). Check nodes in the following sequence:	• Lymph nodes are not easily palpable. Superficial nodes that are palpable but not firm or large enough to be felt are common.	*A palpable fixed node may indicate a cancerous tumor.*
• Occipital nodes at base of skull.		
• Postauricular nodes over mastoid.		
• Preauricular nodes in front of ear.		
• Parotid and retropharyngeal nodes at angle of mandible.		

- Submaxillary nodes
- Submental nodes in midline behind mandibular tip.
- Superficial cervical nodes anterior to the sternocleidomastoid.
- Posterior cervical nodes along border of trapezius.
- Where the skin is more mobile, press lightly at first, and then increase pressure gradually.
- For any palpable nodes, note location, size, shape, tenderness, consistency, moveability or fixation, and discreteness.

Do not use excessive pressure to palpate, because small nodes may be missed. The node may be pressed into or between the muscle.

- Small (less than 1 cm), mobile, soft, nontender nodes are not uncommon.

- Tender, warm, soft, moveable, or fixed nodes.

Assessment	Normal Findings	Deviations From Normal
• Palpate supraclavicular nodes by asking the client to flex the head forward and relax the shoulders (Fig. 8-5). To palpate supraclavicular nodes you may need to hook the index and third finger over the clavicle, lateral to the sternocleidomastoid muscle.	• Nodes are not palpable.	• Enlarged supraclavicular nodes.
• Palpate the trachea for midline position by placing the thumb on one side of the trachea and index finger to other side above suprasternal notch. Compare the space between the trachea and the sternocleidomastoid muscle on each side.	• The trachea is midline at the suprasternal notch.	• Displacement of the trachea.

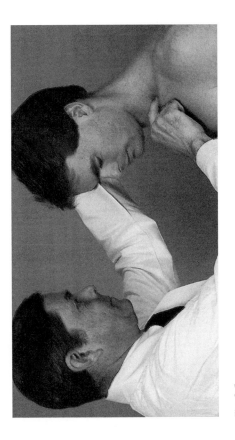

Fig. 8-5
Palpation for supraclavicular lymph nodes.
(From Seidel HM et al: *Mosby's guide to physical examination*, ed 4, St Louis, 1999, Mosby.)

Assessment	Normal Findings	Deviations From Normal
• To palpate the thyroid gland *posteriorly*, stand behind the client. Have the client flex the neck forward slightly and relax the neck muscles. Give the client a glass of water to use when swallowing is required. Place both of your hands around the client's neck, with two fingers of each hand on the sides of the trachea just beneath the cricoid cartilage. As the client swallows, feel for movement of the thyroid isthmus.	• Thyroid moves easily beneath fingers as client swallows.	• Isthmus is enlarged.
• To examine each lobe, have the client swallow while displacing the trachea to the right or left. Palpate the main body of each lobe (Fig. 8-6). For example, while examining the right lobe, move the fingers of the left hand between the trachea and the right sternocleidomastoid muscle. Then	• Thyroid is nonpalpable. If felt, the thyroid nodes should be small, smooth, and free of nodules.	• Enlarged thyroid gland.
	• The thyroid at its broadest base is approximately 1½ to 2 inches (4 cm) (Seidel et al, 1999).	

place fingers of the right hand behind the right sternocleidomastoid muscle and gently press the hands together to palpate the lobe as the client swallows. Repeat for left lobe.

- In thin clients, the thyroid gland is more easily palpable.

- To palpate the thyroid *anteriorly*, stand to the client's side. Use the pads of the index and middle finger and palpate the left lobe with the right hand and the right lobe with the left hand as the client swallows. Gently displace the trachea during palpation.

- Nonpalpable.

- Enlarged thyroid gland.

- When gland appears enlarged, place diaphragm of stethoscope over thyroid.

- No sound audible.

- Enlarged gland causes increase in arterial flow, resulting in fine vibration auscultated as a soft bruit.

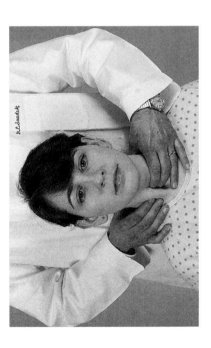

Fig. 8-6
Palpation of the right thyroid lobe from behind the client.
(From Seidel HM et al: *Mosby's guide to physical examination*, ed 4, St Louis, 1999, Mosby.)

UNEXPECTED ASSESSMENT FINDINGS—HEAD AND NECK

Abnormal Finding	Significance	Next Step
• Tilting of head to one side.	• May indicate unilateral hearing or visual loss.	• Assess for hearing and visual changes. • Record and report findings.
• Horizontal jerking of the head.	• May be associated with tremor.	• Review medical history for tremor. • Ask client how long client has been experiencing the head jerking. • Record and report findings.
• Facial asymmetry on an entire side of the face.	• May indicate facial nerve paralysis or cerebral vascular accident (CVA).	• Review neurological assessment (Chapter 20). • Notify physician if new finding. • Record and report findings.

Abnormal Finding	Significance	Next Step
• Facial muscle weakness.	• Facial nerve weakness causes asymmetry of the lower face. Asymmetry of the mouth may result from trigeminal nerve (Cranial nerve V) injury.	• Ask the client to show the teeth, smile, or raise eyebrows. • If a new finding, notify the physician for further evaluation. • May need to complete a neurological assessment (see Chapter 20).
• A rounded or "moon-shaped" face.	• May indicate Cushing's syndrome or obesity.	• Review medical record for history or current therapy with steroids. • Determine if client is obese. • Record and report findings.
• Dull, puffy, yellow skin with periorbital edema and temporal loss of eyebrows.	• Myxedema or hypothyroidism.	• Review laboratory data for elevated thyroid stimulating hormone (TSH). • Record and report findings.

Local skull deformities.	• Typically caused by trauma. • Assess for prior or recent trauma. • Record and report findings.
A large head in adults.	• May result from excessive growth hormone (acromegaly). • Record and report findings.
Indentation or depression of skull.	• May indicate fracture. • Tenderness or swelling may indicate hematoma. • Determine if client has had recent head trauma. • Assess for neurological changes (Chapter 20).
Thickening, hardening, and tenderness of artery.	• May indicate temporal arteritis. • Client presents with complaints of severe headache at the temples. Seen more often in older adults. • Notify physician and record findings.
Edema of neck.	• May be caused by local infections. • Assess for tenderness on palpation and presence of lymphadenopathy. • Record and report findings.
Mass at the base of the neck.	• Masses or nodules may indicate Hashimoto's disease or malignancy. • Review other assessment findings for fever, weight loss or gain, or chronic complaints of pharyngitis.

Abnormal Finding	Significance	Next Step
• Limited ROM of the head and neck.	• Enlarged mass may indicate infection, malignancy, or benign mass (e.g., cyst). • May indicate cranial nerve injury, muscular spasm, or trauma.	• Report findings to physician and record in medical record. • Assess for recent trauma or injury. • Determine if client has any numbness or tingling in the upper extremities. (See Chapter 20)
• Enlargement of the thyroid gland.	• May indicate thyroid dysfunction or tumor. • An enlarged, tender thyroid usually indicates thyroiditis.	• Review laboratory data for history of hypothyroidism. • Review medical record for documentation of enlarged thyroid. • Notify physician if new finding.
• Soft bruit auscultated over thyroid.	• Enlarged gland causes increase in arterial flow, resulting in fine vibration.	• Record and report findings.

• Supraclavicular enlarged nodes	• Frequently sites of metastatic disease (Seidel et al, 1999).	• Report findings to physician if new. • Record and report findings.
• Tracheal displacement.	• Lateral displacement may result from a mass in the neck or mediastinum or pulmonary abnormality such as tension pneumothorax.	• Notify physician as soon as possible if sudden finding. • Assess for mass in neck. • Record and report findings.
• Enlarged lymph nodes.	• Nodes that are warm to the touch indicate inflammation or infection. • Cancerous nodes are usually nontender, hard, and more discrete with unilateral enlargement. • Soft, matted, nontender, and cool-to-touch nodes indicate tuberculosis.	• Review other assessment findings that suggest the cause of the enlarged lymph nodes, such as temperature, history of upper respiratory or sinus infection, whether the client has felt the nodes, or if the client has any risk factors for tuberculosis. • If an enlarged node is a new finding, report to physician and record exact location.

Abnormal Finding	Significance	Next Step
• Enlarged head in an infant.	• An enlarged head, bulging fontanels, dilated scalp veins, and sclerae visible above the iris (Seidel et al, 1999) indicate hydrocephalus (cerebrospinal fluid in the ventricles).	• Evaluate for signs of increasing intracranial pressure (Chapter 20). • Report any positive findings immediately. • Assess for setting sun sign (eyes rotated downward) and bossing (depressed eyes) (Wong, 1999).

Pediatric Considerations

■ The posterior fontanel normally closes by the second month, and the anterior fontanel closes at 12 to 18 months of age.

■ Avoid applying pressure directly over fontanels because of potential for intracranial damage.

■ In a child, Down syndrome is characterized by depressed nasal bridge, epicanthal folds, and mongoloid slant of eyes, low-set ears, and large tongue.

■ In the neonate, palpate anterior and posterior fontanels for size, shape, and texture. Fontanels are normally flattened, smooth, and well demarcated. In infants, a large head may result from congenital anomalies.

■ Presence of small, firm, discrete, and movable lymph nodes that are neither warm nor tender are not uncommon. Lymph nodes can be found in the occipital, postauricular, and cervical chains (Seidel et al, 1999).

■ Do not confuse lymph node enlargement with mumps. Mumps is a painful swelling of the parotid glands, unilateral or bilateral. Swelling can obscure the angle of the jaw.

- Mononucleosis is an acute, self-limiting infectious disease caused by the herpes-like Epstein-Barr virus. Mononucleosis commonly occurs in adolescents and young adults. Affected nodes are generalized but are more commonly felt in the anterior and posterior cervical chains. The client will have fever, acute pharyngitis, fatigue, malaise, and in some cases, a descrete macular rash over the trunk (Wong, 1999).
- The thyroid is difficult to palpate in infants unless it is enlarged. In children, the thyroid may be palpable.

 Gerontologic Considerations

- The size of the head is proportionate to overall body size. Head may be tilted backward slightly.
- Older adults may have reduced neck ROM resulting from arthritic changes. Proceed slowly when evaluating ROM.
- Older adults typically have two prominent wrinkle lines appearing on either side of the midline of the neck. Sagging of surrounding tissue and deposition of fat create a double chin.
- The thyroid may move to a lower position in relation to the clavicles. The gland itself becomes more flexible, which may increase its nodularity on palpation (Lueckenotte, 2000).

- The size of lymph nodes decreases with advancing age because of loss of some lymphoid elements. Nodes become fibrotic and fatty.

 Cultural Considerations

- Thyroid disease is common in Vietnamese clients.
- Filipinos living in Hawaii have been found to have high incidence rates for thyroid cancer.

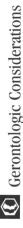 Client Teaching

- Assure parents or caregivers that open fontanels in newborns are normal, and caution them to protect the neonate's skull from pressure and potential trauma.
- Teach client about the lymph nodes and how infection can commonly cause node tenderness.
- Instruct client to call physician or care provider when an enlarged lump or mass is noted in the neck.
- Teach client risk factors for HIV infection.
- Stress the importance of regular compliance with medication schedule to clients with thyroid disease.

Eyes

Anatomy and Physiology

The organs of sight are contained in a bony orbit at the front of the skull, embedded in orbital fat, and innervated by one of a pair of optic nerves from the brain's occipital lobes. Light enters the eye through the transparent cornea (Fig. 9-1). The iris changes the size of the pupil to control the brightness of light entering. The lens changes shape to focus light on a layer of rods and cones constituting the retina. Impulses created by the retina's specialized nerve cells transmit a visual image along the optic nerve to the brain.

The external eyelids protect the eyes from dust and other foreign objects, injury, and strong light. The exposed part of the eye has the transparent conjunctiva for protection. The transparent cornea protects the iris.

Examination of the eye involves the assessment of four areas: Visual acuity, visual fields, extraocular movements, and external structures. The examination includes an ophthalmoscopic examination. You determine the presence of visual symptoms that may indicate the presence of specific eye disorders. Any visual alterations can significantly affect a client's ability to ambulate safely and to remain independent in performing self-care activities.

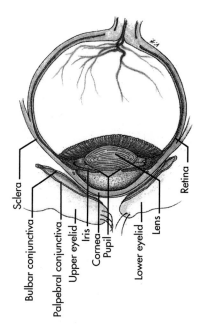

Fig. 9-1
Cross-section of the eye.

Critical Thinking Application—Eyes

Knowledge	Experience	Standards
• Signs and symptoms of eye disorders may represent injury or pathology affecting the visual structures.	• After caring for clients with eye disorders, you will learn that most clients become very independent in the installation of eye drops, cleansing and insertion of contact lenses, and managing any self-care limitations.	During an eye examination, apply the following principles:
• Visual change can indicate neurological injury to the optic nerve, (Cranial nerve II) anywhere along its course from the retina to the occipital lobe of the brain.		• Be very gentle during an eye examination. External and internal eye structures can easily be injured.
• Nerve involvement creates changes in a client's visual fields.	• Learn how your clients adapt to visual alterations in the home.	• Clients are very fearful of loss of vision. Take extra time to explain what will be done during an examination, and explain your findings.
• Consider knowledge of eye and neurological anatomy when conducting an assessment.	• Learn the unique approaches to self-care management clients have developed.	

clients' care, assistive personnel may become aware of subtle changes that may indicate visual disorders such as clients repositioning items within their visual field, being unable to read a diet menu, or continually stumbling over objects in their walking path. Any changes should be reported to you immediately.

Client Preparation

- Explain to the client that you will be touching the client's face and eyes.

- Throughout the examination the client is asked to sit or stand.

- The room may be darkened during the corneal reflex and ophthalmoscopic examination.

History

- Determine if the client has history of eye disease, surgery, eye trauma, diabetes, or hypertension.

- Determine problem that prompted client to seek health care. Ask the client about eye pain, photophobia (sensitivity to light), burning, itching, excess tearing or crusting, diplopia (double vision), blurred vision, awareness of a "film" over

Eye Assessment

Equipment

- Newspaper or magazine
- Index card or plastic eye shield
- Snellen eye chart or lighted screen with chart
- Cotton-tipped applicator
- Penlight
- Ophthalmoscope
- Small ruler
- Disposable gloves (if drainage is present)

Delegation Considerations

The physical examination of the eyes requires critical thinking and knowledge application unique to a professional nurse and should not be delegated to assistive personnel. Assistive personnel can learn the common symptoms of eye disease (see history) and know to report their occurrence. When administering the field of vision, floaters (small black spots that seem to cross the field of vision), flashing lights, or halos around lights.

- Determine whether a family history of eye disorders exists, including glaucoma or retinitis pigmentosa.

- Assess client's occupational history for activities requiring close, intricate work; work involving computers; or activities such as welding and exposure to chemicals that create risk for eye injury. Are safety glasses worn?

- Ask the client whether glasses or contacts are normally worn, and how often.

- Determine date of the client's last eye examination.

- Assess medications client is taking, including eye drops or ointment.

ASSESSMENT TECHNIQUES—EXTERNAL EYE EXAMINATION

Assessment	Normal Findings	Deviations From Normal
Visual Acuity Testing progresses in stages, depending on the response in each stage and the reason for the assessment.		
Stage I • Ask the client to read newspaper or magazine print under adequate lighting. A client who wears glasses should wear them during this stage of assessment. Note distance from eyes where the client holds the print. **Know if the client speaks a language other than English and whether the client is literate. Literacy can be difficult to detect; asking the client to read aloud can be effective.**	• Client is able to read a newspaper or magazine while holding the document eight to ten inches from the face.	• Client holds magazine or newspaper very near the eyes or at arm length.

Assessment	Normal Findings	Deviations From Normal
Stage II		
• Use a Snellen eye chart (available as a chart, pocket chart, or a projected light screen).	• Normal visual acuity is 20/20. Note if visual acuity is measured with correction of glasses or contacts (cc) or without correction (sc).	• A person is considered legally blind in the United States when vision in the better eye, corrected by lenses, is 20/200 or less. The inability to perceive light is indicative of blindness.
• Be sure a paper chart is well lighted.		
• Always test vision with corrective lenses first.	• Able to see with corrective lenses.	• Unable to see with corrective lenses.
• Have the client sit or stand 20 feet (6.1 m) away from the chart or sit in an examination chair specially positioned across from the screen.		
• Ask the client to read all of the letters beginning with the smallest line they can see—once with both eyes open and then with each eye separately (with the opposite eye covered by an index card or eye cover).	• Right eye normally 20/20.	• Vision is less than 20/20.
	• Left eye normally 20/20.	
	• Both eyes 20/20.	

- Have the client avoid applying pressure to the eye.
- Repeat test with client wearing corrective lenses.
- If client is unable to read, use an "E" chart or one with pictures of familiar objects. Have client describe which direction the "E" is pointing or the name of the object.
- Record visual acuity score for each eye and both eyes as two numbers: numerator is the distance from the chart in feet.
- Denominator is the standardized number for the last line read on the chart (e.g., 20/80). This standardized number is the distance from which the normal eye can read the line.

Assessment	Normal Findings	Deviations From Normal
Stage III If a client cannot read even the largest letters or figures of a Snellen chart:		
• Test the client's ability to count up-raised fingers or distinguish light. Hold a hand 30 cm (1 foot) from the face and ask client to count the up-raised fingers.	• Client is able to accurately count up-raised fingers and distinguish light.	• Client is unable to accurately count upraised fingers and distinguish light.
• To check light perception, shine a penlight into the client's eye and then turn the light off. Ask if the client sees the light.	• Client is able to see the light.	• Client is unable to distinguish the light.
Extraocular Movements • Have the client sit or stand 2 feet (60 cm) away, facing you at eye level.		

- Hold a finger at a comfortable distance (6 to 12 inches, or 15 to 30 cm) in front of the client's eyes.

- Hold the client's chin to prevent movement, or ask the client to keep the head in a fixed position facing you and follow the movement of your finger with the eyes only.

- The client follows your finger as it moves through the six cardinal fields of gaze (Fig. 9-2).

- Periodically stop movement of the finger; note if the eye begins to oscillate.

- Eyes follow fields of gaze smoothly with the upper eyelid only covering the iris slightly. A few horizontal nystagmic beats (rhythmic movement of eye) are common in a lateral gaze.

- Note parallel eye movement and presence of abnormal movements.

- Strabismus is a condition in which both eyes do not focus on an object simultaneously because of impairment of muscles or their nerve supply.

- Nystagmus is an involuntary, jerking movement of the eye.

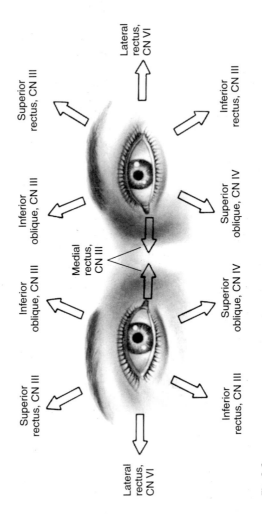

Fig. 9-2
Six directions of gaze. (From Seidel HM et al: *Mosby's guide to physical examination*, ed 4, St Louis, 1999, Mosby.)

Assessment	Normal Findings	Deviations From Normal
• Have client follow your finger in the vertical plane, going from ceiling to floor. Observe the coordinated movement of the globes and the upper eyelid.	• Movement is smooth and without exposure of sclera.	• Jerking nystagmus, which is a faster movement of the eye in one direction, is identified by its rapid phase. If eye moves rapidly to the right and then slowly drifts to the left, the client has nystagmus to the right.
		• Pendular nystagmus occurs when oscillations are equal in both directions.
Corneal Light Reflex		
• Check the alignment of the eyes (balance of extraocular muscles) by shining a penlight onto the bridge of the client's nose from about 12 inches (30 cm) away in a darkened room.	• Light reflects on the cornea in the same spot on both eyes.	• Lid lag, exposure of the sclera above the iris. The upper eyelid covers much of the iris, indicating possible edema or cranial nerve involvement.
• Have the client look at a nearby object but not at the light.		• Light shines on a different spot on each eye indicating, that there is imbalance of the extraocular muscles.

Assessment	Normal Findings	Deviations From Normal
If the corneal light reflex is abnormal, then *perform the cover test.*		
• Have the client stare ahead at a near fixed point (30 cm, or 12 inches, away). Cover one eye and observe for movement of the uncovered eye while the client gazes ahead.	• Uncovered eye does not move and is thus aligned.	• Uncovered eye moves, revealing a misalignment. When the stronger eye is temporarily covered, the weaker eye attempts to fixate on the object.
• Remove the cover and watch for movement of the newly uncovered eye as it fixes on the object.		
• Repeat with the other eye.		
Visual Fields		
• Have the client sit or stand 3 feet (1 m) away, facing you at eye level. Ask the client to gently close or cover one eye	• All objects in the periphery can normally be seen.	• If you see the finger before the client does, a portion of the client's visual field is reduced.

- with index card and look at your eye directly opposite (e.g., client's left eye, your right eye).

- Close or cover your opposite eye so that your field of vision is superimposed on that of the client. Both you and client should be looking at each other's eye.

- Fully extend your arm midway between the client and yourself. Then move the arm forward with fingers moving.

- Both you and the client should see your finger entering the field of vision at about the same time.

- Ask the client to tell you when the moving fingers are first seen. Compare the client's response to the time you first noted the fingers. Move the arm nasally, temporally, superiorly, and inferiorly from outside the field of vision and then slowly back into the visual field.

- A gaze to the far left or right often elicits presence of abnormal eye movements such as nystagmus (rhythmic, involuntary oscillation of the eyes).

- Altered eye movements can reflect injury or disease of eye muscles, supporting structures, or cranial nerves.

Assessment	Normal Findings	Deviations From Normal
• Repeat procedure on the other side, for each field, always comparing the point at which you see the finger coming into your field of vision and the point at which the client sees it.		
External Eye Structures		
⊙ *Standard Precautions Alert If there is crusty drainage on eyelid margins, apply gloves before touching the client's face. Drainage can be infections and easily spread from one eye to the other. Change gloves/hands from one eye to the other.*		
• Stand or sit directly in front of client at eye level and ask the client to look at your face.	• Eyes are normally parallel to each other.	• Bulging (exophthalmos) is usually caused by hyperthyroidism when both eyes are involved.
• Inspect the position of the eyes in relation to one another.		• Tumors or inflammation of the orbit can cause unilateral abnormal eye protrusion.

For the remainder of the examination, the client's contact lenses should be removed.

- Inspect the eyebrows for size, extension, hair texture, and alignment. Note whether eyebrows extend beyond the eye itself or end short of it; if sparse or absent, ask client if waxed or plucked.

  - Eyebrows are normally symmetric.

    - Asymmetry. Coarseness of hair and failure to extend beyond the temporal canthus may indicate hypothyroidism.

    - Loss or absence of hair may indicate a hormonal disturbance or may be a result of waxing or plucking.

- Have the client raise and lower the eyebrows.

  - Brows raise and lower symmetrically. Some clients are able to move one brow at a time.

    - Paralysis of the facial nerve causes impaired movement of the eyebrow.

- Inspect the orbital area for edema, puffiness, or sagging tissue below the orbital ridge.

  - Orbital area is relatively flat with eyes closed.

  - Excess skin folds may appear as eyes open.

- Inspect the eyelids for position. Ask the client to relax with eyes open.

  - Lids do not cover the pupil. The sclera cannot be seen above the iris.

    - Abnormal drooping of the lid over the pupil is ptosis.

Assessment	Normal Findings	Deviations From Normal
• Inspect lid margins (upper and lower). Note blink reflex.	• Lids are flush with the eyeball. The client blinks involuntarily and bilaterally up to 20 times a minute.	• Older adults frequently have lid margins that turn out (ectropion) or in (entropion). Ectropion or entropion can cause irritation to the conjunctiva and cornea. **Absent or infrequent blinking should be reported because it may indicate a problem with Cranial nerve II, III, IV or VI.**
• Note condition and direction of eyelashes.	• Eyelashes are normally distributed evenly and curved outward and upward away from the eye.	• Inward turn of lashes (see entropion, mentioned previously) can cause chronic irritation.
• Inspect surface of upper eyelids by asking client to close the eyes as you raise both eyebrows gently with the thumb and index finger to stretch the skin.	• Lids are normally smooth and the same color as the skin.	• Redness indicates inflammation or infection. Lid edema may be from allergies or heart or kidney failure.

- If lesions are present, note size, shape, distribution, and presence of discomfort and drainage.

- Ask client to relax and close eyes gently.

  - Lids close and meet symmetrically.

    - Unconscious clients or those with facial nerve paralysis have lids that only partially close, thus increasing risk of corneal drying and irritation.

- Inspect lacrimal gland area in upper outer wall of anterior part of orbit for edema and redness (Fig. 9-3).

- Inspect lacrimal duct at the nasal corner (inner canthus) for edema or excess tearing.

  - Tears flow from the gland across the eye's surface to the lacrimal duct, located in the nasal corner or inner canthus of the eye.

    - Edema of gland may indicate infection or tumor. Excess tearing may be caused by blockage in nasolacrimal duct.

- Palpate gland area gently to detect any tenderness.

  - The lacrimal gland area is nontender. The gland cannot usually be palpated.

- If excess tearing is noted, gently palpate nasolacrimal duct at the lower eyelid just inside the lower orbital rim, not on the side of the nose.

    - Continual tearing suggests a blockage.

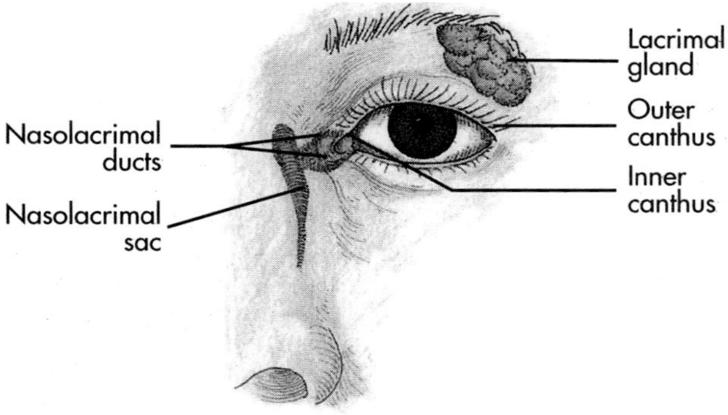

Fig. 9-3
The lacrimal apparatus.

Assessment	Normal Findings	Deviations From Normal
• Gently retract eyelids to inspect the bulbar conjunctiva that covers the exposed surface of the eyeball up to the edge of the cornea.	• Conjunctiva is transparent with light pink color and free of erythema. Tiny underlying blood vessels can be seen.	• Redness may indicate an allergic or infectious conjunctivitis.
• Avoid applying pressure directly on eyeball.		• Bright red blood in a localized area surrounded by normal-appearing conjunctiva usually indicates subconjunctival hemorrhage.
• Retract both lids gently, with the thumb and index finger pressed against the lower and upper bony orbits.		
• Have client look up, down, and side to side. Inspect for color, edema, and lesions.		

Assessment	Normal Findings	Deviations From Normal
• Gently retract lower eyelid with thumb or index finger to examine the palpebral conjunctiva that lines the eyelids (Fig. 9-4). At times the client can depress the eyelid for you. Note the conjunctiva's color, presence of edema, or lesions.	• Conjunctiva is clear and free from erythema.	• Pale conjunctiva results from anemia. Fiery red appearance is result of inflammation (conjunctivitis).
• Inspect upper palpebral conjunctiva lining the upper eyelids by inverting the lid. Do not perform the first time without qualified assistance. **This technique is used only if you suspect a foreign body under the lid.**	• Conjunctiva is clear.	• Foreign object can be seen, embedded in eye. **Do not attempt to remove foreign object. Notify a physician immediately and apply an eye shield.**
• Ask the client to look down, relax eyes, and avoid sudden movements. Gently grasp upper lid, pulling lashes		

down and forward (Fig. 9-5). Place
tip of cotton-tipped applicator ½ inch
(1 cm) above lid margin. Push down
on upper eyelid to turn it inside out;
keep lid inverted by careful grasp of
upper lashes.

- Inspect conjunctiva for edema, lesions, or presence of foreign bodies.
After inspection, return lid to normal
position by gently pulling lashes forward and asking client to look up.
Eyelid will return to normal position.

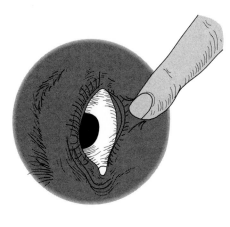

Fig. 9-4
Retraction of the lower eyelid.

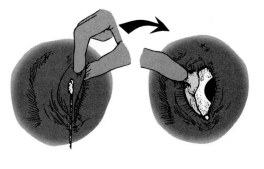

Fig. 9-5
Technique for inspecting the upper palpebral conjunctiva.

Assessment	Normal Findings	Deviations From Normal
• Standing at client's side, using oblique lighting, inspect the cornea for clarity and texture.	• Cornea is normally shiny, transparent, smooth, and dome shaped.	• Irregularity in the surface may indicate an abrasian or tear. Appearance of what looks like blood vessels is a pterygium.
• Test corneal sensitivity by barely touching a wisp of sterile cotton to the cornea.	• Normal response is a blink.	• Absence of blink reflex indicates involvement of either Cranial nerve V or VII.
• Inspect appearance of iris and note any margin defects.	• Iris pattern should be clearly visible. • Color is the same bilaterally.	• A section of the iris missing can result from corrective surgery for glaucoma.

Assessment	Normal Findings	Deviations From Normal
• Inspect pupil for size, shape, and equality.	• Pupils are normally black, round, regular, and equal in size (3 to 7 mm in diameter) (Fig. 9-6). Approximately 20% of healthy people have minor or noticeable differences in pupil size, but reflexes are normal (Seidel et al, 1999).	• Bilateral miosis (pupil constriction in both eyes with pupil less than 2 mm in diameter) is the result of miotic eye drops and systemic drugs (e.g., chloral hydrate, clinidine, guanethidine, opiates). Bilateral mydriasis (dilation usually greater than 6 mm) is caused by use of cycloplegic drops (e.g., atropine) and systemic drugs (e.g., indomethacin) (Seidel et al, 1999). Mydriasis is also caused by midbrain lesions; acute angle glaucoma; and coma resulting from alcohol, uremia, diabetes, and epilepsy. Cloudy pupil indicates a cataract.

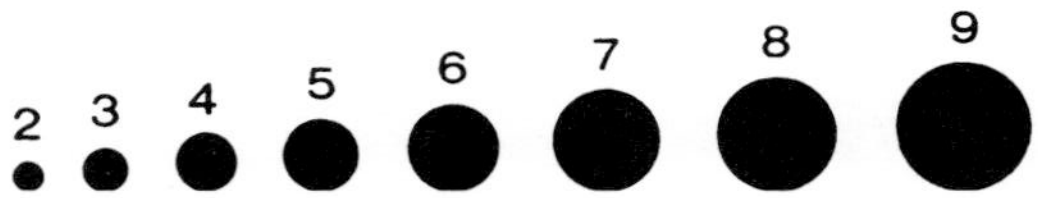

Fig. 9-6
Chart depicting pupillary size in millimeters.

- Test pupillary response to light both directly and consensually. Dim the light in the room to dilate the pupils.

- As the client looks straight ahead, bring penlight from side of client's face and direct light onto pupil.

- Observe the illuminated pupil for quickness of reflex. Also observe opposite pupil for equality of reflex.

- Repeat for opposite eye.

- Test for the accommodation reflex by asking client to gaze at a distant object (far wall) and then at a test object (finger or pencil) held 4 inches (10 cm) from the bridge of the client's nose.

- Delay in pupil response to light can indicate increased intracranial pressure.

- The illuminated pupil should constrict briskly (Fig. 9-7). The opposite pupil constricts consensually.

- Pupils converge and accommodate by constricting when looking at close objects. Pupil responses are equal.

- Test is significant only if there is a defect in the pupillary response to light (Seidel et al, 1999). Delayed or absent light or accommodation reflex may indicate changes in intracranial pressure, nerve lesions, or direct trauma to eye.

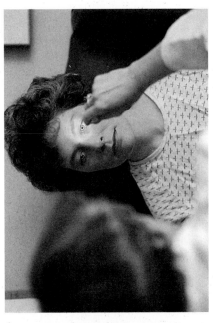

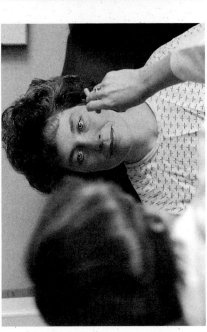

Fig. 9-7
A, Check pupil reflexes by first holding the penlight to the side of the client's face. **B,** Illumination of the pupil causes pupillary constriction.

Internal Eye Structure Examination (Ophthalmoscopic Examination)

Ophthalmoscopic examination is particularly important for clients with diabetes, hypertension, or intracranial pathologic conditions. The examination can detect early stages of disease.

Client Preparation

- Have client remove glasses. Contact lenses may remain in place. (Examiner should remove glasses too.)
- Conduct examination in a darkened room.
- Avoid prolonging the examination without giving the client brief intervals for rest.
- The light is very bright and can cause discomfort.

ASSESSMENT TECHNIQUES—INTERNAL EYE STRUCTURE EXAMINATION

Be familiar with how to handle the ophthalmoscope correctly. Practice holding it in each hand, using the index finger to rotate the lens dial. Turn the white light on; rotate the lens dial to 0; and look through the keyhole, focusing first on a near object such as the palm of the hand. Reading the newspaper is good practice.

Assessment	Normal Findings	Deviations From Normal
• Explain to the client what you are about to do.	• Bright, orange glow in the pupil, called the red reflex, can be seen. The pupil will constrict.	• Absence of red reflex is usually caused by an improperly positioned ophthalmoscope.

Assessment	Normal Findings	Deviations From Normal
• Darken the room.		• A total opacity of the lens from a cataract or hemorrhage into the vitreous humor can also block the light.
• Be sure both you and the client are in comfortable positions, facing each other with eyes at the same height (e.g., both sitting, or client sitting on examination table and you standing).		
• Turn ophthalmoscope light on and rotate lens to clear adjustment to 0.		
• Keep index finger on lens dial to re-focus during examination.		
• Face the client with your eyes at the client's eye level.		
• Ask the client to gaze straight ahead at an object slightly upward, keeping both eyes open. Keep both of your eyes open as well.		

- Use right hand and eye to inspect the client's right eye, and left hand and eye to inspect the client's left eye.

- From a distance of approximately 25 cm (10 inches) from the client and 25 degrees lateral to the client's central line of vision, shine the light on the pupil (Fig. 9-8).

- Move the light slowly toward the pupil while you keep it focused on the red reflex. Remember to stay relaxed and keep both of your eyes open.

- At any one time you will only see a small portion of the retina or fundus (Fig. 9-9).

- Rotate the lens dial to bring the internal structures into focus.

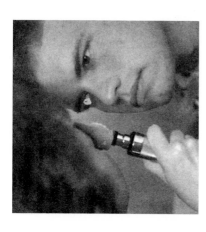

Fig. 9-8
Visualize internal eye structures by moving in toward the pupil with the ophthalmoscope's light focused on the red reflex.

Assessment	Normal Findings	Deviations From Normal
• The first structures commonly seen are blood vessels. Note how they branch. The vessels always branch away from the optic disc and thus can be used as landmarks to locate the disc.	• Arterioles are smaller than venules; 3:5 or 2:3 ratio. Light reflected from arterioles is brighter, and oxygenated blood is brighter.	• Arterioles become smaller in hypertension. Thickening of the arteriolar coat causes a nicking of the venule where the venule passes beneath the arteriole (AV nicking).
• Inspect the vascular supply of the retina. Follow the vessels distally as far as you can see them in each of the four quadrants of the fundus. Note the sites where arterioles and venules cross.		

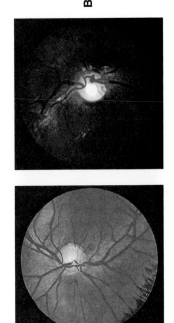

A   **B**

Fig. 9-9
Normal fundus. **A,** White adult. **B,** African American.

- Examine the size, color, and clarity of the disc; integrity of vessels; and presence of retinal lesions (Fig. 9-10).

- Use the diameter of the disc to estimate size of any lesions you observe (e.g., an abnormality of an artery may occur 2 disc diameters from the optic nerve and is 1 disc diameter long, 0.5 diameter wide).

- Examine the macula, or fovea centralis. This is the site of central vision, located about 2 disc diameters temporal to the optic disc. To see the macula, it helps to ask the client to look directly at the light.

The bright light of the ophthalmoscope is irritating and can cause tearing. Do not illuminate the fundus too long. Ask clients to tell you if they become uncomfortable.

- Clear, yellow, sharply well-defined optic disc (reddish-pink in light-skinned clients; darkened retina in dark-skinned clients). Light red arteries and dark red veins. Disc is about 1.5 mm in diameter.

- No blood vessels enter the fovea; it appears as a yellow dot surrounded by a deep-pink periphery.

- Papilledema is loss of definition of the disc. Central vessels may bulge forward, and veins are dilated. Chronic loss of blood supply causes vessels to disappear over the edge of the disc and can be seen again deep within the disc. Disc may also appear whiter.

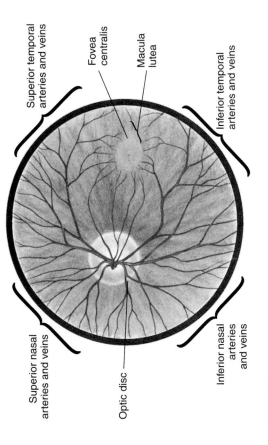

Superior temporal
arteries and veins

Fovea
centralis

Macula
lutea

Inferior temporal
arteries and veins

Superior nasal
arteries and veins

Optic disc

Inferior nasal
arteries and veins

Fig. 9-10
Retinal structures of the eye. (From Seidel HM et al: *Mosby's guide to physical examination,*
ed 4, St Louis, 1999, Mosby.)

UNEXPECTED ASSESSMENT FINDINGS—INTERNAL EYE STRUCTURE EXAMINATION

Assessment Findings	Significance	Next Step
• Blurred vision.	• May be caused by hyperglycemia or ingestion of clomiphene citrate, guanethidine, hydralazine, ibuprofen, or quinine or by use of marijuana (McKenry and Salerno, 2000).	• Ask client if client has ingested any of the aforementioned products. • Determine if the client is seeing multiples of an object or "fuzzy edges." • Record and report findings. • Monitor for improvement or deterioration.
• Decreased visual fields.	• May indicate degenerative cataract changes, optic nerve injury, or retinal disease.	• Complete eye assessment. Determine if there are other assessment findings that support optic nerve injury, retinal disease, or cataract. • Record and report findings.

Assessment Findings	Significance	Next Step
• A *sudden* reduction in visual fields.	• May indicate a detached retina. The client is at risk for injury because of inability to see all objects in front of client.	**Requires referral to an ophthalmologist as soon as possible. Clients with visual field alterations may be at risk for injury, because they cannot see all objects in front of them.**
• Bright red, inflamed conjunctiva.	**Viral conjunctivitis is a highly contagious infection.**	**Crusty drainage that collects on eyelid margins can easily spread from one eye to the other. Wear gloves during an examination. Wash hands thoroughly before proceeding.**
	• Conjunctivitis can also be caused from ingestion of excess amounts of aspirin and use of marijuana (McKenry and Salerno, 2000).	
	• Yellowish drainage may indicate a bacterial infection. An allergy may produce a whitish drainage.	
• Ptosis.	• Caused by edema or impairment of the third cranial nerve, sign of myasthenia gravis.	• Determine if this is a new finding for this client. Ask about episodes of generalized weakness or falls.
		• Record and report finding.

- Hordeolum or sty.

  - An acute inflammation of the follicle of an eyelash causing an erythematous or yellow lump.
    - Encourage client to keep hands from eye.
    - Do not try to remove eyelash.
    - Apply warm, moist compresses to client's eye every 2-4 hours while client is awake.

- Scratched or abraded cornea.

  - Condition is very painful and requires medical intervention.
    - Provide eye patch and tape lightly in place. **Do not cover eye with a non-woven cover. Dressings such as 4 × 4's can cause additional damage to the cornea.**
    - Condition requires referral to an ophthalmologist, who will treat with antibiotic drops or ointment and local anesthetic for pain relief.

- Jerking nystagmus.

  - Can indicate barbiturate intoxication or vestibular, vascular, or neurological disease.
    - Review toxicology screen if available.
    - Report findings to physician, especially if suspicion of drug intoxication or sudden change in neurological condition.

Assessment Findings	Significance	Next Step
• Pendular nystagmus.	• Occurs in various diseases of the retina and in miners who have worked in darkness.	• Record and report findings. • Correlate with occupational history.
• AV nicking.	• Seen in clients with hypertension.	• Review blood pressure (BP) and current BP management. Determine if BP is currently within recommended guidelines. • Record and report findings. • Referral to ophthalmologist for examination and evaluation.
• Papilledema.	• Caused by increased intracranial pressure along the optic nerve.	• Record and report findings. Initially, vision is not altered (Seidel et al, 1999). • Referral to an ophthalmologist is indicated.
• Retinal hemorrhage.	• Poorly controlled or undiagnosed glaucoma.	• Determine client's last visit to ophthalmologist.

- Cupping of the disc.

- Seen in clients with glaucoma. Results from increased intraocular pressure and interruption of the blood supply to the optic nerve. Causes constriction of peripheral visual fields (Seidel et al, 1999).

- Record and report findings.
- Referral to ophthalmologist or neurologist if the client has an increased intracranial pressure (ICP).
- Record and report findings.

Pediatric Considerations

- Infants shut their eyes tightly during an eye examination. A dimly lit room may encourage the infant to open the eyes. Holding an infant upright, suspended under the arms, also encourages the eyes to open (Seidel et al, 1999).
- The Snellen symbol chart and the Blackbird Preschool Vision Screening System are used to assess visual acuity in children (Wong, 1999).
- Abnormalities in placement or position of the eyes may indicate congenital alterations. Look for an epicanthal fold, a vertical fold of skin nasally that covers the lacrimal duct area. This fold is common in Asian children but may suggest Down syndrome. Draw an imaginary line through the medial canthus of each eye and extend the line past the outer canthus. The medial and outer canthus should be horizontal.
- Widely spaced eyes, or hypertelorism, is a finding associated with mental retardation. The distance between the inner canthus of each eye is normally 1.2 inches (3 cm).
- Lacrimal apparatus may not function properly until 3 months of age.

- The National Society for the Prevention of Blindness recommends the following criteria for referring children with visual acuity problems:
  - 3-year-old child with vision in either eye of 20/50 or less;
  - all other ages with vision in either eye of 20/40 or less;
  - a two-line difference in visual acuity between the eyes in the passing range (e.g., 20/20 in one eye and 20/40 in the other).

- Because a child may be fearful of the equipment and the dark, you should show the ophthalmoscope to the child and explain the procedure before beginning.

- Children should be screened for color blindness. School-age children can have difficulty performing academic skills if they are unable to detect color variations in instructional materials.

Gerontologic Considerations

- Eyebrows may become more coarse in males and thin at the temporal sides in males and females (Lueckenotte, 2000).
- With aging, the lacrimal glands decrease their production of tears. Tears also evaporate quickly, causing the conjunctivae to be drier.

- A common change of aging is the presence of arcus senilis, a white ring that appears around the iris. It is caused by the deposit of lipids in the periphery of the cornea. If present in clients under age 40, the condition may indicate hyperlipidemia.
- Other changes include scleral discolorations, decrease in pupil size and the ability to constrict in response to light, decrease in peripheral vision, and an increase in the rate of adaptation to the dark. The lens yellows and becomes opaque, resulting in cataract formation. The pupil may have an irregular shape unilaterally or bilaterally in older adults.
- With aging the conjunctiva thins and takes on a yellowish appearance.
- With aging the retinal vessels become narrowed and straighter. Arteries may appear more opaque and somewhat gray in color (Lueckenotte, 2000). Dark spots may interrupt the red or orange glow of the red reflex or black shadows indicating opacities.
- The fovea centralis is less bright with advanced age.

 ## Cultural Considerations

- The sclera has the color of white porcelain in white clients and is light yellow in African-American clients.

- African-American men have a 2-mm greater protrusion of the eye than white males. African-American females have a 2.4 mm greater protrusion of the eye than white females (Seidel et al, 1999).
- Clients at risk for hypertension include African Americans, Russian Americans, and Filipino Americans (Giger, 1999). Screening for retinal changes is important.
- American Eskimos are susceptible to primary narrow-angle glaucoma (Giger, 1999).

Client Teaching

- School-age children require visual screening by age 3 or 4 and every 2 years thereafter.
- Inform adult clients that persons younger than 40 years of age should have complete eye examinations every 3 to 5 years (or more often, if family history reveals risks such as diabetes or hypertension).
- Instruct clients older than 40 years of age to have eye examinations every 2 years to screen for glaucoma. Screening should also be done for presbyopia, which is a reduction in near vision and far-sightedness.

- Persons older than 65 years of age should have yearly eye examinations.
- Instruct clients to seek medical care as soon as possible for any changes in vision.
- Clients with burning or itching of the eyes should avoid rubbing them to prevent transmitting infection from one eye to the other.
- Instruct clients on proper administration of eye drops and ointments. Instruct clients never to share medications with another person. Cleanse the eye by wiping from the inner to the outer canthus.
- Instruct older adults to take the following precautions because of normal visual changes:
  - Use caution when driving at night. Because the pupil becomes less responsive to changes in light, the older adult may need to limit driving to the daylight hours.
  - Increase nonglare lighting in the home to reduce risk of falls.
  - Paint the first and last steps of a staircase and the edge of each step in between in a bright color to aid depth perception.
  - Look to the sides before crossing streets.

10

Ears

Anatomy and Physiology

The organ of hearing consists of the external, middle, and inner ear (Fig. 10-1).

External ear structures consist of the auricle or pinna, outer ear canal, and tympanic membrane (eardrum). The ear canal is normally curved and about 1 inch (2.5 cm) long in an adult. The ear canal is lined with skin containing fine hairs, nerve endings, and glands secreting cerumen (ear wax). The middle ear is an air-filled cavity containing the three bony ossicles (malleus, incus, and stapes). The eustachian tube connects the middle ear to the nasopharynx. Pressure between the outer atmosphere and middle ear is stabilized through the eustachian tube.

Sound waves transmitted by way of the external auditory canal cause the sensitive tympanic membrane to vibrate and conduct sound waves through the bony ossicles of the middle ear to the sensory organs of the inner ear. The semicircular canals, vestibule, and cochlea within the inner ear are the sensory structures for hearing and balance. Sound waves are transduced into nerve impulses, which travel from the inner ear along the acoustic nerve (the VIII cranial nerve) to the brain.

Clients may experience three types of hearing loss: conduction, sensorineural, and mixed. A conduction loss interrupts sound waves as they travel from the outer ear to the cochlea of the inner ear, because the sound waves are not transmitted through the outer and middle ear structures. Swelling of the auditory canal or tears in the tympanic membrane can be causes. A sensorineural loss involves the inner ear, auditory nerve, or hearing center of the brain. Sound is conducted through the outer and middle ear, but the continued transmission of sound becomes interrupted at some point past the bony ossicles. A mixed loss involves a combination of conduction and sensorineural loss.

Ear disorders may result from mechanical dysfunction (blockage by ear wax or foreign body), trauma (foreign bodies or noise exposure), neurological disorders (auditory nerve damage), acute illnesses (viral infections), or toxic effects of medications.

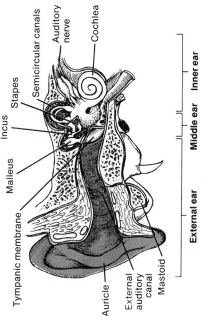

Fig. 10-1
Structures of the external, middle, and inner ear.

Critical Thinking Application—Ears

Knowledge	Experience	Standards
Hearing is critical for a person to interact successfully within the environment. To assess a client accurately, refer to your knowledge regarding communication techniques for clients with hearing deficits. Clients with existing hearing deficits may not always acknowledge a hearing problem. Also be aware that hearing deficits may result from localized problems of the ear itself or neurological abnormalities affecting the course of the eighth cranial nerve to the pons and medulla.	Caring for clients with hearing deficits in the home environment will allow you to learn how these clients adapt to their sensory losses. Use this experience when teaching clients with relatively recent deficits. Your experience with clients in an institutional or hospital setting will allow you to teach other clients about background noise and adaptive techniques.	During an ear examination, apply the following principles: The external auditory canal is very sensitive, because little subcutaneous tissue is present between skin and underlying cartilage. Use care when palpating or inserting the otoscope. Speak to the client in a normal tone of voice.

Ear Assessment

Equipment

- Otoscope
- Ear speculum (choose largest one that fits comfortably into ear canal)
- Tuning fork (256, 512, or 1024 Hz)
- Disposable gloves (if drainage is present)

Delegation Considerations

The examination of the ear requires critical thinking and knowledge application unique to a professional nurse. The examination should not be delegated to assistive personnel. Be sure staff who care for clients with hearing deficits are familiarized with appropriate communication techniques.

Client Preparation

- Have the adult client sit during the examination.
- Explain steps of the procedure, particularly when the otoscope is inserted, and assure client that procedure is normally painless.

History

- Has the client experienced earaches, itching, discharge, tinnitus (ringing in ears), vertigo (sensation of spinning), or change in hearing? Note onset and duration. Assess risks for hearing problem:
- Infants/children: Hypoxia at birth, meningitis, birth weight less than 1500 g, family history of hearing loss, congenital anomalies of skull or face, nonbacterial intrauterine infections (e.g., rubella, herpes), maternal drug use, excessively high bilirubin, head trauma.

- Adults: Exposure to industrial or recreational noise, genetic disease (Meniere's disease), neurodegenerative disorders. For armed service veterans, exposure to explosions during wartime.
- If client has had recent hearing loss, note affected ear, onset, contributing factors, such as a repeated history of cerumen impaction, and the effect on activities of daily living.
- Determine whether the client uses a hearing aid.
- Determine the client's exposure to loud noises at work and the availability of protective devices.

- Determine the client's exposure to loud noise (e.g., music, workplace noise), or the use of earphones.
- Note behaviors indicative of hearing loss, including failure to respond when spoken to, leaning forward to hear, inattentiveness in children, use of monotonous or loud voice tone, or repetition of the question, "What did you say?"
- Determine whether the client is taking or has taken large doses of aspirin or other ototoxic medications such as aminoglycosides, furosemide, streptomycin, cisplatin, and ethacrynic acid.
- Ask how the client normally cleans the ears.

ASSESSMENT TECHNIQUES—EARS

Assessment	Normal Findings	Deviations From Normal
External ear		
• Inspect the auricle's position, color, size, shape, symmetry, and landmarks and compare with normal findings.	• Auricles are of equal size and level with each other. The upper point of attachment is in a straight line with the outer canthus or corner of the eye.	• Ears that are low set or at an unusual angle are a sign of chromosome abnormality such as Down syndrome.
• Be sure to examine lateral and medial surfaces and the surrounding tissue.	• The auricle also sits vertically. • Color is same as the face, without cysts, moles, deformities, or nodules.	• Redness is a sign of inflammation or fever. • Extreme pallor indicates frostbite.
• Gently palpate the auricle for texture, tenderness, swelling, and lesions (Fig. 10-2).		
• Gently pull the auricle; press on the tragus; and palpate behind the ear over the mastoid process for tenderness, swelling, and nodules.	• The auricle is smooth, firm, mobile, and without nodules. If folded forward, the auricle returns to its normal position upon release.	• A cauliflower ear (multiple enlarged cartilaginous nodules along the helix) is a sign of blunt trauma and necrosis of the underlying cartilage.

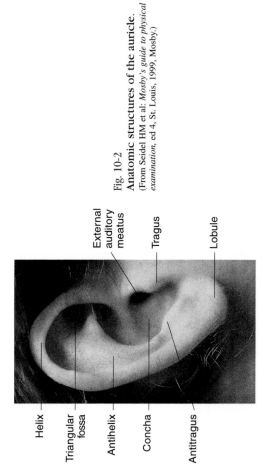

Fig. 10-2
Anatomic structures of the auricle.
(From Seidel HM et al: *Mosby's guide to physical examination*, ed 4, St. Louis, 1999, Mosby.)

Assessment	Normal Findings	Deviations From Normal
	• A Darwin tubercle (thickening along the upper ridge of the helix) is a normal variation (Seidel et al, 1999).	
	• Tragus and mastoid are smooth, without nodules, and nontender.	
• Inspect opening of the ear canal for size and discharge.	• Absence of swelling at meatus; no discharge. A small amount of earwax (cerumen) is normal.	• Yellow or green, foul-smelling discharge. If the client has a history of head trauma, bloody or serous drainage in the external canal suggests a skull fracture.
Ear Canals and Eardrums The otoscope is used to examine deeper ear structures. Specula come in different sizes to conform to the size of ear canals.	• Canal is clear.	
• Before inserting the speculum, check for foreign bodies in the opening of the canal.		• Foreign object in ear canal (e.g., marble, bug, food, small toy piece).

Assessment	Normal Findings	Deviations From Normal
• Instruct client to not move the head during the otoscopic examination. • Turn on the otoscope by rotating the dial at the top of the battery tube. • Have the client tip the head slightly toward the opposite shoulder. • Hold the handle of the otoscope in the space between the thumb and index finger (like a pencil), supported on the middle finger (right hand for right ear; left hand for left ear).		If a foreign body is present in the ear canal, be careful not to impact the body farther into the ear canal with the otoscope. A physician or other specialist should remove the foreign body.

- Use the ulnar side of the hand to rest against the side of the client's head to stabilize the otoscope.

- For the adult: Pull the auricle upward, backward, and slightly out to straighten the ear canal (Fig. 10-3).

- Insert the speculum slightly down and forward 1.0 or 1.5 cm (½ inch) into the ear canal. Do not abrade the lining of the ear canal. Avoid any sudden movement.

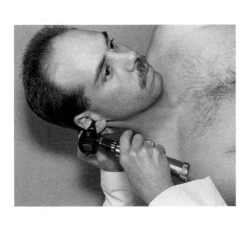

Fig. 10-3
Insertion of the otoscope.

Assessment	Normal Findings	Deviations From Normal
• Inspect auditory canal from meatus to tympanic membrane for color, lesions, scaling, foreign bodies, and cerumen (earwax) or discharge.	• Canal has little cerumen and is uniformly pink with tiny hairs in the outer third of the canal.	• A reddened canal with discharge is a sign of inflammation or infection.
	• Cerumen is usually dry, light brown to gray, and flaky in Oriental and Native Americans. Cerumen is moist, dark yellow, or brown and sticky in Caucasians and African Americans (Seidel et al, 1999). Cerumen is odorless. Absence of lesions, discharge, or foreign body.	**If the otoscope touches the bony walls of the auditory canal (inner two thirds), the client will sense pain.**
		• Excessive cerumen can contribute to hearing loss.
• Inspect eardrum (tympanic membrane) by slowly moving the otoscope to see the entire eardrum and its periphery. Moving the otoscope helps to vary the direction of the otoscope light.	• The eardrum is translucent, shiny, and pearly gray. It is free from tears or breaks (Fig. 10-4, *B*). A ring of fibrous cartilage surrounds the oval membrane. The umbo is near the center of the membrane, and the attachment of the malleus is behind it. A cone of light appears on the membrane. The membrane moves during swallowing.	• A pink or red bulging membrane indicates inflammation.
Know the anatomic landmarks (Fig. 10-4, *A*). Inspect the color, integrity, position of bony ossicles, and presence of cone of light.		• Blood may be behind the eardrum if it appears dull with a bluish color or if the cone of light is distorted.
		• A white color reveals pus behind it.
		• Perforations or scarring is abnormal.

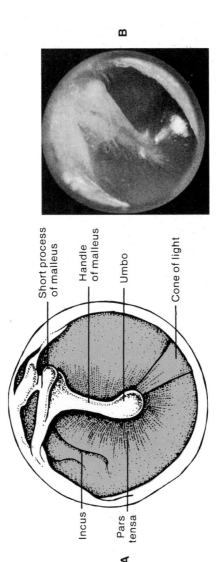

Short process
of malleus

Handle
of malleus

Umbo

Cone of light

Incus

Pars
tensa

A

B

Fig. 10-4
A, Anatomic landmarks of tympanic membrane. **B,** Normal tympanic membrane.

Assessment	Normal Findings	Deviations From Normal
Hearing Acuity		
• Have the client remove hearing aid if worn. Note the client's response to questions during normal conversation.	• Client responds without excessive requests to have you repeat questions.	• Client frequently asks you to repeat questions.
• If you suspect a hearing loss, check the client's response to the whispered voice.		
• Test one ear at a time while the client occludes the other ear with his or her finger.		
• Have the client gently move the finger up and down during the test.		
• While standing 1 to 2 feet (30 to 60 cm) from the ear being tested, cover your mouth so that the client is unable to read lips. After exhaling fully, whisper softly toward the unoc-	• Client correctly repeats the numbers. Responds correctly at least 50% of the time (Seidel et al, 1999).	• Client is unable to repeat numbers.

cluded ear, reciting random numbers (e.g., "nine-four-ten") with equally accented syllables.

- If necessary, gradually increase the loudness of the whisper. Test other ear and note any difference.

- If a client has difficulty hearing, test further with tuning fork tests:

- **Weber's test** (Fig. 10-5): Hold tuning fork at its base and tap it lightly against heel of palm. Place base of vibrating fork on midline vertex of client's head or middle of forehead. Ask client if sound is heard equally in both ears or better in one ear.

  - Sound heard equally well in both ears.

  - Sound lateralizes to either ear. Conduction deafness: sound is heard best in impaired ear. Unilateral sensorineural loss: sound is identified only in normal ear.

- **Rinne test** (Fig. 10-6): Place stem of vibrating tuning fork against client's mastoid process.

  - Air-conducted sound is heard twice as long as bone-conducted sound.

  - Conduction deafness: bone-conducted sound can be heard longer. Sensorineural loss: sound is reduced and heard longer through air.

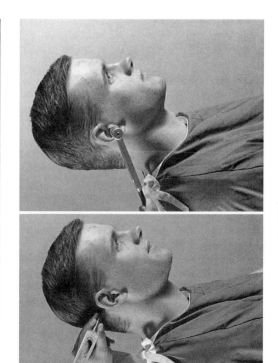

Fig. 10-6
Rinne test.

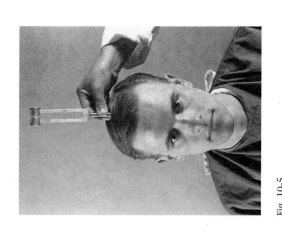

Fig. 10-5
Weber's test.

Assessment	Normal Findings	Deviations From Normal
• Begin counting the interval with your watch. Ask client to tell you when sound is no longer heard; note number of seconds. Quickly place the still-vibrating tines 1 to 2 cm ($\frac{1}{2}$ to 1 inch) from the ear canal, and ask client to tell you when the sound is no longer heard. Continue counting time the sound is heard by air conduction. Compare number of seconds sound is heard by bone versus air conduction.		Clients with impaired hearing should be referred to their physician for further evaluation. To minimize communication problems, stand to the side of the client's better ear; speak in a clear, normal tone of voice; and face the client so that your lips and face can be seen.

UNEXPECTED ASSESSMENT FINDINGS—EARS

Assessment Findings	Significance	Next Step
• Pain on manipulation of the pinna and tragus of the ear.	• Increased pain suggests an external otitis media. • Tenderness in mastoid area can indicate mastoiditis.	• Examine the ear canal. Note any exudate or pus. Note any periauricular nodes. • Notify physician of findings.
• Yellow, green, or foul-smelling drainage.	• May indicate infection or a foreign body.	• Try to visualize the tympanic membrane (TM). Determine if there is a foreign body or a perforated eardrum. Do not try to retrieve the foreign body. If the eardrum is perforated, do not lavage the ear canal. • Notify physician of findings.
Abnormal TM Findings		
• Bulging.	• Fluid or pus in the middle ear.	• All of these findings require recording and reporting. Notify the physician of the findings and confirm assessment.
• Retracted or mobile.	• Eustachian tube obstruction.	
• Yellow or amber.	• Serous fluid in the middle ear.	
• Deep red or bluish.	• Blood in the middle ear.	

- Redness.
- Chalky white.
- Dullness.
- Dense white plaques or white flecks.
- Air bubbles.
- Excess mobility in small areas.

Abnormal Weber Test

- Lateralization to deaf ear unless sensorineural loss.
- Lateralization to better ear unless conductive loss.
- Sudden hearing loss or decline.

- Infection in the middle ear; prolonged crying.
- Infection in the middle ear.
- Fibrosis.
- Healed inflammation.
- Serous fluid in the middle.
- Healed perforation.

- Conductive hearing loss.
- Sensorineural hearing loss.

- May be the result of excessive cerumen blocking the ear canal.

- Record and report findings.
- Notify physician of findings.
- Client will need a hearing evaluation/referral to audiology.
- If tympanic membrane is blocked by cerumen, a warm-water irrigation will safely remove the wax.

BOX 10-1 Expected Hearing Response (Newborn to 1 Year)

Birth to 3 Months: Startle reflex, crying, cessation of breathing in response to sudden noise

4 to 6 Months: Turns head toward source of sound but may not locate sound; responds to parents' voice

6 to 10 Months: Responds to own name, telephone ringing, person's voice; begins to localize sound above and below

10 to 12 Months: Recognizes and lateralizes sources of sound

Modified from Seidel HM et al: *Mosby's guide to physical examination*, ed 4, St Louis, 1999, Mosby.

Pediatric Considerations

- Infant's ability to hear is assessed by noting behaviors and responses to sound (Box 10-1).

- Before otoscopic examination, be sure the child has not placed a foreign body in the ear. Young children may need to be restrained or held by the parent, with child's head immobile. Infants should lie supine with the head turned to one side and arms held securely at the sides.

- Invert the otoscope and brace it against the side of the child's head or cheek to prevent accidental movement when the scope is in the ear canal.

- When inserting the scope into the meatus, move it around the outer rim to accustom the child to the feel of something in the ear. If the ear is painful to the child, touch a non-painful part first, then examine the unaffected ear, and finally return to the painful ear (Wong, 1999).

- In children less than 3 years of age, pull the pinna down and back to straighten the ear canal. Introduce the speculum into the meatus in a downward and forward position.

- Allow older children to play with the otoscope before insertion. This lessens their anxiety.

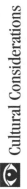

Gerontologic Considerations

- Because of changes in sebaceous glands, itching of the ear canal may be a problem for some older adults. Excessive scratching or rubbing, which may lead to inflammation, should be avoided.
- The lobule of the external ear may become elongated with creases.
- With aging, the external ear canal narrows as a result of inward collapsing of the canal wall. Cilia become coarser and stiffer (Lueckenotte, 2000).
- Tympanic membrane may have a dull, retracted, and white or gray appearance.
- Degenerative changes in the cochlea and neurons of higher auditory pathways result in presbycusis, a bilateral, progressive, sensorineural hearing loss that begins in middle age.
- Older adults often have a reduced ability to hear high-frequency sounds and consonant sounds such as S, Z, T, and G. In addition, they typically are able to hear softly whispered words with 50% accuracy at a distance of 1 to 2 feet (Lueckenotte, 2000).

Cultural Considerations

- Whites have earlobe creases much earlier than Navajo Indians (Giger, 1999).
- Oriental and Native Americans usually have dry, light brown to gray, and flaky cerumen. The cerumen in Caucasians and African Americans is usually moist, dark yellow or brown, and sticky (Seidel et al, 1999).
- Mexican Americans believe that certain diseases are caused by a hot and cold imbalance. Illness is thought to be caused by prolonged exposure to hot or cold. Earaches are believed to be the result of cold air entering the body. When a person has an earache with a fever, a hot poultice is administered to the legs to draw the fever out of the head to the cool legs (Giger, 1999).

Client Teaching

- Instruct the client about the proper way to clean the outer ear with a damp cloth and to avoid the use of cotton-tipped applicators and sharp objects such as hairpins.

- Tell the client to avoid inserting pointed objects into the ear canal. Parents should caution children against placing any kind of object into the ears.
- Children should have routine ear screenings. Clients over 65 years of age should have their hearing checked regularly. Explain that a reduction in hearing is a normal part of aging.
- Instruct family members of clients with hearing losses to speak in normal lower tones, to not shout, and to face the client while speaking.

- Instruct hearing-impaired clients to install safety devices in the home, such as wake-up and burglar alarms, doorbells, smoke detectors, or telephones connected to a flashing light.
- Explore use of a hearing aid with the client. If the client has an aid, explain how to care for the device: routine cleansing, proper storage, and care of batteries.

Nose and Sinuses

11

Anatomy and Physiology

The nose consists of an external and an internal portion. The external portion is formed by bone and cartilage and is covered with skin. The external portion of the nose is considerably smaller than the internal portion, which lies over the roof of the mouth. The internal portion is hollow and separated by a partition, the septum, into a right and a left cavity. Each nasal cavity is divided into three passageways (superior, middle, and inferior meatus) by the projection of the turbinates (conchae) from the lateral walls of the internal portion of the nose. The external openings into the nasal cavities (nostrils) are called *anterior nares*. The *posterior nares* (choanae) are openings from an area of the internal nasal cavity above the superior meatus, called the *sphenoethmoidal recess*, into the nasopharynx (Fig. 11-1).

The internal nose is covered by a vascular mucous membrane lined with small hairs and mucous secretions. The membrane collects and carries debris and bacteria from inspired air to the nasopharynx for swallowing or expectoration.

The nose serves as a passageway for air going to and from the lungs. The purpose of the nose is to filter air of impurities and warm, moisten, and chemically examine air for substances that might prove irritating to the mucous lining of the respiratory tract. The nose is the organ of smell, because olfactory receptors are located in the nasal mucosa, and it aids in phonation.

The paranasal sinuses are air-filled extensions of the nasal cavities. The nasal cavity is lined by mucosa and cilia that move secretions through the nasal cavity and nasopharynx.

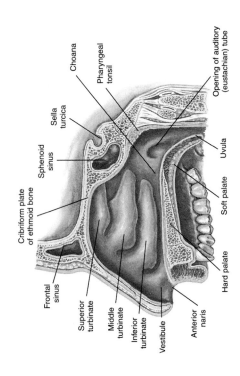

Fig. 11-1
Cross-section of nose and nasopharynx.
(From Seidel HM et al: *Mosby's guide to physical examination*, ed 4, St. Louis, 1999, Mosby.)

Critical Thinking Application—Nose and Sinuses

Knowledge	Experience	Standards
• Be familiar with what the chronic use of nasal decongestants and drugs such as intranasal cocaine and opioids can do to the nasal mucosa. • Habitual use of these drugs is a common health problem.	• Your experience with clients that have chronic nasal and sinus problems or artificial nasal airways will help in your assessment and care planning.	During an examination of the nose, apply the following principles: • Remember that the nasal mucosa is sensitive tissue. • For any client with a nasogastric or nasotracheal tube, frequent inspection is necessary to recognize early signs of tissue irritation.

Nose and Sinus Assessment

Equipment

- Nasal speculum
- Examination light
- Penlight
- Gloves (optional; if drainage is present)

Delegation Considerations

Examination of the nose and sinuses requires critical thinking and knowledge application unique to a professional nurse. The examination should not be delegated to assistive personnel. Do instruct staff to observe for nasal irritation in clients with nasogastric or intestinal tubes and to report such changes immediately. Assistive personnel can report the amount and color of nasal drainage.

Client Preparation

- The client will usually be seated.

History

- Ask the client about recent trauma or surgery to the nose.
- Ask the client about prior trauma or surgery to the nose and/or sinuses.
- Ask whether the client has a history of allergies, nasal discharge (character, odor, amount, duration), epistaxis (nosebleeds), or postnasal drip.
- If there is a history of nasal discharge, ask the client about character, amount, odor, duration, and associated symptoms (for example, sneezing, nasal congestion, obstruction, or mouth breathing).
- If there is a history of epistaxis, ask the client about past and recent nosebleed. Assess site, frequency, amount of bleeding, treatment, and difficulty stopping bleeding. The most common causes include trauma, medication use, and excessive dryness.
- Ask whether the client uses a nasal spray or drops and the type, amount, frequency, and duration.
- Ask whether the client snores at night or has difficulty breathing.
- Determine if client has a history of cocaine use or inhalation of aerosol fumes.

ASSESSMENT TECHNIQUES—NOSE AND SINUSES

Assessment	Normal Findings	Deviations From Normal
• Inspect external nose for shape, size, skin color, and presence of deformity or inflammation.	• Nose is smooth and symmetric with same color as face. Columella is directly midline, and its width does not exceed diameter of a naris. Naris is oval and symmetrically positioned.	• Recent trauma may cause edema and discoloration.
• If swelling or deformities exist, gently palpate the ridge and soft tissue of the nose by placing one finger on each side of the nasal arch and gently moving fingers from the nasal bridge to the tip. Note any tenderness, masses, and underlying deviations.	• Nasal structures are firm and stable.	• Localized tenderness is a result of trauma or inflammation.

Assessment	Normal Findings	Deviations From Normal
• Observe nares for discharge and flaring.	• No discharge or flaring.	• Watery, purulent, or bloody drainage.
⊙ *Standard Precautions Alert If discharge is present, apply gloves for remainder of examination.*		
• If discharge is present, describe its character (watery, mucoid, purulent, crusty, or bloody), amount, color, and whether unilateral or bilateral.		
• Assess patency of each naris by placing a finger on side of the nose and occluding the naris.	• Nasal breathing is noiseless and equal bilaterally, with free exchange of air.	• Nasal breathing is noisy; client has difficulty with air exchange, indicating blockage.
• Ask the client to breathe with mouth closed. Repeat for other naris.		
• Use examination light to illuminate each naris. Inspect visible mucosa for color, lesions, discharge, swelling, and evidence of bleeding.	• Mucosa is pink and moist, without lesions, discharge, swelling, or evidence of bleeding.	• Pale mucosa with clear discharge indicates allergy.
		• Habitual use of intranasal cocaine and opioids can cause puffiness and increased vascularity of mucosa.

- For client with nasogastric, nasopharyngeal, or nasointestinal tube, routinely check for local skin breakdown (excoriation) of each naris.

- Naris is clear, without inflammation.

- Mucosa of naris is inflamed, with sloughing skin and tenderness.

  Sloughing of tissue requires immediate removal and replacement of tube, either in opposite naris or via a different route. Tissue sloughing may be unavoidable because of the critical nature of the client's condition. Meticulous skin care must be used to preserve the tissue of the nares. The family should be aware of possible tissue damage, because permanent scarring can occur.

Assessment	Normal Findings	Deviations From Normal
• To view the septum and turbinate, have the client tip the head back slightly for a clear view.	• Septum is close to midline and is thicker anteriorly than posteriorly.	• Deviated septum, perforated septum, or nasal polyps.
• Inspect for alignment, perforation, and bleeding.	• Turbinates are covered with mucus that is pink, moist, and clear.	
• For a more thorough examination of the nasal cavity, use a nasal speculum.		
• Hold the speculum (connected to otoscope) in the palm of the hand and use the index finger for stabilization.		
• Use the other hand to change the client's head position.		
• Have the client tip the head backward. Insert the speculum gently and carefully about $1/2$ inch (1 cm) to dilate the naris.		

- Do not overdilate the naris.

- Inspect for color, discharge, masses, lesions, and edema.

- Keep client's head erect to see the vestibule and inferior nasal turbinate. Tilt the client's head back to see the middle meatus and middle turbinate. Move the speculum tip midline to view the septum.

- Repeat for other naris.

Sinus Palpation

- Externally palpate the frontal and maxillary facial areas to detect tenderness of sinuses.

- Palpate frontal sinus by exerting pressure with the thumb up and under the client's eyebrow.

- Nasal mucosa is deep pink and glistening.

- Turbinates are same color as surrounding area and are firm.

- Clear discharge is present on septum.

- Erythema of mucosa.

- Bluish-gray or pale pink turbinates.

Assessment	Normal Findings	Deviations From Normal
• Palpate maxillary sinuses by pressing thumb up under the zygomatic process (Fig. 11-2).	• Sinuses are nontender.	• Tenderness indicates inflammation from infection and/or allergy.
Avoid applying pressure to the eyes.		
• If sinus tenderness is present or infection is suspected, **transilluminate** the sinuses.	• Light is transmitted through tissues.	• Absence of glow in sinus indicates sinus either contains secretions or is underdeveloped.
• Conduct examination in a darkened room using a sinus transilluminator or small bright penlight. To view the frontal sinuses, place the light against the medial aspect of each supraorbital rim. Look for a dim red glow of light just above the eyebrow (Fig. 11-3, A).		

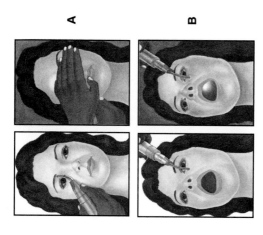

Fig. 11-2
Palpation of maxillary sinus.

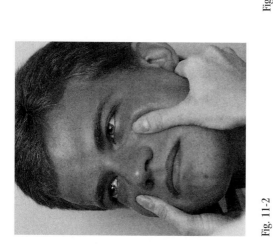

Fig. 11-3
A, Transillumination of frontal sinus. **B,** Transillumination of maxillary sinus.
(From Seidel HM et al: *Mosby's guide to physical examination,* ed 4, St. Louis, 1999, Mosby.)

Assessment	Normal Findings	Deviations From Normal
• To view the maxillary sinuses, place the light lateral to the client's nose, just beneath the medial aspect of the eye (Seidel et al, 1999).	• Air normally found within the sinuses is outlined by a dim red glow.	
• Have the client open the mouth and look to see if the hard palate is illuminated (Fig. 11-3, *B*).		
• Notice the outline of the sinus, and observe for color variations.		

UNEXPECTED ASSESSMENT FINDINGS—NOSE AND SINUSES

Assessment Findings	Significance	Next Step
• Bilateral watery discharge.	• Usually associated with sneezing and congestion, caused by an allergy.	• Assess for symptoms of allergy (e.g., exposure to allergen, watery eyes, duration), and what, if anything, makes it better.
• Unilateral watery discharge in a client with head trauma.	• May be caused by spinal fluid leaking from a fracture.	• Assess for recent head trauma. • Complete a neurological assessment (see Chapter 20). • Notify physician of findings; record and report data.
• Bloody discharge.	• Results from epistaxis (nose bleed), dry nasal mucosa, or trauma.	• Assess for amount of bleeding, frequency, spontaneous bleeding, or the result of blowing the nose. • Assess for use of anticoagulants (e.g., aspirin, coumadin [warfarin], Lovenox, heparin).

Assessment Findings	Significance	Next Step
• Bilateral purulent discharge.	• Usually the result of a sinus or upper respiratory infection.	• Assess for fever and other symptoms of an upper respiratory tract infection. Record and report findings.
• Deviated septum.	• Can be congenital or acquired as a result of nasal trauma.	• When placing a nasogastric tube, do not force the tube.
	• Can obstruct breathing and passage of nasogastric or other nasally placed tubes.	• If resistance is encountered, gently try to advance the tube. If significant resistance is met, try the other naris.
		• Consult with physician if both nasal passages are obstructed.
• Perforated septum.	• Can be the result of repeated use of intranasal cocaine.	• Question client about drug use. Report and record findings.
• Nasal polyps.	• May obstruct breathing. Can contribute to chronic sinus problems.	• Estimate size of polyps. Record and report findings.
• Erythematous nasal mucosa.	• May indicate infection or allergic response.	

- Bluish-gray or pale pink turbinates with mucosal edema.

- May indicate allergic reaction.

- Question client about other symptoms that suggest an allergy (see history, p. 238).

- Question client about other symptoms that suggest an allergy (see history, p. 238).

- A foreign body may cause discharge from one naris and a foul odor.

- Examination of the maxillary and ethmoid sinuses is unnecessary.

 Gerontologic Considerations

- Nasal mucosa may appear drier.

- Older adults have a decrease in their ability to differentiate odors (Lueckenotte, 2000).

- Older adults may experience xerostomia, a dry mouth caused by medications, systemic diseases, heavy smoking, or head and neck radiation (Seidel et al, 1999).

 Pediatric Considerations

Flaring of nostrils is a sign of respiratory difficulty in children.
External nose should be symmetric and positioned in vertical midline of the face. The nares should move minimally with breathing.

- A saddle-shaped nose with a low bridge and broad base or a short, small nose may indicate congenital anomalies (Seidel et al, 1999).

- While examining infants or young children, tilt the nose tip upward with a thumb to view internal nose structures. Use a speculum only if closer examination of the nasal membranes is necessary.

- If a child has been crying, a watery nasal discharge is normal.

Cultural Considerations

- The bridge of the nose is sometimes flat in Oriental and African-American children.
- Otitis media occurs more frequently in Caucasians, Native Americans, Alaskan natives, and Canadian natives (Seidel et al, 1999).
- The incidence of cleft lip and palate is higher in Caucasians and Japanese, and is lower in African Americans (Seidel et al, 1999).

 Client Teaching

- Caution clients against overuse of over-the-counter nasal sprays, which can lead to rebound effect, causing excess nasal congestion.
- Instruct parents on the care of children with nosebleeds. Have the child sit up and lean forward to avoid aspiration of blood. Apply pressure to the anterior of nose with thumb and forefinger as the child breathes through mouth. Apply ice or cold cloth over bridge of nose. If pressure fails to stop bleeding, notify a physician.
- Instruct older adults with reduced sense of smell to always check dated labels on food to ensure against spoilage.

12

Mouth, Pharynx, and Throat

Anatomy and Physiology

The mouth, containing the tongue, teeth, and gums, is the anterior opening of the oropharynx (Fig. 12-1). The bony arch of the hard palate and the fibrous soft palate form the roof of the mouth. The floor of the mouth consists of loose, mobile tissue. The tongue is anchored to the back of the oral cavity at its base and to the floor of the mouth by the frenulum.

Salivary glands are located in tissues surrounding the oral cavity. Saliva initiates digestion and moistens the oral mucosa. The gingivae, or gums, are fibrous tissue covered by mucous

membrane. The roots of the teeth are anchored to alveolar ridges, and the gingivae cover the neck and roots of each tooth. Adults have 32 permanent teeth.

The mouth and oropharynx provide a passageway for food, liquid, and saliva; initiate digestion through mastication and salivary secretion; detect the sense of taste; and emit air for vocalization and nonnasal expiration. The oropharynx is continuous with the nasopharynx and separated from the mouth by the anterior and posterior tonsils.

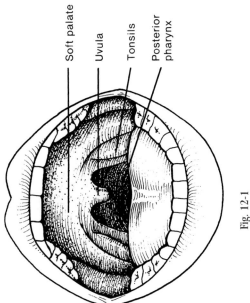

Soft palate

Uvula

Tonsils

Posterior
pharynx

Fig. 12-1
Oral cavity.

Critical Thinking Application—Mouth, Pharynx, and Throat

Knowledge	Experience	Standards
• Apply what you know regarding oral hygiene principles.	This type of examination is easily integrated into routine nursing care.	During an oral and pharyngeal examination, apply the following principles:
• The assessment will reveal a great deal about the client's hygiene habits and pattern of routine dental visits.	• When a client receives oral hygiene, conduct a thorough examination of the mouth, gums, teeth, and tongue.	• Oral lesions can be very uncomfortable; use care when examining tissues.
• Also recognize that changes in oral mucosa can be associated with alcohol, drug, and tobacco abuse, and can indicate nutritional status.	• Clients at high risk for mucosal dehydration include those who are NPO and who have intranasal or interoral tubes that cause mouth breathing and/or irritation to oral mucosa.	• Clients become very self-conscious during removal of dentures.
		• Conduct the examination as quickly as possible.
		• Be thorough in examining all surfaces of the oral cavity.
		• Unconscious clients may have a bite reflex elicited during stimulation of the mouth. Use a padded tongue blade to keep the mouth open and to prevent injury to your hands.

Mouth, Pharynx, and Throat Assessment

Equipment

- Penlight
- Tongue depressor
- Gauze square
- Clean gloves

Delegation Considerations

The examination of the mouth and pharynx requires critical thinking and knowledge application unique to a professional nurse. The examination should not be delegated to assistive personnel. Staff will be involved in administering oral hygiene and in assisting with feeding. Instruct them on types of abnormalities to report (for example, lesions, bleeding, difficulty swallowing, and pain).

Client Preparation

- Client may sit or lie.
- Ask the client to remove dentures and retainers.

History

- Determine whether dentures or retainers the client wears are comfortable and snug. What is the condition of braces, dentures, bridges, or crowns?
- Has the client had a recent change in appetite or weight?
- Assess the client's dental hygiene practices, including use of fluoride toothpaste, frequency of brushing and flossing, and frequency of dental visits.
- Does the client have risks for oral or pharyngeal cancer, including cigarette, cigar, or pipe smoking; use of smokeless tobacco; or excessive consumption of alcohol?
- Does the client have any pain or lesions of the mouth; a lump or thickening; a red or white patch that persists; or difficulty chewing, swallowing, or moving the tongue or jaws? These are signs and symptoms of oral and pharyngeal cancer (NIH 1996, NIH 2001) (www.NIH.gov).
- Does the client have history of streptococcal infection, tonsillectomy, or adenoidectomy?
- Does the client have a history of cancer of the tongue, lips, oral mucosa, or throat?

ASSESSMENT TECHNIQUES—MOUTH, PHARYNX, AND THROAT

Your assessment of the oral cavity determines the client's ability to enunciate words, masticate, salivate, swallow, and taste. Examine the oral cavity for the presence of local or systemic changes that can interfere with a client's nutritional intake and predispose the client to more serious health alterations. Assessment may be done during participation in clients' oral hygiene. Inspect the mouth and pharynx to determine oral hygiene needs and develop a plan of care for clients with dehydration, restricted intake, oral airway obstruction, or oral trauma, and for clients who will undergo or have recently undergone surgery.

Assessment	Normal Findings	Deviations From Normal
◉ *Standard Precautions Alert* *Apply gloves for the examination.*		
• Begin by inspecting the lips for color, texture, hydration, contour, and lesions.	• Lips are pink, moist, symmetric, and smooth, with surface free from lesions.	• Pallor, cyanosis, cherry red color.
		• Lesions such as nodules or ulcerations.
• Have client close mouth, and view the lip end to end.		• Dry, cracked lips.
• Clients should remove lipstick or any other kind of lip substance before the examination.		
• Ask client to clench the teeth and smile.		

Assessment	Normal Findings	Deviations From Normal
• Assess for teeth occlusion.	• Upper molars rest directly on the lower molars, and the upper incisors slightly override the lower incisors.	• Malocclusion (protrusion of the upper or lower incisors, failure of upper incisors to overlap with lower teeth, and failure of back teeth to meet) (Seidel et al, 1999).
• Inspect the condition of teeth, including posterior surfaces. • Ask client to open and relax mouth slightly. A tongue depressor may be needed to retract the lips and cheeks to view the molars.	• Teeth are smooth, white, and shiny.	• Yellow, discolored teeth, tartar at the gumline, black spots on teeth (dental caries).
• Count the number of teeth.	• Normal adult has 32 teeth.	• Multiple missing teeth.
• Ask client to smile.	• Symmetric smile reveals normal facial nerve (Cranial nerve VII) function.	• Droop or half smile.
To view the anterior mucosa and gums: • Ask the client to open and relax the mouth slightly. Gently retract the client's lower lip away from the teeth (Fig. 12-2). Repeat process for upper lip.		

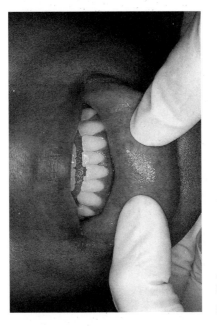

Fig. 12-2
Inspection of inner oral mucosa.

Assessment	Normal Findings	Deviations From Normal
• Inspect mucosa for color, texture, hydration, and lesions.	• Mucosa is pinkish-red, smooth, moist, and without lesions.	• Stomatitis, inflammation of gums and/or oral mucosa.
• If lesions are present, palpate them gently with a gloved hand for tenderness, size, and consistency.		• Gingivitis (inflammation of the gums).
• Inspect buccal mucosa by asking client to open mouth; retract cheek with a tongue depressor or a gloved finger covered with gauze (Fig. 12-3).	• Mucosa is glistening pink, soft, smooth, and moist.	• Dry mucosa, palpable masses or lumps, lesions.
• Buccal mucosa is a good site to inspect for jaundice and pallor.	• Small yellow-white raised lesions commonly seen on the buccal mucosa and lips are Fordyce's spots, which are ectopic sebaceous glands (Seidel et al, 1999).	
• View the surface of the mucosa from right to left and top to bottom.		
• Use a penlight to view posterior mucosa.		
• Palpate the cheek. Insert one finger along the inner mucosa and the thumb along the outside cheek to check for deep-seated lumps or ulcerations.	• Mucosa is smooth, without lesions.	• White patchy lesions (leukoplakia).

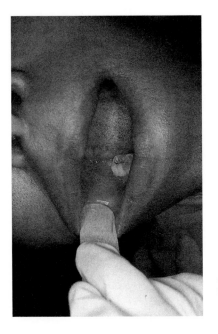

Fig. 12-3
Retraction of the buccal mucosa.

Assessment	Normal Findings	Deviations From Normal
• Retract the cheeks to inspect the gums (gingivae).	• Gums are a slightly stippled pink color, moist, and smooth, with a tight margin at each tooth.	• Gums are swollen, tender, and separated from teeth.
• Inspect for color, edema, retraction, bleeding, and lesions. Take care to view the gums around the back molars.		
• Palpate the gums to assess for thickening or masses.	• No tenderness or lesions. • Gum enlargement occurs with pregnancy, puberty, and phenytoin (Dilantin) use (Seidel et al, 1999).	• Spongy gums that bleed easily.
• Probe each tooth gently with a tongue blade.	• Teeth are firmly set.	• Loose or mobile teeth, swollen gums, or pockets containing debris at tooth margins.
• Have the client relax mouth and protrude tongue halfway. Note any deviation, tremor, or limitation in movement.	• Tongue protrudes midline, without fasciculation. • Tongue moves freely.	• Deviation or limitation of movement.

Procedure		Abnormal Findings
• Ask client to raise the tongue up and move it side-to-side.	• Test the function of glossopharyngeal and hypoglossal nerves (Cranial nerves IX and XII) (see Chapter 20).	
Use a penlight to illuminate the dorsum of the tongue.		• Thickened secretions, coating, swelling, and inflammation or smooth or elongated papillae of the tongue.
• Inspect the tongue for color, size, hydration, texture, position, coating, lesions, and piercings.	• Tongue is medium or dull red in color and size, moist, slightly rough on top surface, and smooth along lateral margins. Without coating or lesions.	
• To view the ventral surface of the tongue and floor of the mouth, ask the client to lift the tongue by placing its tip on the palate behind the upper incisors (Fig. 12-4).	• Ventral surface of tongue is pink and smooth.	• Swollen mass in the floor of the mouth.
	• There are large veins between the frenulum and folds, no edema or lesions.	
	• Wharton ducts should appear on either side of the frenulum (Seidel et al, 1999).	• A swollen, bluish or blackened mass.
• Inspect for color, texture, swelling, and lesions such as nodules or cysts.		
• Palpate the tongue: ask the client to protrude the tongue halfway out.	• Varicosities (swollen, torturous veins) are not uncommon.	• Leukoplakia.
		• Elevated papillae.

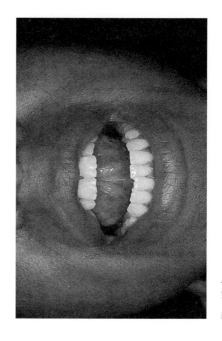

Fig. 12-4
Ventral surface of the tongue.

Assessment	Normal Findings	Deviations From Normal
• Grasp the tip gently with a gauze square. Gently pull the tongue to one side.	• Tongue has smooth, even texture, and is firm and without lesions.	• Mass. • Lesions. • Ulceration.
• Palpate the full length of the tongue and the base for any areas of hardening or ulceration.		
• Have the client tip head back and hold mouth open as you inspect the hard and soft palates for color, shape, texture, and extra bony prominence or defects (Fig. 12-5).	• Hard palate or roof of mouth is located anteriorly.	• Lesions. • Mass or nodule.
	• The whitish-pink hard palate is dome shaped, with transverse ridges.	
	• Bony growth (exostosis) between the two palates is common.	
	• The soft palate, best seen while depressing the tongue with a tongue blade, extends posteriorly toward the pharynx. It is light pink and smooth.	

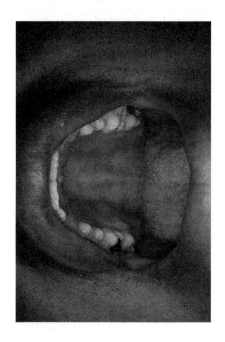

Fig. 12-5
Soft and hard palates.

Assessment	Normal Findings	Deviations From Normal
Explain the pharyngeal examination to client. Ask client to tip head back, open mouth, and say "Ah." Have tongue depressor on middle third of tongue. Use penlight to inspect pharynx.		
• Inspect the uvula and soft palate as the client says "Ah." **Do not place tongue depressor too far anteriorly, or posterior tongue will mound up to obstruct view. Do not place depressor too far posteriorly, or gag reflex will be elicited.**	• Both structures rise centrally. Uvula varies in length and thickness. Tests vagus nerve (Cranial nerve X).	• Deviation or immobility.
• Inspect the arch formed by the anterior and posterior pillars, soft palate, and uvula.	• Tonsils are oval with infoldings of tissue.	• Edema, ulceration, or inflammation indicates infection or abnormal lesions.
• The tonsils can be seen in the cavities between the pillars.	• Pharyngeal tissues are pink and smooth.	• Absence of tonsils indicates previous surgical removal.

Assessment	Normal Findings	Deviations From Normal
• View the posterior pharynx behind the pillars.	• Tissues are smooth, glistening pink, and well hydrated. • Small, irregular spots of lymphatic tissue and small blood vessels are normal.	• Clear exudate may be found with chronic sinus problems. Yellow or green exudate indicates an infection. A typical sore throat is evidenced by reddened, swollen uvula and tonsillar pillars with possible exudate. Client will express discomfort.

UNEXPECTED ASSESSMENT FINDINGS—MOUTH, PHARYNX, AND THROAT

Assessment Findings	Significance	Next Step
Abnormal color of oral mucosa		
• Pallor.	• Can be caused by anemia.	• Assess for other signs of anemia.
• Cyanosis.	• Result of respiratory or cardiovascular problems.	• Cyanosis is a late sign of oxygenation deficit. Assess for vasoconstriction (see Chapter 14), acid-base status, and history that may suggest exposure to carbon monoxide (e.g., victim of a fire).
		• Record and report findings.
• Cherry red color.	• Caused by acidosis and carbon monoxide poisoning (Seidel et al, 1999).	**Acidosis and carbon dioxide poisoning should be reported to the physician as soon as possible.**
• Dry, cracked lips.	• May be caused by dehydration, wind chapping, or excessive lip licking.	• Determine cause. Apply petroleum jelly, or lip moisturizer. Check to see if physician order is required.

Assessment Findings	Significance	Next Step
		• Assess fluid status. Increase oral intake if not contraindicated by medical condition.
Abnormal Color of Teeth		
• Yellow or darkened.	• May indicate poor oral hygiene or lack of regular dental care.	• Record and report findings.
• Chalky, white discoloration of the enamel.	• Tobacco smoking or chewing tobacco.	• Review history for prior use of medications that may affect the teeth.
• Tartar at the base of the teeth.	• Intrauterine medications (e.g., tetracycline).	
• Multiple extraction sites.	• Chemotherapeutic agents.	
• Blackened spots (dental caries).		
• Droop in smile or only able to smile with one side of the mouth.	• Indicates facial nerve paralysis (Cranial nerve VII).	**If acute finding, report to physician immediately.**
• Stomatitis (inflammation of gums and/or oral mucosa).	• May be caused by bacterial infection, herpes simplex virus (HSV I, HSV II), vitamin deficiency (B_6), or side effects of chemotherapeutic drugs.	• Assess for signs of infection, review current and prior medications, evaluate nutritional status.

Findings		Actions
• Gingivitis (inflammation of the gums).	• Caused by poor oral hygiene, lack of regular dental care and infection, pregnancy, puberty, medication (e.g., Dilantin), and leukemia (Seidel et al, 1999).	• Record and report findings. • May need blood drawn to identify vitamin deficiency. • Notify physician of findings. • Record and report findings noting client's pattern of oral hygiene and dental care.
• Blue-black line 1 mm above gum line.	• May indicate chronic lead or bismuth poisoning.	• Record and report findings. • Notify physician. • Evaluate for risk of lead or bismuth ingestion.
• Leukoplakia (white patchy lesions).	• Precancerous lesion.	• Notify physician. • Record and report findings.
• Oral, hairy leukoplakia.	• Often seen as an oral manifestation of HIV infection.	• Identify risk factors for oral cancer.

Assessment Findings	Significance	Next Step
• Angular cheilitis.	• May indicate deficiency in riboflavin. • May be caused by over-closing of the mouth, allowing saliva to macerate the tissue (Seidel et al, 1999). • Oral manifestation of HIV infection (Seidel et al, 1999).	• Record and report finding to physician. • Requires prescription for antifungal cream.
• Smooth tongue.	• May be the result of a vitamin B_{12} deficiency or niacin deficiency.	• Record and report findings. • Discuss with care provider. • Client may require blood work to identify abnormality.
• Raised papillae on posterior tongue.	• May indicate vitamin B_6 deficiency.	• Record and report findings. • Discuss with care provider. • Client may require blood work to identify abnormality.

• Glossitis (swelling and inflammation of the tongue).	• May result from a burn, bite, or an infectious disease or infected tongue piercing.
	• Record and report findings.
	• Review assessment data for findings that support infection, elevated temperature, mucopurulent drainage, elevated white blood count (WBC).
	• Notify physician of findings.
	• Determine when and where tongue piercing took place and under what conditions (e.g., sterile, clean).
• Tongue deviates or has limited movement.	• May indicate involvement of the hypoglossal nerve (Cranial nerve XII).
	• Record and report findings.
	• Notify the physician.
• Black, hairy tongue.	• May be caused by antibiotic therapy.
	• Record and report findings.
	• Review medication record for recent or past antibiotics.
	• Notify physician of findings.
• Spongy gums that bleed easily.	• Indicates periodontal disease and vitamin C deficiency.
	• Record and report findings, noting client's pattern of oral hygiene and dental care.

Assessment Findings	Significance	Next Step
• Soft palate does not rise uniformly.	• May indicate involvement of the vagus nerve (Cranial nerve X).	• Record and report findings. • Notify physician.
• Aphthous ulcers (canker sore or ulcerative stomatitis).	• Recurrent circumscribed ulcers with erythematous margins. Cause is unknown. Occurs more often in women than men (Seidel et al, 1999).	• Assess risk factors for oral HSV I or HSV II infection. • Have client rinse mouth with warm water. May use anesthetics such as viscous lidocaine to relieve pain. • Obtain physician orders for anesthetics, antibiotics, suspensions, or corticosteroids.

Pediatric Considerations

- Children have 20 deciduous teeth that erupt between 8 and 30 months of age, depending on the tooth. Permanent teeth begin to appear around 6 years of age, with final molars in place at 12 to 17 years of age.
- Inspection of the oral cavity is easier while an infant is crying.
- Nonadherent white patches on the tongue or buccal mucosa are usually milk deposits. Adherent patches may indicate *candidiasis* (thrush).
- Drooling is common in infants up to 6 months of age but may indicate neurological disorder or swallowing difficulty after 12 months of age.
- Inspect infant's hard and soft palates carefully for presence of clefts.
- Children may need to be gently restrained in a parent's lap during the examination. The parent reaches around to restrain the child's arms with one arm and controls the child's head with the other.

Gerontologic Considerations

- In older adults, the mucosa is normally dry because of reduced salivation, and the gums are pale.
- The tongue may appear more fissured.
- Loose or missing teeth are common, because bone breakdown increases.
- An older adult's teeth often feel rough when tooth enamel calcifies. Yellow or darkened teeth are also common because of the general wear and tear that exposes the darker, underlying dentation.
- The teeth may appear longer because of resorption of the gum and bone underneath.

Cultural Considerations

- Dark-skinned clients will have increased pigmentation on the buccal mucosa and gums.
- When comparing clients from different cultures, whites have the smallest teeth, African Americans have somewhat larger teeth, and Orientals and Native Americans have even larger teeth. The Australian Aborigines have the largest teeth in the world, as well as extra molars (Giger, 1999).
- Hyperpigmentation of the buccal mucosa is normal in 10% of whites and 90% of African Americans over 50 years of age.
- Smoking patterns differ by culture. White students are more likely than black or Hispanic students to smoke. Smoking prevalence is highest among American Indian and Alaskan Natives. Smokeless tobacco is used more widely by American Indian, Alaskan Native, and white men than black, Hispanic, or Asian/Pacific Islander men (American Cancer Society, 2001).

Client Teaching

- Discuss proper techniques for oral hygiene, including brushing and flossing.
- Explain that oral cancer is more common in clients who chew tobacco or smoke a pipe. Lip cancer is seen more often in men and people with light-colored skin who have had a great deal of sun exposure (National Cancer Institute, 2002).
- Explain early warning signs of lip and oral cancer (Box 12-1).
- Caution clients about the risk for cheek and gum cancer. The use of smokeless tobacco (plug, leaf, and snuff) is on the increase in the United States. The 1997 Youth Risk Behavior Survey by the Centers for Disease Control and Prevention (CDC) reported that 15.8% of male high school students currently use smokeless tobacco or snuff (MMWR, 1999). Explain warning signs of gum (periodontal) disease, including gums that bleed easily; red, swollen gums that pull away from teeth; and pus between teeth or around a loose tooth.

- Encourage yearly dental examinations for children and adults.
- Older adults should visit a dentist every 6 months.
- Older adults should eat soft foods and cut food into small pieces because of difficulty in chewing.
- Warn parents not to put a child to bed with a bottle containing formula, milk, or juice, because these liquids may pool and cause tooth decay.

BOX 12-1 Early Signs of Lip and Oral Cancer

A sore in the mouth doesn't heal in 2 to 3 weeks, bleeds easily, or is painful.

A lump or thickening in the mouth.

Numbness or pain in mouth and throat.

Persistent red or white patches on oral mucosa.

Dentures no longer fit well.

From National Cancer Institute: *Lip and oral cavity cancer,* CancerNet, www.cancernet.nci.nih.gov, 2002.

13

Thorax and Lungs

Anatomy and Physiology

The two primary physiological functions of the lungs are the exchange of respiratory gases and maintenance of acid-base balance. The process of oxygenation has three steps: ventilation, perfusion, and diffusion. For the exchange of gases to occur, the organs, nerves, and muscles of respiration must be intact.

The thorax is a cage of bone, cartilage, and muscle that moves as the lungs expand. The anterior thorax consists of the sternum, manubrium, xiphoid process, and costal cartilages. Twelve pairs of ribs form the lateral chest. Posteriorly, the tho-

rax consists of the 12 thoracic vertebrae, eight of which extend behind the bony scapulae. All of the ribs connect to the thoracic vertebrae; the upper seven attach to the sternum by the costal cartilages.

The primary muscles of respiration are the diaphragm and intercostal muscles. During inspiration the diaphragm contracts and moves downward, lowering the abdominal contents to increase intrathoracic space. The external intercostal muscles increase the anteroposterior chest diameter during inspiration. On expiration, the diaphragm relaxes and the internal intercostals decrease the transverse diameter of the thoracic cage.

The interior chest contains the right and left pleural cavities and the mediastinum. The mediastinum, situated between the lungs, contains all of the thoracic organs except the lungs. The pleural cavities are lined with parietal and visceral pleura, serous membranes that enclose the lungs. The elastic, spongy lungs are paired, asymmetric organs located within the pleural cavities. The right lung has three lobes, and the left has two. Each lung is cone shaped with the rounded apex extending about 1½ inches (4 cm) above the first rib. The base of each lung is broad and concave. Each lobe contains blood vessels, lymphatics, nerves, and an alveolar duct connecting with the alveoli.

The tracheobronchial tree is a tubular system that forms a pathway for air to travel from the upper airway to the alveoli. The trachea is 10 to 11 cm (4 to 4½ inches) long and about 2 cm (¾ inch) in diameter. The trachea lies anterior to the esophagus and posterior to the thyroid isthmus. The trachea divides into the right and left main bronchi at the level of thoracic vertebra T4 or T5.

During assessment, you will use key landmarks to describe findings (Fig. 13-1). The angle of Louis (manubriosternal junction), suprasternal notch, costal angle, clavicles, and vertebral prominens (spinous process of C7) are key landmarks for anterior and posterior chest assessment. The clavicle is divided into two sections by the midclavicular line. The lateral landmarks include the anterior, mid, and posterior axillary lines (Fig 13-1, C). On the anterior chest, the anterior axillary lines are used to denote the outer edge of the anterior chest wall. Keep in mind the underlying position of the lungs and the position of each rib.

The angle of Louis is located on the anterior chest wall at the manubriosternal junction (Fig. 13-1, A). The angle is a visible and palpable angulation of the sternum below the suprasternal notch, at the point at which the second rib articulates with the sternum. Count the ribs and the intercostal spaces (between the ribs) from this point to locate findings, such as the position of the lobes of the lung. The number of each intercostal space corresponds to that of the rib just above it. The spinous process of the third thoracic vertebra and the fourth, fifth, and sixth ribs help to locate the lung's lobes posteriorly (Fig. 13-1, B).

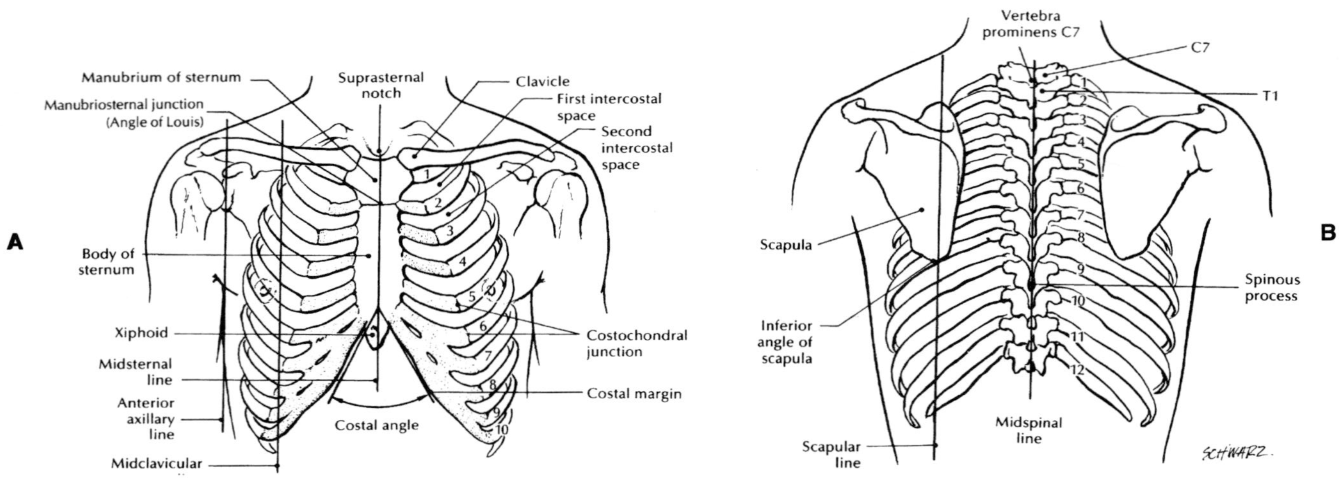

Fig. 13-1
Topographic landmarks. **A**, Anterior thorax. **B**, Posterior thorax.
(From Malasanos L, et al: *Health assessment*, ed 4, St Louis, 1990, Mosby.)

Continued

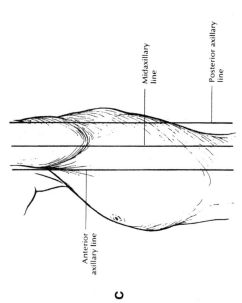

Fig. 13-1, cont'd
C, Lateral thorax.
(From Malasanos L et al: *Health assessment*, ed 4, St Louis, 1990, Mosby.)

The upper and middle lobes are found on the anterior chest wall (Fig. 13-2). The apex of the upper lobes extends 2 cm above the clavicles. The anterior lobes extend to the seventh rib. The left side of the lung is slightly longer than the right. There is a small portion of the lower lobe on the anterior chest wall at and below the seventh rib.

Laterally, the lung extends from the T3 spinous process to the sixth rib at the anterior axillary line and the seventh rib at the posterior axillary line (Fig. 13-3).

The lower lobes project laterally and anteriorly. Posteriorly, the tip or inferior margin of the scapula lies approximately at the level of the seventh rib (Fig. 13-4). By identifying the seventh rib the examiner can count upward to locate the third thoracic vertebra and align it with the inner borders of the scapula to locate the posterior lobes. The vertebral prominens can be more readily seen and felt when the client bends the head forward. If two prominences are felt, the upper is that of C7 and the lower is that of T1.

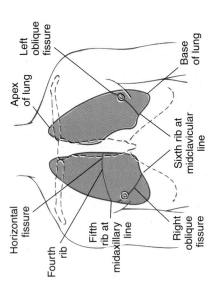

Fig. 13-2
Anterior position of lung lobes.

Left oblique fissure

Apex of lung

Base of lung

Horizontal fissure

Fourth rib

Fifth rib at midaxillary line

Right oblique fissure

Sixth rib at midclavicular line

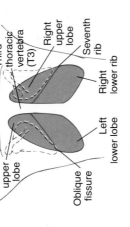

Fig. 13-4
Posterior position of lung lobes.

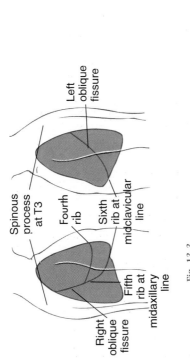

Fig. 13-3
Lateral position of lung lobes.

Critical Thinking Application—Thorax and Lungs

Knowledge	Experience	Standards
• Refer to the knowledge you have regarding the anatomy of the lung.	• To accurately assess the lungs and thorax, you must be competent in use of the stethoscope.	During the examination of the lungs and thorax apply the following principles:
• Refer to the knowledge you have about the physiology of respiratory control.		• Clients in respiratory distress are anxious and restless. Keep the history brief and use simple questions that require "Yes" and "No" answers.
• Refer to the knowledge you have regarding pulmonary pathologies. Findings may be caused by abnormal collections of air or fluid, or by solid tumors within the pleural space.		• Be sure the client is in as comfortable a position as possible to allow for full chest expansion.
• Oxygen is a basic human need to sustain life.		• Be systematic in the examination. Always compare right side to left side. Proceed in exactly the same order every time you examine the lung. Examine all lung lobes bilaterally (anteriorly, laterally, and posteriorly).
• Pulmonary disease can be acute or chronic.		

- Assess for long-term disabilities related to pulmonary disease.

- Clients can be screened early for potential disorders.

- If the lungs are affected by disease, other body systems will reflect alterations. For example, reduced oxygenation can cause changes in mental alertness because of the brain's sensitivity to lowered oxygen levels.

- Be sensitive to asking the client to breath deeply frequently because of dizziness and light-headedness.

Thorax and Lung Assessment

Equipment

- Stethoscope
- Centimeter ruler and tape measure
- Marking pencil

Delegation Considerations

The examination of the lungs and thorax requires critical thinking and knowledge application unique to a professional nurse. Delegation of the examination is inappropriate. Assistive personnel can learn to monitor respirations and changes in sputum and report any abnormalities to you.

Client Preparation

- Client must be undressed to the waist.
- Make sure lighting is good.
- Client sits (when possible) for assessment of posterior and lateral chest. Assessment in the side-lying position is possible but not desirable. Client may sit or lie with head of bed raised for assessment of anterior chest. (If client cannot sit up alone, provide assistance.)

History

- Review the client's family history for cancer, tuberculosis, cystic fibrosis, allergies, and chronic obstructive pulmonary disease such as asthma and emphysema.
- Assess client's history of allergies to pollens, dust, or other airborne irritants, as well as to foods, drugs, or chemical substances.
- Assess client's history of tobacco or marijuana use. Include type of tobacco, duration, and amount (pack years = number of years smoking × number of packs per day), age started, and efforts to quit. Be sure to include cigar or pipe smoking. What is the extent of smoking by others at work or home (passive smoking)?
- Does the client have a *persistent cough* (productive or non-productive), *sputum production, chest pain,* shortness of breath, orthopnea, dyspnea during exertion or at rest, poor activity tolerance, or *recurrent attacks of pneumonia or bronchitis?* (Italicized symptoms are warning signals for lung cancer.)
- Does the client have a history of chronic pulmonary disease, such as tuberculosis (TB) (date, treatment, compliance), asthma, emphysema, bronchitis, or cystic fibrosis)?

- Does or did the client work in an environment that contains pollutants, such as asbestos, arsenic, coal dust, exhaust fumes, or chemical irritants? Does the client use protective devices?
- Identify risk for TB. Determine if client has history of any of the following:

  Known or suspected human immunodeficiency virus/acquired immunodeficiency disease (HIV/AIDS) infection.

  Substance abuse.

  Living in an overcrowded area.

  Low income.

  Malnourishment.

  Homelessness.

  Recent immigration.

  Residence in a nursing home.

- Clients with other serious disorders, such as alcoholism, chronic renal failure, diabetes mellitus, or neoplastic diseases are at higher risk of developing TB (American Thoracic Society, 2000).

- Does client have history of cough, weight loss, fatigue, night sweats, fever, and/or hemoptysis?
- When did the client last have a chest x-ray examination or tuberculosis test?
- If a client, especially a young adult, complains of acute chest pain, consider drug use, particularly cocaine. Cocaine can cause pneumothorax with severe acute chest pain (Seidel et al, 1999).
- What is the client's exercise tolerance? How far can the client walk on the level without becoming short of breath? How many flights of stairs can the client climb without stopping?
- Does client have history of chronic hoarseness (indicative of laryngeal disorder or abuse of cocaine and opioids from sniffing)?
- Has the client had the pneumococcal (pneumonia) or influenza vaccine? Determine the length of time since the last pneumovax. If greater than 5 years in clients ≥ 6 months with underlying conditions, revaccination is recommended (CDC, 1997). Influenza vaccine is recommended annually (CDC, 1999).
- What medications is the client taking?

ASSESSMENT TECHNIQUES—THORAX AND LUNGS

Reduced oxygenation can affect body systems other than that of the lungs. For example, a lowering of oxygenation can cause reduced mental alertness and changes in skin color. Be alert to subtle cues. For example, note the client's breath. Malodorous breath can indicate pulmonary infection. Compare findings from the assessment of the skin, nails, and oral mucosa, noting if cyanosis or pallor is present.

Assessment	Normal Findings	Deviations From Normal
• Observe the client's breathing pattern	• Normal breathing is quiet and barely audible near the open mouth.	• Client may use accessory muscles of respiration, pursed-lip breathing, or labored breathing.
	• Respiration of males is more diaphragmatic (more movement of abdominal muscles), and respiration of females is more costal (more movement of ribs).	• Client may make grunting sounds with each breath.
• Observe the accessory muscles of breathing: trapezius, sternocleidomastoid, and abdominal muscles.	• The accessory muscles move little with normal passive breathing.	• The use of accessory muscles of respiration indicates an increased work of breathing.
• Observe for bulging of the intercostal spaces on expiration.	• No bulging or active movement should occur in the intercostal spaces with respiration.	• Bulging of intercostal spaces with respiration, indicating a great effort to breathe.

- Inspect the chest wall movement during respiration.

- Expansion is symmetric.

- Chest asymmetry can be from unequal expansion of the lungs.
- Unilateral or bilateral bulging can be a reaction of the ribs and interspaces to respiratory obstruction (Seidel et al, 1999).

- Observe the shape and symmetry of the chest from the back and front. Note the anteroposterior diameter.

- Chest contour is relatively symmetric. The bony framework is obvious, the clavicles are prominent, and the sternum is flat.
- The anteroposterior diameter (AP diameter) is normally one third to one half of the transverse (side-to-side) diameter.
- The angle is usually larger than 90 degrees.

- Barrel-shaped chest. AP diameter equals transverse and ribs are more horizontal.

- Observe the width of the costal angle as measured between the two costal margins anteriorly.

- Inspect anterior thoracic skeleton.

- Sternum and xiphoid are relatively inflexible.

- Abnormal contours are caused by congenital and postural alterations.

Assessment	Normal Findings	Deviations From Normal
Posterior Chest Wall		
• Standing at a midline position behind the client, look for deformities, position of the spine, slope of the ribs, and symmetry of scapulae.	• Spine is normally vertically straight without lateral deviation.	• A pigeon chest (pectus carinatum) is a prominent sternal protrusion.
	• Posteriorly, the ribs tend to slope across and downward at a 45-degree angle.	• A funnel chest (pectus excavatum) is an indentation of the lower sternum above the xiphoid process.
	• Scapulae are symmetric and closely attached to the chest wall.	• Spine may be deviated posteriorly (kyphosis), or laterally (scoliosis).
• Palpate the posterior thoracic muscles and skeleton for lumps, masses, pulsations, tenderness, bulges, and unusual movement or position.	• Chest wall is not tender.	• Localized pain.
	• Rib cage is somewhat elastic.	• Crepitus (a crackly sensation that feels like cellophane under the skin)
	• Thoracic spine is rigid.	

- If pain or tenderness presents, avoid deep palpation because fractured rib fragments may displace against vital organs.

Measure posterior chest excursion

- Stand behind the client and place your thumbs along the spinal processes at the level of the tenth rib (Fig. 13-5, *A*), with your palms lightly in contact with the posterolateral surfaces.

- Your thumbs should be about 2 inches (5 cm) apart, pointing toward the spine and fingers pointing laterally.

- Press your hands (do not slide) toward spine to create a small skin fold between the thumbs.

- Ask the client to take a deep breath after first exhaling; observe the movement of your thumbs (Fig. 13-5, *B*).

is the result of air leaking into the subcutaneous tissues from a rupture or tear in the lung.

- Reduced chest excursion can be caused by pain, postural deformity, or fatigue.

- Chest excursion should be symmetric, separating the thumbs 1 $\frac{1}{4}$ to 2 inches (3 to 5 cm).

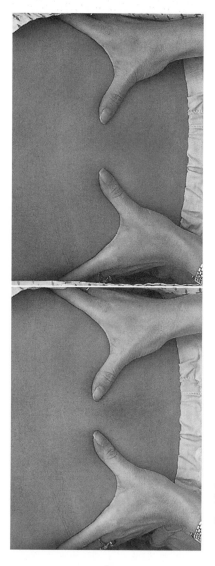

Fig. 13-5
Position of nurse's hands for palpation of excursion. **A,** Before client inhales. **B,** After client inhales.

Assessment	Normal Findings	Deviations From Normal
• Palpate for symmetry of respiration.		• Decreased or increased fremitus.
• Palpate for tactile (vocal) fremitus (the palpable vibration of the chest wall during speech).	• Tactile fremitus is felt as a faint vibration.	
• If fremitus is faint, ask client to speak louder or in a lower tone.	• Tactile fremitus is symmetric and strongest at the apex of the lung, near the tracheal bifurcation.	
• Place the ball or lower palm of your hand over symmetric intercostal spaces, beginning at the lung apex (Fig. 13-6).	• Tactile fremitus decreases in the periphery of the chest.	
• Use a firm, light touch.	• Increased fremitus feels rougher.	
• At each position ask client to say "99," note if you feel a vibration.		

Assessment	Normal Findings	Deviations From Normal

- For comparison, palpate both sides simultaneously and symmetrically, or use one hand very quickly while alternating sides.

- Be sure to palpate the lateral chest wall as well. It may be difficult to palpate posteriorly, because the scapula can obscure fremitus.

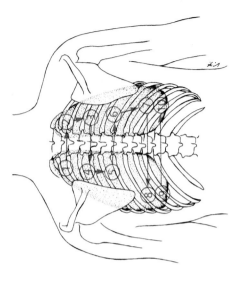

Fig. 13-6
Nurse follows a systematic pattern when comparing fremitus, percussion, and auscultation. Posterior thorax.

- Percuss the chest wall to determine whether lung tissue is air filled, fluid filled, or solid:

- Ask the client to fold arms across chest with head bent forward.

- With indirect percussion technique, percuss intercostal spaces at 1 1/2- to 2-inch (4- to 5-cm) intervals, following a systematic pattern to compare both sides (see Fig. 13-6).

- Measure the diaphragmatic excursion (Seidel et al, 1999):

  - Have client breathe deeply and hold.

  - Percuss along the scapular line until you locate the lower border where resonance turns to dullness.

  - Mark the point with the skin pencil at the scapular line.

- The posterior thorax is normally resonant on percussion.

- Percussion over scapula, ribs, or spine is dull.

- Normal excursion distance is 1 1/4 to 2 inches (3 to 5 cm). The diaphragm is normally higher on the right than the left.

- A lung mass causes a flat sound.

- Hyperresonance may be from emphysema, pneumothorax, or asthma.

- Dullness may be caused by atelectasis, pleural effusion, or asthma.

- Diaphragmatic descent may be limited by pulmonary lesions (emphysema), abdominal lesions (tumor or ascites), or superficial pain.

Assessment	Normal Findings	Deviations From Normal
• Allow client to breathe and repeat on the other side.		
• Have client take several breaths and then exhale as much as possible and hold.		
• On each side, percuss up from the marked point and make a mark at the change from dullness to resonance.		
• Have client resume breathing.		
• Measure with the ruler and record the distance in centimeters between the marks on each side.		
Auscultate the Lung		
• Use the stethoscope diaphragm for adults and bell for children.	• Normal breath sounds include bronchial, vesicular, and bronchovesicular breath sounds (Table 13-1).	• Abnormal breath sounds (Table 13-2).
		• Absence of lung sounds.

Table 13-1 Normal Breath Sounds

	Description	Location	Origin
Vesicular	Vesicular sounds are soft, breezy, and low pitched. Inspiratory phase is three times longer than expiratory phase.	Best heard over lung's periphery (except over scapula).	Created by air moving through smaller airways.
Bronchovesicular	Bronchovesicular sounds are medium-pitched and blowing sounds of medium intensity. Inspiratory phase is equal to expiratory phase.	Best heard posteriorly between scapulae and anteriorly over bronchioles lateral to sternum at first and second intercostal spaces.	Created by air moving through large airways.
Bronchial	Bronchial sounds are loud and high pitched with hollow quality. Expiration lasts longer than inspiration (3:2 ratio).	Best heard over trachea.	Created by air moving through trachea to chest wall.

Table 13-2 Adventitious Sounds

Sound	Site Auscultated	Cause	Character
Crackles (previously called *rales*)	Are most commonly heard in dependent lobes; right and left lung bases.	Random, sudden reinflation of groups of alveoli*; disruptive passage of air.	Fine crackles are high-pitched, fine, short, interrupted crackling sounds heard during end of inspiration, usually not cleared with coughing.* Moist crackles are lower, more moist sounds heard during middle of inspiration; not cleared with coughing.
Rhonchi	Are primarily heard over trachea and bronchi; if loud enough, can be heard over most lung fields.	Muscular spasm, fluid, or mucus in larger airways, causing turbulence.	Are loud, low-pitched, rumbling, coarse sounds heard most often during inspiration or expiration; may be cleared by coughing.
Wheezes	Can be heard over all lung fields.	High-velocity air flow through severely narrowed bronchus.	Are high-pitched, continuous musical sounds like a squeak heard continuously during inspiration or expiration; usually louder on expiration, do not clear with coughing.†
Pleural friction rub	Is heard over anterior lateral lung field (if client is sitting upright).	Inflamed pleura, parietal pleura rubbing against visceral pleura.	Has dry, grating quality heard best during inspiration; does not clear with coughing, heard loudest over lower lateral anterior surface.

*Data from Forgacs P: The functional basis of pulmonary sounds, *Chest* 73:399, 1978.
†Data from Wilkins RL, Hodgkin JE, Lopez B: *Lung sounds: a practical guide,* St Louis, 1988, Mosby.

Assessment	Normal Findings	Deviations From Normal
• Ask the client to breathe slowly and deeply with the mouth slightly open.		
• Listen to an entire inspiration and expiration at each position.		
• If sounds are faint, as in the obese client, ask the client to breathe deeper with the mouth open.		
• Follow the same systematic pattern as with percussion, comparing side-to-side (see Fig. 13-6).		
• If client has signs of congestive heart failure, auscultate from the base of the lung for crackles. Note the level to which they rise.		
Voice Sounds		
• Place stethoscope over same locations to hear voice sounds.	• Sounds are normally muffled, faint and indistinct.	• Sounds are distinct, clear and easily distinguished. "ee" sounds like "aa".

Assessment	Normal Findings	Deviations From Normal
• Have the client say "99" (bronchophony, whisper "One, two, three" (whispered pectoriloquy), or "ee" (egophony).		
Differences in techniques of inspection, palpation, percussion and auscultation are described in the following sections on the lateral and anterior thorax.		
Lateral Thorax		
With client seated and arms raised above the head, extend assessment to lateral thorax.		
• Inspect, palpate, percuss, and auscultate lateral thorax in same manner as with posterior thorax. Use a systematic method to compare both sides (Fig. 13-7).		• Deviations are same as with posterior thorax.
• Excursion cannot be assessed laterally.		

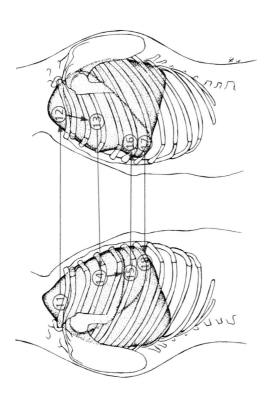

Fig. 13-7
Lateral thorax.

Assessment	Normal Findings	Deviations From Normal
Anterior Chest Wall		
• Measure anterior chest excursion:	• Chest excursion should separate the thumbs 1 ¼ to 2 inches (3 to 5 cm).	• See p. 304 for unexpected assessment findings.
• Place hands over each lateral rib cage along the costal margin. Place thumbs parallel 2 ½ inches (6 cm) apart and angled along the costal margins.		
• Push thumbs toward midline to create a skin fold.		
• Ask client to inhale deeply.		
• Observe separation of thumbs.		
• Palpate for tactile fremitus (Fig. 13-8), with the same technique used for the posterior thorax.	• Fremitus is normally decreased over the heart, lower thorax, and breast tissue.	• See p. 304 for unexpected assessment findings.
• Fremitus is best felt next to the sternum at the second intercostal space, at the level of the bifurcation of the bronchi (Seidel et al, 1999).		

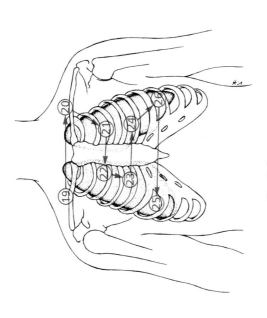

Fig. 13-8
Anterior thorax.

Assessment	Normal Findings	Deviations From Normal
You will not be able to sense vibrations over breast tissue and thus must gently retract the breasts.		
• With client sitting or supine, percuss the anterior thorax and compare both sides (see Fig. 13-8), considering the locations of the underlying liver, heart, and stomach (Fig. 13-9).	• Percussion over the heart and liver are dull. • The gastric air bubble is percussed as a tympanic sound. (See Chapter 16.)	Dullness percussed over the anterior chest may suggest consolidation or fluid-filled alveoli.
• Percuss in a systematic pattern from above the clavicles, moving across and down; always comparing right side to left side.		
• Displace female breasts as needed.		
• With client sitting erect and shoulders back, auscultate the anterior thorax using the same pattern as with percussion (see Fig. 13-8).	• Breath sounds are clear.	• See Tables 13-1 and 13-2, pp. 295-296.

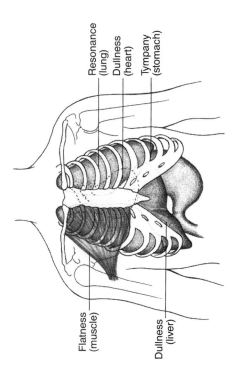

Resonance
(lung)

Dullness
(heart)

Tympany
(stomach)

Flatness
(muscle)

Dullness
(liver)

Fig. 13-9
Variations in percussion notes in the normal thorax and upper abdomen.

Assessment	Normal Findings	Deviations From Normal
• Pay particular attention during auscultation of the right lung where mucous secretions are commonly aspirated and can accumulate.		

UNEXPECTED ASSESSMENT FINDINGS—THORAX AND LUNGS

Assessment Findings	Significance	Next Step
Abnormal Respiratory Patterns	• See Fig. 13-10.	• Record and report findings. Discuss any changes or new breath sound heard with the physician.
• Bradypnea		
• Tachypnea		

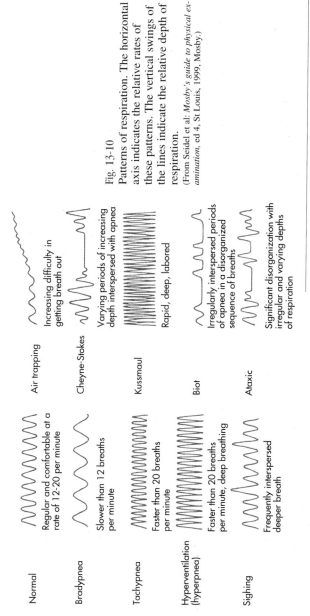

Normal

Regular and comfortable at a
rate of 12-20 per minute

Bradypnea

Slower than 12 breaths
per minute

Tachypnea

Faster than 20 breaths
per minute

Hyperventilation
(hyperpnea)

Faster than 20 breaths
per minute, deep breathing

Sighing

Frequently interspersed
deeper breath

Air trapping

Increasing difficulty in
getting breath out

Cheyne-Stokes

Varying periods of increasing
depth interspersed with apnea

Kussmaul

Rapid, deep, labored

Biot

Irregularly interspersed periods
of apnea in a disorganized
sequence of breaths

Ataxic

Significant disorganization with
irregular and varying depths
of respiration

Fig. 13-10

Patterns of respiration. The horizontal
axis indicates the relative rates of
these patterns. The vertical swings of
the lines indicate the relative depth of
respiration.

(From Seidel et al: *Mosby's guide to physical examination*, ed 4, St Louis, 1999, Mosby.)

Assessment Findings	Significance	Next Step
• Kussmaul's respirations		• Evaluate need for suctioning, coughing and deep breathing or chest physiotherapy.
• Cheyne-Stokes respiration		
• Hyperventilation (hyperpnea)		• Be prepared to support respirations if necessary.
• Biot		
• Sighing		
• Ataxic		
• Air trapping		
• Apnea	• Periods of no respiration.	**Immediately notify physician skilled in intubation. Assess for adequate air movement, (e.g. level of consciousness, use of accessory muscles of respiration).**
• Respiratory stridor	• Narrowed or obstructed airway.	**Be prepared to administer racemic epinephrine if requested.**

		Be prepared for airway support with suction, assistance with ventilation or possible intubation.
• Tactile fremitus	• May indicate increased density of underlying lung tissue due to fluid, atelectasis or consolidation of lung tissue.	• Auscultate for altered voice sounds. Percuss for dullness. Correlate with other assessment findings. Record and report findings.
• Localized pain	• Can indicate fractured rib. May result from excessive coughing or trauma.	• Assess for paradoxical chest wall movement or crepitus. This finding requires immediate medical attention (Seidel et al, 1999).
• Crepitus	• Crepitus is the result of leaking air into the subcutaneous tissues from a rupture in the lung.	
• Suspicious mass or swollen area on chest wall.	• May indicate a sebaceous cyst, lipoma or tumor.	• Lightly palpate for size, shape, and typical qualities of a lesion. Record and report findings.
• Use of accessory muscles of respiration or pursed-lip breathing.	• Use of accessory muscles indicates an effort to breathe. May be caused by chronic obstructive pulmonary disease.	• Assess client for oxygenation.

Assessment Findings	Significance	Next Step
	• Pursed-lip breathing is used to control exhalation and is an adaptive measure that increases arterial oxygen saturation.	• Position client to provide optimal chest wall expansion. Notify MD that client is in respiratory distress.
	• Some clients produce a grunting sound.	
• Decreased fremitus	• From excess air in the lungs, e.g., emphysema, pleural effusion, pulmonary edema.	• Record and report findings.
• Increased fremitus	• Occurs in the presence of fluids or a solid mass within the lungs (Seidel et al, 1999).	• Notify physician if new findings.
• Abnormal breath sounds (see Table 13-2, p. 296).	• Result from air passing through moisture, mucus, or narrowed airways; from alveoli suddenly popping open; or from inflammation of the pleura.	• Record and report findings. If new or changed assessment notify physician.

- Bronchophony or egophony

- The absence of lung sounds may indicate collapsed lung or surgically removed lobes.

- Suggest consolidation of lung tissue, as in pneumonia or atelectasis.

- Correlate with other assessment findings, breathlessness, tenderness on palpation, crackles and difficulty with deep breathing.

- Record findings.

- Notify MD if new finding or client in significant distress.

 Pediatric Considerations

- The chest circumference is almost round in infants.
- In newborns, try to conduct the examination without disturbing the baby. Percussion is usually unreliable (Seidel et al, 1999).
- Measure an infant's chest circumference; it is normally 11¾ to 14¼ inches (30 to 36 cm) in a healthy full-term infant.
- Irregular respirations are common among preterm infants at birth.

- In children younger than 6 years of age, ventilatory movement is mainly abdominal or diaphragmatic rather than costal. Infants have a thin chest wall with a bony and cartilaginous rib cage that is soft and pliant. Lungs are usually hyperresonant throughout in infants and young children. Breath sounds are louder and harsher.
- See Chapter 6 for normal respiratory rates for children.

Gerontologic Considerations

- Because of calcification of the vertebral cartilages, reduced mobility of the ribs, partial contraction of the intercostal muscles, and kyphosis that frequently occurs with aging, older adults do not breathe as deeply as younger adults.
- An older client is not able to cough as effectively because of a more rigid thoracic wall and weaker respiratory muscles. Loss of lung resiliency, coupled with the loss of skeletal muscle strength in the thorax and diaphragm, results in a characteristic barrel chest (Leuckenotte, 2000).
- Older adults have difficulty breathing deeply and holding their breath.
- Alveoli become less elastic and more fibrous, which decreases the body's exertional capacity (Lueckenotte, 2000).
- Drier mucous membranes impede removal of secretions and pose a risk for respiratory infection (Lueckenotte, 2000).

 Cultural Considerations

There are many countries in which tuberculosis is endemic. Ethnic minorities account for more than two thirds of all of the reported cases of tuberculosis in the United States.

American Indians have had a tuberculosis incidence as much as 7 to 15 times that of non-Indians, whereas African Americans have had a tuberculosis incidence three times higher than whites. Tuberculosis is also five times more prevalent among American Eskimos than in the general U.S. population (Giger, 1999).

Immigrants from Haiti and Mexico have a high incidence of tuberculosis (Giger, 1999).

Russians typically receive an immunization of bacillus Calmette-Guérin (BCG) 2 days after birth. The bacillus is an effective treatment when a high prevalence of tuberculosis exists. The immunization causes tuberculin reactions to read positive and makes tuberculin readings unclear (Giger, 1999).

Lung cancer is the second most common cancer. Incidence rates per 100,000 are lowest in American Indians highest among African Americans. The lowest rates for females is seen in Japanese woman and the highest among Alaska

Natives (CancerNet, 2001). The highest death rates per 100,000 population from lung cancer occur in Hungary, the Czech Republic, the Russian federation, Poland, and Estonia (American Cancer Society, 2001).

Client Teaching

- Explain risk factors for chronic obstructive lung disease and lung cancer, including cigarette smoking; history of cigarette smoking for over 20 years; exposure to environmental pollution (e.g., arsenic, asbestos); and radiation exposure from occupational, medical, and environmental sources. Residential radon exposure may increase risk for lung cancer, especially in cigarette smokers (American Cancer Society, 2001).

- Clients who are overweight will experience an exacerbation of pulmonary symptoms. The extra weight impairs normal ventilatory movement.

- Discuss warning signs of lung cancer, including persistent cough, sputum streaked with blood, chest pains, and recurrent attacks of pneumonia or bronchitis.

- Instruct clients with excessive mucus about the need for deep-breathing exercises, coughing, intake of fluids, postural drainage, and chest percussion.

- Instruct older adults regarding benefits of annual influenza and pneumonia vaccinations to reduce chances of respiratory infection.

- Refer interested clients to smoking-cessation programs.

- Nonsmokers may be more at risk for lung cancer from exposure to passive smoke.

Heart and Vascular System

14

Heart disease is the leading cause of death in the United States and Canada. Clients are assessed for the presence of cardiac risk factors and cardiac disease.

Anatomy and Physiology

The heart is located in the thoracic cavity toward the middle of the mediastinum, left of the midline, just above the diaphragm and bounded on both sides by the lungs (Fig. 14-1). It lies behind the sternum and the contiguous parts of the third to the sixth costal cartilages. The base of the heart is the upper portion, and the apex is the bottom tip. The apex actually touches the anterior chest wall at approximately the fourth to fifth intercostal space just medial to the left midclavicular line. This point is known as the *apical impulse*, or *point of maximal impulse (PMI)*. The area of the chest overlying the heart is the precordium.

Heart

The heart is a muscular, four-chambered pump that delivers blood to the lungs and the arterial system. It is the shape of a blunt cone and about the size of a closed fist. The pericardium is a tough, double-walled sac encasing and protecting the heart. The fibrous pericardium is the tough outer layer that prevents overdistention of the heart. The serous pericardium is the thin, transparent inner layer. It forms a space around the heart that is filled with a thin layer of pericardial fluid. The fluid helps reduce friction as the heart moves within the pericardial sac.

Cardiac Blood Flow

The four chambers of the heart are the two ventricles and two atria. The right atrium and right ventricle form the right heart, which receives deoxygenated blood from the systemic circulation. Blood enters the right atrium and passes into the right ventricle as the ventricle relaxes following a contraction. When the right atrium contracts, blood is propelled forward into the ventricle. Contraction of the right ventricle pushes blood against the tricuspid valve, forcing it closed. At the same time, blood is pushed against the semilunar pulmonary valve, forcing it open and sending blood into the pulmonary artery. The pulmonary artery carries deoxygenated blood to the lung, where carbon dioxide is exchanged for oxygen. Oxygenated blood returning from the lung enters the left atrium through the pulmonary vein. The blood passes from the left

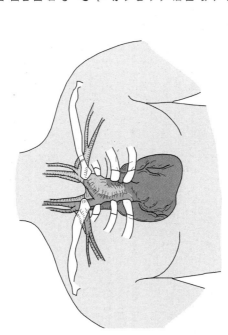

Fig. 14-1
Anatomic position of the heart.
(From Potter PA, Perry AG: *Fundamentals of nursing*, ed 5, St Louis 2001, Mosby.)

contractions maintain an average cardiac output of 5 L of blood per minute.

Cardiac Cycle

To assess heart function, you must understand the cardiac cycle and the physiological signs of each event. Both sides of the heart function in a coordinated fashion. Events occurring on the left side of the heart have the most dramatic effect on assessment findings. Pressure is greatest on the left side, creating longer and louder sounds. Events on the left side slightly precede those on the right.

The cardiac cycle has two phases, systole and diastole. During systole the ventricles contract and eject blood from the right and left ventricles. During diastole the ventricles relax and the atria contract to move blood into the ventricles and fill the coronary arteries.

Heart sounds occur as follows in relation to the cardiac cycle:

- As systole begins, the ventricles contract and raise pressure that closes the mitral and tricuspid valves. Valve closure causes the **first heart sound (S₁)**, known as **"lub."**
- The ventricles continue to push blood through the aortic and pulmonic valves into the aorta and pulmonary circulation.

atrium to the left ventricle through the mitral (bicuspid) valve during atrial contraction. Contraction of the left ventricle then forces blood against the mitral valve, closing it, and against the semilunar aortic valve, opening it and allowing blood to enter the aorta. The arterial system is a branching network of blood vessels that maintains a pressure necessary to deliver blood to distant peripheral tissues. The ability of the arterial system to compensate for changes in heart function, blood volume, and blood flow ensures the delivery of oxygen and nutrients to the body's cells.

Cardiac Conduction

The heart's unique electrical conduction system relays electrical impulses through the heart. All cardiac muscle cells generate action potentials (electrical impulses), but the sinoatrial (SA) node does so with greater frequency. Impulses originating from the SA node spread through cardiac muscle fibers of the atrium to the atrioventricular (AV) node where there is a brief delay in conduction. Delay at the AV node allows atrial contraction to be completed before ventricular contraction begins, thus maximizing cardiac output. From the AV node the impulse travels through conduction bundles and Purkinje's fibers that penetrate the ventricles. Rhythmic

- After the ventricles empty, the pressure in the ventricles falls below that in the aorta and pulmonary artery, allowing the aortic and pulmonic valves to close. Valve closure causes the **second heart sound (S₂)**, known as *"dub."*

- If the mitral and tricuspid valves open for rapid ventricular filling and there are noncompliant ventricles, a **third heart sound (S₃)** is created.

- As the atria contract to enhance ventricular filling, a **fourth heart sound (S₄)** is produced, if they contract against noncompliant ventricles.

- Both S₃ and S₄ heart sounds are abnormal when heard in adults.

Vascular System

When the left ventricle pumps blood into the aorta, a pressure wave is transmitted throughout the arterial system in the form of the arterial pulse. The arterial blood pressure is the force exerted by the blood against arterial walls. Pressure waves are manifested as palpable pulses in arteries close to the skin or areas that lie over bones. Pressure within the carotid arteries correlates with that of the aorta because of the close proximity to the heart. Both carotid arteries supply blood to the brain. Occlusion of either can cause serious neurological deficits.

The most accessible veins to assess are the internal and external jugular, which empty into the superior vena cava. The external vein lies superficially and can be seen just above the clavicle. The internal jugular lies deeper, along the carotid artery. Both veins reflect the activity of the right side of the heart. Jugular venous pressure reflects pressure within the right atrium.

The peripheral arteries deliver oxygenated blood to the extremities. Hand function is impaired by reduced circulation in the brachial artery but not necessarily by impairment of the radial or ulnar artery because of its interconnected circulation. Similarly, the foot is protected by interconnections between the posterior tibial and dorsalis pedis arteries.

Critical Thinking Application—Heart and Vascular System

Knowledge	Experience	Standards
• Be very familiar with the anatomy and physiology of the heart. • Be familiar with the heart's anatomy and relationship to the chest wall. • Apply knowledge that you have regarding fluid and electrolyte balance and its effect on myocardial function. • When clients experience signs and symptoms of heart disease, they may become very anxious. Apply good therapeutic communication techniques as you question and examine the client.	• Be comfortable in using the diaphragm and bell of the stethoscope. • As you care for different clients you will find that the position of the heart may vary somewhat. In tall, slender persons the heart tends to hang more vertically and is positioned more centrally. With increased stockiness and shortness, the heart tends to lie more to the left and horizontally.	As you examine the heart apply the following principles: • Be methodical in the examination. • Follow the same sequence every time to ensure each area of the heart is examined properly. • Listen for 30-60 seconds at each point of auscultation (see p. 321). Explain to the client that you are listening carefully and not to be concerned. • Palpate the radial pulse while listening to the apical pulse to help differentiate between S_1 and S_2.

- Do not show concern (nonverbally) if you detect abnormal findings.

- If you are uncertain about heart sounds, ask a more experienced practitioner to confirm your findings.

- Caution against misinterpreting findings in an anxious client who might have mild tachycardia.

Heart and Vascular Assessment

Equipment

- Stethoscope
- Ultrasound stethoscope (optional) or Doppler stethoscope
- Conductance gel
- Penlight
- 2 centimeter rulers

Delegation Considerations

The heart examination requires critical thinking and knowledge application unique to a professional nurse. Delegation is inappropriate. If assistive personnel are assisting in the care of a client with cardiac risk factors or known cardiac disease, in-

struct them to report immediately any incidence of chest pain, unusual fatigue, or changes in heart rate and blood pressure.

Client Preparation

The client should initially lie supine with the head of the bed elevated at a 45-degree angle. The client will be asked to change positions throughout the examination.

- Client sits during examination of the carotid arteries.
- Client lies supine during assessment of the jugular veins and peripheral arteries and veins.
- Stand at the client's right side to begin.
- Ask the client not to talk during the assessment, especially during auscultation of heart sounds.

- Be sure the client is relaxed and comfortable.
- Have good lighting in the room, including an examination light.

History

- Assess for cardiovascular disease risk factors, such as history of smoking, alcohol intake, use of drugs (e.g., cocaine, amyl nitrite), exercise habits, and dietary patterns and intake (including fat and sodium intake). Ask whether the client wears tight garters or hosiery or sits or lies in bed with legs crossed.
- Assess the client's family history for heart disease, diabetes, hypertension, stroke, high cholesterol levels, and rheumatic heart disease.
- Does the client have a stressful lifestyle? What physical demands or emotional stress exists?
- Does the client participate in any relaxing activities, such as hobbies or recreational exercise? What is the frequency, intensity, duration of exercise?
- Assess the client's eating habits, including fat and sodium intake. Is the client obese? Determine if the client consumes excessive amounts of caffeine-containing beverages such as soft drinks, coffee, or tea.

- Does the client have known hypertension; diabetes or heart disease, including congestive heart failure; congenital heart disease; coronary artery disease; or cardiac dysrhythmia or murmurs? What is the client's understanding of the disease? Has the client had previous heart surgery? What was the client's age at the time?
- Is the client taking medications for cardiovascular function or hypertension? If so, what medications? Does the client know the purpose, dosage, and side effects of the each medication?
- Assess for chest pain, including onset and duration, character, location, severity, associated symptoms, frequency, and treatment. Do symptoms occur at rest or during exercise? Does the pain radiate to the shoulder, neck, or arms? Has the pain been associated with diaphoresis? Assess for episodes of light-headedness or fainting.
- Assess for dyspnea at rest, on exertion, or positional.
- Assess for fatigue, including effect on activities of daily living, associated symptoms, and any medication that may contribute to fatigue, such as antihypertensives.
- Assess for cough, including onset, duration, character, frequency, and time of day most often occurs.

• Does the client experience leg cramps; numbness or tingling in the extremities; sensation of cold hands or feet; pain in the legs; or swelling or cyanosis of the feet, ankles, or hands? If leg pain or cramps are present, does walking or standing for long periods or during sleep aggravate them?

ASSESSMENT TECHNIQUES—HEART AND VASCULAR SYSTEM

Perform the assessment of the heart and vascular system together. Alterations in either system may be manifested as changes in the other. Assessment of cardiovascular function involves a thorough evaluation of apical and peripheral pulses, the events that occur in relation to the cardiac cycle, and the overall integrity of the heart and major arteries.

Assessment	Normal Findings	Deviations From Normal

Heart

Inspection and Palpation

Perform inspection and palpation together at each of the following landmarks (Fig. 14-2).

Assessment	Normal Findings	Deviations From Normal
• The **aortic area**—2nd ICS Right sternal border (RSB).		
• The **pulmonic area**—2nd ICS Left sternal border (LSB).		
• The **tricuspid area**—4th ICS Left sternal border (LSB).		
• The **mitral area**—5th ICS Midclavicular line (MCL).		
• The **epigastric area**—at the tip of the sternum.		
• View each landmark over the chest at an angle to the side.		
• Look for the appearance of pulsations.	• No pulsations seen.	• Visible pulsation to the left of the midclavicular line may indicate cardiac enlargement.
• Use the penlight held at an angle to aid in identifying pulsation.	• The apical impulse should not be visible in more than one space.	
	• Pulsation may be seen at the PMI or epigastric area in thin clients.	
• Have client sit up and lean forward.	• Increases ability to visualize apical pulse.	

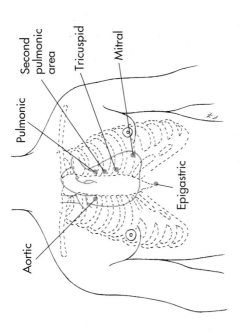

Fig. 14-2
Anatomical sites for assessment of cardiac function.
(From Potter PA, Perry AG: *Fundamentals of nursing*, ed 5, St Louis, 2001, Mosby.)

Assessment	Normal Findings	Deviations From Normal
• Be sure your hands are warm.	• No pulsations, vibrations, or thrills are normally felt in the second, third, or fourth intercostal spaces.	• Thrill (fine, palpable, rushing vibrations) indicates a disruption of blood flow from a defect in closure of the aortic or pulmonary valves (e.g., pulmonary hypertension, atrial septal defect).
• With the client supine, palpate each landmark.		
• Use the first metacarpophalangeal joints of the four fingers together, then alternate with the ball of the hand.	• Aortic pulsation is palpable at the epigastric area.	
• Touch gently and allow movements to lift your hand.		
• Palpate for the apical impulse (PMI) and identify its location and the distance from the midsternal line.	• The PMI is the point at which the apical pulse can be seen or palpated as most intense. The PMI is a light tap felt in an area 1 to 2 cm ($\frac{1}{2}$ inch) in diameter at the apex of the heart, usually at the fifth intercostal space at the left sternal border (LSB) (Fig. 14-3).	
• Determine the width of the arc in which the PMI is felt.	• Palpable within a small radius, no more than 1 cm (>$\frac{1}{2}$ inch). Impulse is gentle and brief.	• Apical impulse to the left of the mid-clavicular line indicates cardiac enlargement.
	• Obesity, muscularity, and large breasts can obscure the apical impulse.	

- Feel for lifts and thrills.

- If the apical impulse cannot be found with the client in the supine position, ask the client to roll onto the left side (left lateral recumbent) (Fig. 14-4, C) to move the heart closer to the chest wall.

- If pulsations or vibrations are palpated, time their occurrence in relation to systole or diastole by auscultation of heart sounds or palpation of the carotid artery simultaneously.

- Describe the carotid pulse in relation to the cardiac cycle.

- While palpating over the heart, use the other hand to palpate the carotid artery.

- Vigorous pulsation that is forceful and widely distributed is described as a heave or lift.

- An absence of an apical impulse accompanied with faint heart sounds indicates pleural or pericardial fluid.

- Apical impulse is easily palpable.

- The carotid pulse and S_1 (first heart sound) are practically synchronous.

- Carotid pulse and S_1 are almost synchronous.

- Lack of synchrony can indicate valvular dysfunction.

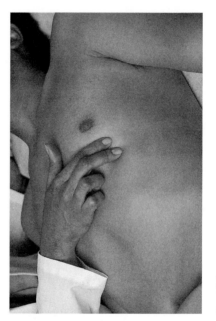

Fig. 14-3
Palpation of PMI.

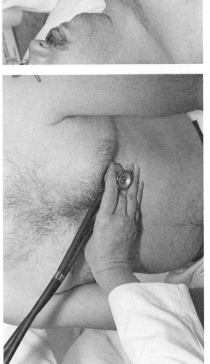

Fig. 14-4
Sequence of client positions for heart examination. **A**, Sitting up, leaning slightly. **B**, Supine. *Continued*

Assessment	Normal Findings	Deviations From Normal

- Percussion of heart borders to determine heart size is limited. Chest x-ray examinations are preferred.

Auscultation of Heart Sounds

- Eliminate room noise.

- Explain to the client it will take several seconds to hear heart sounds.

- The client will assume three different positions during auscultation: 1) sitting up and leaning forward (good to hear all areas and high-pitched murmurs), 2) supine (good for all areas), and 3) left lateral recumbent (good for all areas and best to hear low-pitched sounds) (Fig. 14-4, *A-C*).

- Follow a pattern, moving systematically and slowly inching the stethoscope across the anatomic sites (see

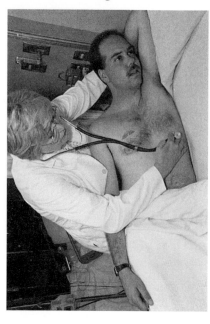

C

Fig. 14-4, cont'd
C, Left lateral recumbent.

Fig. 14-2, p. 321). Be sure to proceed in the same pattern every time you listen to the heart. Lift a female client's left breast to hear over the chest wall better.

- Begin by using the diaphragm of the stethoscope to hear high-pitched sounds. Listen to each sound and each phase in the cardiac cycle.

- Take time to hear each sound and each pause in the cardiac cycle.

- Listen for the first (S_1) heart sound.

- Sounds differ in pitch, loudness, and duration, depending on the auscultatory site (Table 14-1).

- S_1 sounds like "*lub*" and occurs after the long diastolic pause and preceding the short systolic pause. S_1 is high-pitched, dull in quality, and heard best at the apex.

- Increased or decreased intensity of S_1.

- Splitting of S_1 (two distinct sound components to S_1) is usually not heard.

Table 14-1 Heart Sounds According to Auscultatory Area

	Aortic	Pulmonic	Second Pulmonic	Mitral	Tricuspid
Pitch	$S_1 < S_2$	$S_1 < S_2$	$S_1 < S_2$	$S_1 < S_2$	$S_1 < S_2$
Loudness	$S_1 < S_2$	$S_1 < S_2$	$S_1 < S_2$*	$S_1 > S_2$†	$S_1 < S_2$
Duration	$S_1 > S_2$	$S_1 > S_2$	$S_1 > S_2$	$S_1 > S_2$	$S_1 > S_2$
S_2 split	>Inhale	>Inhale	>Inhale	>Inhale‡	>Inhale
	<Exhale	<Exhale	<Exhale	<Exhale	<Exhale
A_2	Loudest	Loud	Decreased		
P_2	Decreased	Louder	Loudest		

*S_1 is relatively louder in second pulmonic area than in aortic area.
†S_1 may be louder in mitral area than in tricuspid area.
‡S_2 split may not be audible in mitral area if P_2 is inaudible.

Assessment	Normal Findings	Deviations From Normal
• Listen for the second (S_2) heart sounds.	• S_2 sounds like "*dub*" and follows the short systolic pause and precedes the long diastolic pause.	• The usual S_2 will have two audible components.

After both sounds are heard clearly as "*lub dub*," count each combination of S_1 and S_2 as one heartbeat. Count rate of beats for 1 minute.	• High-pitched and heard best at the aortic area.	• Splitting of S_2 is expected and best heard on inspiration at the pulmonic area (Lewis et al, 2000).
		• Wide splitting is abnormal and can be caused by delayed activation of contraction or valve stenosis (Seidel et al, 1999).
• Assess heart rate.	• Normal rate is 60 to 100 beats/minute in an adult.	• Sinus bradycardia: regular rhythm but decreased rate (less than 60 beats/minute); sinus tachycardia: regular rhythm but increased rate (more than 100 beats/minute).
• Assess heart rhythm.	• Regular rhythm involves regular intervals between each sequence of beats.	• Irregular heart rhythm.

Assessment	Normal Findings	Deviations From Normal
• Note the time between S_1 and S_2 (systolic pause) and then the time between S_2 and the next S_1 (diastolic pause).	• A distinct pause is heard between S_1 and S_2.	
• Auscultate for S_3 and S_4 sounds. Best heard at the apex with the client lying on the left side.	S_3 and S_4 heart sounds are quiet and difficult to hear. Increasing venous return may accentuate the sounds. Commonly heard in pediatric clients (Seidel et al, 1999).	S_3 and S_4 heart sounds are easily distinguished and resemble a gallop.
• Auscultate for extra heart sounds (clicks and rubs).	• Extra heart sounds are normally absent with cardiac valves opening noiselessly.	• Clicks and rubs.
• Clicks are short, high-pitched extra sounds.		
• Rubs are squeaky or rubbing sounds.		
Auscultate for murmurs: best heard at Erb's point (3rd ICS LSB). Because murmurs are low pitched sounds, use the bell of the stethoscope.		

- Note timing (in relation to systole or diastole), location heard best, radiation, loudness, pitch, and quality.

- No murmurs are usually heard.

- A murmur is heard as a swishing or blowing sound at the beginning, middle, or end of the systolic or diastolic phase.

- A murmur occurring between S_1 and S_2 is a systolic murmur.

- A murmur occurring between S_2 and S_1 is a diastolic murmur.

Note intensity of murmur:

- Grade I/VI. Barely audible.

- Grade II/VI. Audible immediately but faint.

- Grade III/VI. Loud without thrust or thrill.

- Grade IV/VI. Loud with thrust or thrill.

Assessment	Normal Findings	Deviations From Normal
		• Grade V/VI. Very loud, with lift/heave or thrill; audible with stethoscope only partially applied.
		• Grade VI/VI. Louder; may be heard without stethoscope.
Vascular System	**Vascular System**	**Vascular System**
• Auscultate blood pressure (BP) at the brachial artery in the antecubital space in both arms.	• Blood pressure should be 130/80 mm Hg or less (USDHHS, 1997).	• Systolic reading that differs by 15 mm Hg or more suggests atherosclerosis or aortic disease.
	• Readings between the arms may vary by as much as 10 mm Hg and tend to be higher in the right arm (Seidel et al, 1999). The higher reading is accepted as closest to the client's BP.	
• Compare sitting BP with pressures measured while client is in lying and standing positions.	• When client changes position from supine or sitting to standing, there is a slight or no drop in systolic pressure and a slight rise in diastolic pressure.	• Orthostatic hypotension is indicated by a drop in systolic BP of 15 mm Hg or more and a fall in diastolic pressure.

Clients most at risk for orthostatic hypotension are those who have just donated blood, have autonomic nervous system disease, are hypovolemic, have had recent surgical procedures, take certain vasodilator medications, or have stayed a prolonged time in a recumbent position.

- Assess the carotid arteries with the client seated.

- Inspect the neck on both sides for obvious artery pulsation.

- Ask the client to turn the head slightly away from the side being examined during inspection.

Examine only one carotid artery at a time.

Do not vigorously palpate the carotid artery to prevent carotid sinus stimulation, which produces a drop in heart rate and BP.

Assessment	Normal Findings	Deviations From Normal
• During palpation have the client turn the head slightly toward the side being examined. Palpate gently with index and middle fingers around medial edge of sternocleidomastoid muscle (Fig. 14-5).		• Diminished or unequal carotid pulsations can indicate atherosclerosis or aortic arch disease. Change in carotid pulse during inspiration may indicate a sinus dysrhythmia.
• Note if pulse changes as client inspires and expires.	• The carotid pulse is localized, strong, thrusting, and unchanged by inspiration, expiration, or position changes.	
	• Rotation of the neck or a shift from a sitting to a supine position does not change the carotid's quality.	
• Compare rate, rhythm, and strength of pulse on each side.	• Both pulses are equal in rate, rhythm, and strength bilaterally.	
	• Rate is the same as apical pulse.	

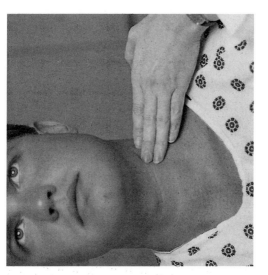

Fig. 14-5
Palpation of internal carotid artery.

Assessment	Normal Findings	Deviations From Normal
• Place the bell of the stethoscope over the carotid artery at the lateral end of the clavicle and the posterior margin of the sternocleidomastoid muscle. Have the client turn the head slightly away from the side being examined. Then ask the client to hold the breath for a moment so that breath sounds do not obscure vascular sounds.	• No sound is heard over the carotid arteries on auscultation.	• A bruit or blowing sound is osculated.
• If a bruit is auscultated, palpate the artery lightly for a thrill.	• No thrill or bruit is palpable.	• A palpable bruit (thrill) can be felt in severe arterial narrowing.
• Examine the right internal jugular to indirectly determine pressure in the right atrium. Be sure there is no tight clothing around the client's neck. First, have the client sit upright at a 45- to 90-degree angle. A pillow may be used for client comfort (Fig. 14-6).	• Normal veins are flat; pulsations are not evident.	• Distended veins while sitting indicate heart disease.

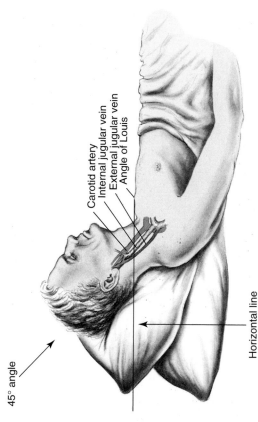

45° angle

Carotid artery
Internal jugular vein
External jugular vein
Angle of Louis

Horizontal line

Fig. 14-6
Position of client to assess jugular vein distention.
(From Thompson JM et al: *Mosby's clinical nursing,* ed 5, St Louis, 2001, Mosby.)

Assessment	Normal Findings	Deviations From Normal
• Have the client slowly lean backward into a supine position. Avoid hyperextension or flexion of the neck. Be sure penlight is tangential to illuminate neck area.	• Level of venous pulsations begins to rise above level of manubrium, 1 to 2 cm when client reaches 45-degree angle (Seidel et al, 1999).	
• Measure venous pressure by measuring the vertical distance between the angle of Louis and the highest level of the visible point of the internal jugular vein pulsation.		
• Use two rulers. Line up the bottom edge of a regular ruler with the top of the pulsation in the jugular vein.		
• Then take a centimeter ruler and align it perpendicular to the first ruler at the level of the sternal angle.		
• Measure in centimeters the distance between the second ruler and the sternal angle (Fig. 14-7).		

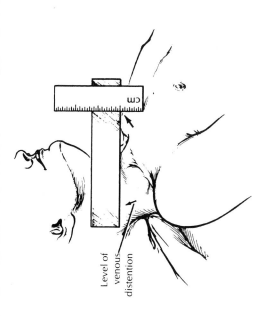

Level of venous distention

Fig. 14-7

Measurement of jugular vein distention.
(From Seidel HM et al: *Mosby's guide to physical examination*, ed 4, St Louis, 1999, Mosby.)

Assessment	Normal Findings	Deviations From Normal
• Repeat measurement on the other side.	• Measurement of 2 cm or less is considered normal.	• Bilateral pressures higher than 2.5 cm (1 inch) are considered elevated and are a sign of right heart failure.
• Observe the right and left jugulars for symmetry.	• Equal bilaterally.	• Distention on one side suggests a localized abnormality (e.g., obstruction). Bilateral distention suggests an intracardiac problem.
• Examine each peripheral artery using the distal pads of the second and third fingers. The thumb may be used to assess larger arteries such as the femoral.		
• Apply firm pressure, but do not occlude the pulse. When it is difficult to find a pulse, try to vary pressure and feel all around the pulse site. Be sure you are not palpating your own pulse.		
• Radial artery: located along the radial side of the forearm, at the wrist.		

- In thin individuals, a groove is formed lateral to the flexor tendon of the wrist (Fig. 14-8).

- Ulnar artery: located on the opposite side of the wrist from the radial artery. Feels less prominent than the radial (Fig. 14-9).

- Brachial artery: located in groove between biceps and triceps muscles above the elbow at the antecubital fossa. The artery runs along the medial side of the extended arm (Fig. 14-10).

- Femoral artery: primary artery in the leg. Have client lie supine with inguinal area exposed. Artery is located below the inguinal ligament, midway between the symphysis pubis and the anterosuperior iliac spine (Fig. 14-11). Bimanual pulsation, with fingertips of both hands on opposite sides of the pulse site, may be necessary in obese clients.

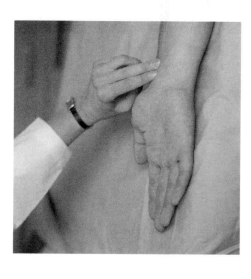

Fig. 14-8
Radial pulse site.

Heart and Vascular System **341**

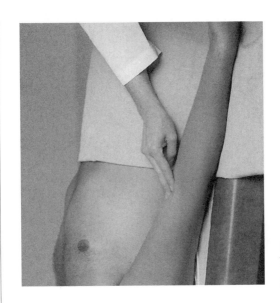

Fig. 14-10
Brachial pulse site.

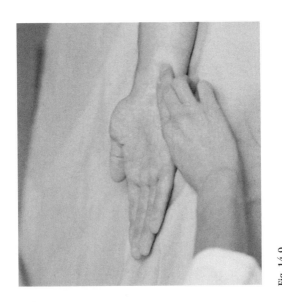

Fig. 14-9
Ulnar pulse site.

Assessment	Normal Findings	Deviations From Normal

- Popliteal pulse: located behind the knee. Have client flex the knee, with the foot resting on the examination table, or assume a prone position with the knee slightly flexed (Fig. 14-12). Palpate deep into the popliteal fossa, just lateral to the midline.

- Dorsalis pedis pulse: located along the top of the foot in line with the groove between the extensor tendons of the great toe and first toe (Fig. 14-13). Be sure client's foot is relaxed.

- Posterior tibial pulse: located on the inner side of each ankle (Fig. 14-14). Place fingers behind and below the medial malleolus (ankle). Have foot relaxed and slightly extended.

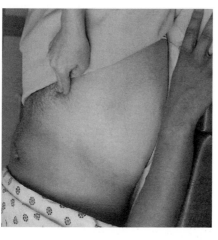

Fig. 14-11
Femoral pulse site.

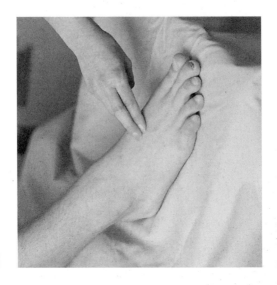

Fig. 14-12
Popliteal pulse site.

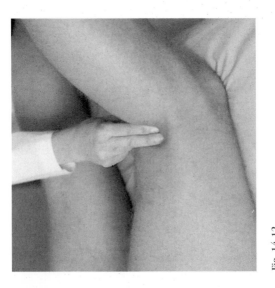

Fig. 14-13
Dorsalis pedis pulse.

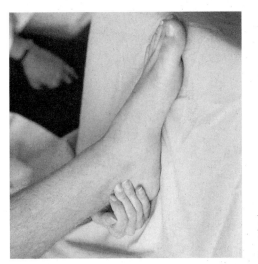

Fig. 14-14
Posterior tibial pulse.

Assessment	Normal Findings	Deviations From Normal
• The radial pulse may be used to assess heart rate and rhythm (see Chapter 6). To check local circulatory status of tissues, palpate each peripheral artery long enough to note that a pulse is present and assess its character.		
• Assess each peripheral pulse for strength and equality (Box 14-1).	• Normal pulse is 2+ and equal bilaterally.	• Absent or diminished pulse may be from a pathological process interfering with blood flow or obstruction caused by application of external device (e.g., cast, tight bandage).
• Assess each artery for elasticity of vessel wall.	• Wall of artery is easily palpable. After depressing artery, it will spring back to shape when pressure is released.	• Sclerotic artery is hard, inelastic, or calcified.

- If arterial insufficiency is expected in the hand, perform Allen's test. Have client make a fist as you compress the ulnar and radial arteries simultaneously. Then have the client open the hand while you release the ulnar artery.

- When difficult to palpate a pulse or the pulse is not palpable, use an ultrasound stethoscope over the pulse site.

- Connect stethoscope headset to ultrasound probe.

- Apply ample amount of conductance gel to client's skin over the pulse site.

- Turn stethoscope's volume control to on.

- Gently apply probe at a 45- to 90-degree angle, pointed in the opposite direction of blood flow, on the skin at the pulse site.

- Hand should quickly turn pink if ulnar artery is patent.

- Failure of color to return indicates arterial occlusion.

  Allen's test should always be performed before drawing an arterial blood sample from the radial artery.

BOX 14-1 Scale for Measuring Pulse Strength

0	Absent
1+	Pulse is diminished, barely palpable, easy to obliterate
2+	Easily palpable, normal pulse
3+	Full pulse, increased
4+	Strong, bounding pulse, cannot be obliterated

Assessment	Normal Findings	Deviations From Normal
• Adjust volume as needed.	• Pulse creates a regular "swooshing" sound.	• Pulse is not auscultated.
• Assess the skin, nail beds, and lower extremities for color, temperature, and condition.	• Skin is warm to slightly cool, intact, without obvious varicosities. • Pulses are present.	• Unable to obtain audible pulse.
• If arterial occlusion is suspected, have the client lie supine and elevate a leg. Observe for blanching. Then have client sit on edge of bed to lower the extremity.	• Slight pallor occurs with elevation. • Full color returns when leg again becomes dependent.	• Delay in return of full color indicates arterial occlusion.
• Examine lower extremities for hair distribution and scars or lesions.	• Hair growth is evenly distributed. • Male clients may have hair loss around calf from tight-fitting pants or socks.	• Absence of hair growth over legs may indicate circulatory insufficiency. Chronic recurring ulcers of the feet or lower legs are signs of circulatory insufficiency.

- Assess status of peripheral veins by asking client to assume sitting and standing positions. Inspect and palpate for varicosities.

- Palpate lower extremities around feet and ankles for dependent edema. Use your thumb to press firmly 1 to 2 seconds and then release over the medial malleolus or the shins.

- Assess for phlebitis in leg veins. Inspect calves for localized redness, tenderness, and swelling over vein sites. Also check for Homans' sign by supporting the leg, keeping the knee slightly flexed while quickly flexing the foot upward (dorsiflexion).

- Extremities are clear, without edema or inflammation.

- Edema is absent.

- Absence of pain during calf flexion. Achilles' tendon pain, common in athletes and in women who repeatedly wear high-heel shoes, should not be confused with thrombosis. Calf will feel tender in these clients.

- Varicosities are superficial veins that become dilated, especially when legs are in dependent position. Varicosities in the anterior or medial part of the thigh and the posterolateral part of the calf are abnormal.

- Depression left in the skin indicates edema and can be a sign of venous insufficiency and right-sided heart failure. (For grades of edema, see Chapter 7).

- Complaint of calf pain during flexion indicates thrombosis.

  Do not continuously massage a tender or painful calf; massaging may increase the risk of an embolus.

Assessment	Normal Findings	Deviations From Normal
• Assess the lymphatic drainage of the lower extremities. Palpate the area of the superficial inguinal nodes beginning in the groin area and moving down toward the inner thigh.	• A few soft, nontender nodes may be palpable.	• Enlarged, hardened, or tender nodes can indicate infection or metastatic disease.

UNEXPECTED ASSESSMENT FINDINGS—HEART AND VASCULAR SYSTEM

Assessment Findings	Significance	Next Step
• Loud S₁ heart sound.	• May be caused by anemia, fever, hyperthyroidism, or effects of vigorous exercise. • May indicate stenotic mitral valve (Seidel et al, 1999).	• Review assessment data for evidence of fever. Review laboratory data for elevated thyroid stimulating hormone (TSH), low hematocrit and hemoglobin (H & H). Question client about activity.

Finding	Description	Nursing Action
Faint S_1 heart sound.	Increase in fat, tissue, or fluid overlying the heart (e.g., obesity, emphysema, pericardial effusion). Diminished valve flexibility such as those seen in clients who have experienced rheumatic heart disease.	If new finding in person with appropriate height and weight, report to primary care provider.
Loud S_2 heart sound.	Heard in clients with systemic hypertension, aortic valve syphilis, exercise, pulmonary hypertension, mitral stenosis, or congestive heart failure.	Record and report findings. Correlate with client history and other assessment findings.
Diminished S_2 heart sound.	Increase in fat, tissue, or fluid overlying the heart, aortic or pulmonic stenosis.	Review chart for prior findings of aortic or pulmonic stenosis. Report finding to physician. Document findings in the client's chart.
Split S_2 heart sound.	Closure of the aortic valve slightly ahead of the pulmonic valve. Valve heard best during inspiration, disappears during inhalation or breath holding.	Ask client to hold breath to validate that sound heard is a split S_2 heart sound. Record and report finding.

Assessment	Normal Findings	Deviations From Normal
• S_3 gallop.	• The combination of S_1, S_2, and S_3 sounds like "Ken-tuc-**ky**".	• Does not require intervention.
• S_4 gallop.	• S_4 is an atrial gallop, occurring just before S_1 or ventricular systole. It sounds like "**Ten**-nes-see".	• A new finding of an S_3 or S_4 gallop should be reported to the primary care provider.
	• When S_3 or S_4 becomes easy to hear, it may be from increased resistance to filling because of loss of ventricular wall compliance (e.g., hypertension, coronary artery disease) or increased stroke volume (e.g., anemia, pregnancy, thyrotoxicosis).	• Be prepared for a complete cardiovascular assessment. • Review fluid volume status and vital signs. • Record and report findings.
• Quadruple gallop (S_1, S_2, S_3, and S_4 all heard separately).	• S_3 and S_4 occurring together indicate severe myocardial disease.	• Notify physician of finding. • Assess client's fluid balance, BP, and heart rate. • Record and report findings.

- Murmur.
  - Can be asymptomatic or indicative of heart disease.
  - A murmur usually indicates a disruption of blood flow into, through, or out of the heart.
  - Record and report finding, noting intensity, location, and radiation.
  - To assess for radiation, listen over areas besides where the murmur is heard best, such as the neck or back.

- Clicks.
  - May be caused by old artificial heart valves inserted during cardiac surgery.
  - Record and report finding.
  - Extra heart sounds may also occur with murmurs and usually indicate pathology such as mitral valve prolapse or aortic stenosis.

- Rub.
  - Results from a rubbing of inflamed pericardial tissues.
  - Report finding to primary care provider.
  - Record assessment finding.

- Lift or heave.
  - May indicate increased cardiac output or left ventricular hypertrophy.
  - Review medical record for previous assessment of heave or lift.

Assessment	Normal Findings	Deviations From Normal
• Lift or heave along left sternal border.	• May be caused by right ventricular hypertrophy.	• Record and report findings. • If new finding, report to physician.
• Carotid bruit.	• Indicates disturbance in blood flow because of arterial narrowing.	**A bruit should be reported immediately to the client's primary care provider.**
• Irregular heart rhythm.	• Compare apical and radial pulse rates to determine whether a pulse deficit exists. • Auscultate the apical pulse first and then immediately assess the radial pulse. • If a deficit exists, the radial pulse is usually less than the apical pulse.	**Presence of a deficit requires further evaluation; usually an electrocardiogram is performed.**
• Sinus dysrhythmia.	• Pulse rate changes during respiration, increasing at the peak of inspiration and declining during expiration.	• Record and report findings. Benign rhythm.

• Sinus bradycardia.	• Associated with hypothermia, hypothyroidism, and drug intoxication; common in well-conditioned athletes.	• Identify cause of bradycardia. May be benign.
• Sinus tachycardia.	• Common after exercise or caffeine or alcohol ingestion; also associated with fever, pain, hyperthyroidism, shock, heart disease, and anxiety.	• Determine underlying cause. • Notify physician if sudden onset and client is symptomatic (e.g., short of breath, dizzy, diaphoretic, complaining of chest pain). • Review the need to decrease intake of caffeine and alcohol. • Record and report findings.
• Premature ventricular contractions.	• Results from abnormal electrical stimulation and conduction in the ventricular tissue. • May be caused by hypoxemia.	**Ventricular premature contractions can be dangerous and should be reported to the physician. Count and report their frequency per minute.**

Assessment	Normal Findings	Deviations From Normal
• Arterial occlusion.	• Pain, pallor, and pulselessness characterize arterial occlusions. An acute occlusion may also cause paresthesias (Seidel et al, 1999). Pain from arterial insufficiency occurs during exercise and is quickly relieved by rest.	**Acute arterial occlusions are medical emergencies. The primary care provider should be notified immediately.**
• Venous congestion.	• Characterized by normal or cyanotic color, normal temperature, normal pulse, marked edema, and brown pigmentation around ankles.	• Determine how far the client can ambulate before experiencing pain.
	• Pain from venous insufficiency and musculoskeletal problems occurs during or often hours after exercise.	• Assess pedal and dorsalis pedis pulses.
		• Assess temperature and color of feet and toes.
	• Rest relieves the pain; however, the pain can be constant.	• Assess distribution of hair.
		• Record and report findings.

Pediatric Considerations

- The PMI can be found just lateral to the left midclavicular line and fourth intercostal space in children under 7 years of age and at the left midclavicular line and fifth intercostal space in children over 7 years of age. A child's thin chest wall makes it easy to see and palpate the PMI (Wong, 1999).

- The heart rates of children are more variable than those of adults, reacting with wider swings to stress such as exercise, fever, or tension (Seidel et al, 1999). A heart rate of 200 beats per minute is not uncommon.

- Sinus arrhythmia, variation of the heart rate, (faster on inspiration and slower on expiration) is common in childhood.

- Fixed splitting, a condition in which the split in S_2 does not change during inspiration, is an important diagnostic sign of atrial septal defect.

- To assess cardiac function in infants, be sure to inspect the color of skin and mucous membranes. A well newborn is pink. An ashy white color indicates shock, and cyanosis of the skin and mucous membranes can indicate congenital heart disease.

- Murmurs are relatively frequent in newborns until about 48 hours of age. Most murmurs are benign (Seidel et al, 1999).

- The brachial, radial, and femoral pulses are easy to palpate in newborns. Reduced cardiac output or peripheral vasoconstriction may cause a weak or thready pulse. A bounding pulse can be caused by patent ductus arteriosus (Seidel et al, 1999).

- Absence of femoral pulse can be a sign of coarctation of the aorta.

Gerontologic Considerations

- With aging the heart rate slows, stroke volume decreases, and cardiac output is reduced by 30% to 40% (Lueckenotte, 2000).

- Locating the PMI in the older adult may be more difficult because the chest deepens in its anteroposterior diameter and there may be scoliosis or kyphosis.

- The elderly experience reduced cardiac output and thus the heart reacts less efficiently to stress. Heart failure is a common disorder. Fatigue, restlessness, syncope, and confusion may be early signs of congestive heart failure.

- Heart sounds are not as loud in older adults.
- Carotid arteries normally become tortuous and dilated because of changes in arterial elasticity.
- Vasomotor tone decreases and baroreceptor sensitivity decreases. Vagal tone increases, which slows heart rate.
- Systolic blood pressure increases in response to loss in elasticity in peripheral vessels and an increase in peripheral vascular resistance.
- Auscultation of the carotid artery is especially important for clients in whom cerebrovascular disease is suspected.
- Dependent edema of the lower extremities is common in older clients.

Cultural Considerations

- Studies suggest that the incidence of cardiovascular disease is highest among non-Hispanic blacks, followed by Mexican Americans and whites (AHA, 2001). Heart disease is significantly higher among Jews from Israel, although the fatality rates are low (Giger, 1999).
- Cardiovascular risk factors are higher among black and Mexican-American women than among white women of the same socioeconomic status (SES) (AHA, 2001). Both

- American Indian and Alaska Native men and woman have at least one or more cardiovascular risk factor (CDC, 1997).
- African Americans have a higher incidence of hypertension than whites. The age of onset is earlier and the hypertension is more severe. The prevalence of hypertension tends to be low among persons of Asian descent, with the exception of Filipinos.
- African Americans are less susceptible to varicose veins than whites.

Client Teaching

- Explain risk factors for heart disease, including high dietary intake of saturated fat or cholesterol, lack of regular aerobic exercise, smoking, excess weight, stressful lifestyle, hypertension, and family history of heart disease.
- Refer client (if appropriate) to resources for controlling or reducing risks (e.g., nutritional counseling, exercise class, stress-reduction programs).
- Explain that research shows benefit from reducing dietary intake of cholesterol and saturated fats. Instruct the client in risk factor reduction such as:

- weight loss to ideal body weight or body mass index of 25 or less (See Chapter 21, p. 576).
- limit alcohol intake; 1 oz (30 ml) of ethanol, 10 ounces of beer, 300 ml of wine or 2 ounces of 100-proof whiskey per day.
- 0.5 ounces (15 ml) of ethanol/day for women and lighter weight clients (less than 150 lbs.).
- increased aerobic activity of 30-45 minutes 3-4 days of the week.
- reduce sodium intake to 2.4 g of sodium or 6 g sodium chloride per day.
- maintain adequate dietary intake of 20 mEq of potassium per day.
- maintain dietary intake of calcium (1000 mg per day for men and menstruating women and 1500 mg for post-menopausal women) and magnesium.
- stop smoking.
- reduce intake of dietary saturated fat to 7% of calories and no more than 200 mg of cholesterol per day (NHLBI, 2001).
- Encourage clients to have regular measurement of total blood cholesterol levels and triglycerides.

- Desirable level for cholesterol is <200 mg/dL (AHA, 2000, NHLBI, 2001). More than one cholesterol measurement is needed to assess the blood cholesterol level accurately.
- Low-density lipoprotein (LDL) cholesterol is the major component of atherosclerotic plaque. The LDL cholesterol level should be <100 mg/dl. LDL cholesterol of ≥190 mg/dl is very high risk.
- The high-density lipoprotein (HDL) level should be ≥40 mg/dl with levels ≥60 considered protective. HDL cholesterol <40 mg/dl indicates a high risk for heart disease (NHLBI, 2001).
- The cholesterol ratio should be below 5/1, with an ideal of 3.5/1 (AHA, 2000).
- Triglyceride level should be less than 150 mg/dl. Clients with levels between 150-199 should be treated aggressively with weight reduction and exercise. A level >200 mg/dL indicate underlying diseases or genetic disorders and requires lipid lowering medications (AHA, 2000; NHLBI, 2001).
- Women have a higher HDL cholesterol level due to estrogen. The HERS trial in women showed that hormone replacement therapy (HRT) does not appear to reduce the risk

of cardiovascular disease and stroke in postmenopausal women (AHA, 2000; King, 2000). The NCEP (2001) recommends that HRT is not an alternative for statin therapy.

- For clients with heart disease, explain the importance of compliance with the treatment program.
- Teach clients who take heart medication how to measure their own pulse.
- Clients who have known angina may benefit from taking a daily low dose of aspirin. Consult physician before starting therapy.
- Inform clients of their blood pressure reading. Explain normal readings for the client's age and implications of any abnormalities.

- Instruct clients with risk or evidence of vascular insufficiency in the lower extremities to avoid tight clothing over the lower body or legs, avoid sitting or standing for long periods, avoid crossing legs, walk regularly, and elevate feet when sitting.
- Elderly clients with hypertension may benefit from regular monitoring of blood pressure (daily, weekly, or monthly). Home monitoring kits are available. Teach clients how to use them.
- Advise client with vascular disease to avoid tobacco products because nicotine causes vasoconstriction.

15

Breasts

Breast cancer is the second leading cause of cancer deaths in women (American Cancer Society, 2000). Early detection is the key to cure. You play a major role in assessment of the breasts as well as the education of clients about breast cancer and the need to screen for masses or irregularities in breast tissue.

Anatomy and Physiology

The breasts are paired mammary glands located on the anterior chest wall. The female breasts normally extend in an area from the second or third rib to the sixth or seventh rib and from the sternal margin to the midaxillary line. Each breast consists of glandular and fibrous tissue and subcutaneous and retromammary fat. The glandular tissue is arranged in lobes that radiate about the nipple of each breast. Layers of subcutaneous fibrous tissue provide the breasts with support. An extensive series of lymphatic vessels and channels drain lymphatic fluid from the breast into the axillary, supraclavicular, and subclavicular nodes. In the axillae the mammary tissue is in direct contact with the axillary lymph nodes.

The male breast consists of a small nipple and areola overlying a thin layer of breast tissue that is indistinguishable by palpation from surrounding tissue (Seidel et al, 1999).

Critical Thinking Application—Breasts

Knowledge	Experience	Standards
• Apply the knowledge you have regarding therapeutic communication techniques and human sexuality.	• You will need to practice to be able to recognize changes in breast tissue.	During examination of the breast apply the following principles:
• The possibility of breast cancer raises considerable anxiety and fear for the female client.	• Premenopausal female clients frequently have fibrocystic breast disease, a benign condition that involves changes in the breasts such as cyst formation, adenosis, fibrosis, and fibroadenoma formation.	• Teach client about breast self-examination as you conduct the examination.
• Understanding and support is critical for a successful examination.	• Use the client as a resource if she has performed breast self-examinations (BSEs) regularly.	• Be methodical as you examine each quadrant and tail of the breast.
• Refer to knowledge you have regarding developmental and pregnancy-related changes in the female breast.		

Breast Assessment

Equipment

- Small pillow or folded towel
- Disposable gloves (only when open lesions are present)
- Ruler
- Hand mirror
- Adequate lighting

Delegation Considerations

The examination of the breast requires critical thinking and knowledge application unique to a professional nurse. Delegation of the examination is inappropriate. However, have assistive staff report to you any client-reported breast mass.

Client Preparation

- Initially the client may sit or stand with arms at side. Remove gown down to waist for simultaneous viewing of both breasts. Use a composed and respectful approach during the examination.
- Optionally, use a mirror to assist the woman in learning how to perform breast self-examination.
- During palpation have client sit and then lie supine with small pillow placed under upper back.

History

Determine risk factors for breast cancer.

- Over age 40.
- A personal or family history of breast cancer.
- Biopsy confirmed atypical hyperplasia.
- Long menstrual history (menarche before age 12 or late-age menopause, after age 50.
- Recent use of oral contraceptives or postmenopausal estrogens.
- Never had children or gave birth to first child after age 30.
- Consumes two or more alcoholic drinks daily.
- Higher education and socioeconomic status (American Cancer Society, 2000).

Ask if client has noticed a lump, thickening, pain, or tenderness of breast; discharge, distortion, retraction, or scaling of nipple; or change in size of breast. Have the client point out any masses.

If client reports a breast mass, ask about length of time since lump was first noted, whether lump comes and goes or is always present, and whether there have been changes in the lump (for example, size, relationship to menses, other symptoms).

Does the client have breast implants?

Ask the female client whether she performs a monthly BSE. If so, determine time of month she performs it in relation to her menstrual cycle. Have client describe or demonstrate techniques used.

Does client take oral contraceptives, digitalis, diuretics, steroids, estrogen, or foods high in caffeine? How long have medications been taken?

Determine date of first day of last menstrual period.

If client has experienced menopause, review onset, course, and associated problems.

For pregnant woman determine history of breast sensations, use of supportive brassiere, and preparation procedures for breast-feeding. For a lactating woman determine use of nursing brassiere, nursing routine, use of breast pump, cleansing procedures for breasts, and history of discomfort or other problems involving the nipples.

The incidence of breast cancer in men is low. In the year 2000 approximately 1400 new cases of breast cancer in men was expected (American Cancer Society, 2000).

ASSESSMENT TECHNIQUES—BREASTS

Assessment	Normal Findings	Deviations From Normal
Female Breast Assessment		
• Make observations in relation to imaginary lines that divide the breast into four quadrants and a tail (Fig. 15-1).		
• With client sitting and arms hanging loosely at the sides, inspect the size and symmetry of both breasts.	• Breasts extend from the third to the sixth ribs, with the nipple at the level of the fourth intercostal space. One breast is often larger.	• Inflammation or a mass may cause a difference in breast size.
• Inspect the contour and shape of the breasts and note any masses, flattening, retraction, or dimpling.	• Breasts vary in shape from convex to pendulous or conical.	• Retraction, or dimpling, results from invasion of underlying ligaments by tumors. Edema may change breast contour.

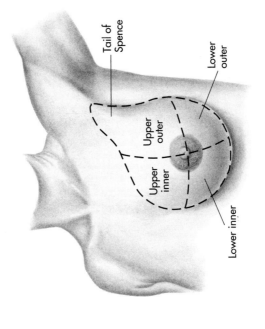

Fig. 15-1
Quadrants of the left breast.

Assessment	Normal Findings	Deviations From Normal
• To bring out retraction or changes in the shape of the breasts, have the client assume three positions: 1) Raise arms above the head. 2) Press hands against the hips. 3) Extend arms straight ahead while sitting and leaning forward.	• No retraction present.	• If retraction is present, maneuvers will accentuate the retraction.
• Inspect overlying skin for color; texture; venous patterns and presence of edema, lesions, or inflammation.	• Breasts are smooth and the color of neighboring skin. Any venous patterns are the same bilaterally. Venous patterns are easily seen in thin clients, those with light complexion, and in pregnant women.	• Unequal contour when comparing both breasts may be caused by an underlying lesion.
• Lift the breasts to observe the undersurface and lateral aspects for color or texture changes.	• Smooth and the color of neighboring skin.	• Rubbing of skin surfaces causes redness and excoriation.

Assessment	Normal Findings	Deviations From Normal
• Inspect nipple and areola for size, color, shape, discharge, and the direction nipples point.	• Areolae are round or oval and nearly equal bilaterally. Color ranges from pink to brown.	• Rashes or ulcerations, bleeding or discharge from nipple.
	• In light-skinned women the areola turns brown during pregnancy and remains dark.	
	• In dark-skinned women the areola is brown before pregnancy.	
	• Nipples are bilaterally equal or nearly equal in size and point in symmetric directions.	• If not symmetrical, may indicate underlying mass.
	• Nipples are everted and without drainage. Clear yellow discharge 2 days after childbirth is common.	
• Assess for normal developmental changes.	• *Preadolescent (Tanner 1 stage):* Only the nipple is raised above the level of the breast (Seidel et al, 1999).	

- *Puberty (Tanner 2 stage):* Breast buds appear, nipples darken, areola diameter increases, and one breast may grow more rapidly.

- *Adolescence (Tanner 3 stage):* Breast and areola enlarged. No contour separation.

- *Young adulthood (Tanner 4 stage):* Breasts reach full normal size, shape is usually symmetric, one breast may be larger. The areola forms a secondary elevation above that of the breast (Seidel et al, 1999).

- *Full adulthood (Tanner 5 stage):* The areola is usually part of general breast contour and is strongly pigmented. Nipple projects.

Assessment	Normal Findings	Deviations From Normal
	• *Pregnancy:* Breasts enlarge to two or three times their normal size. Nipples enlarge and may become erect. Areolae darken. Superficial veins in the breasts become prominent, and a yellowish fluid (colostrum) may be expelled from the nipples.	
	• *Menopause:* Breasts shrink, tissue becomes softer, and becomes flabby.	
• Palpate the axillary lymph nodes with client sitting.		
• With a female client's arms at her sides, ask her to relax her muscles.		
• Face the client; stand on the side being examined.		

- Support the arm in a flexed position while abducting that same arm from the chest wall.

- Place your hand against the client's chest wall and high in the axilla hollow.

- With the fingertips, press gently down over the surface of the ribs and muscles. Know the location of axillary lymph nodes (Fig. 15-2).

- Gently roll soft tissue against the chest wall and muscles.

Palpate the following areas:

- External mammary (anterior pectoral) lymph nodes. Edge of the pectoralis major muscle along the anterior axillary line.

- Brachial lymph nodes. Chest wall in the midaxilla.

- Lymph nodes are not palpable.

B

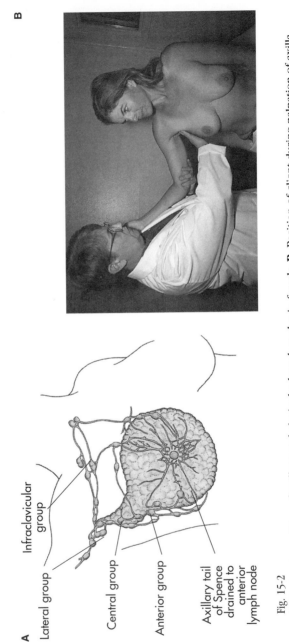

Fig. 15-2
A, Anatomic position of axillary and clavicular lymph nodes in female. **B**, Position of client during palpation of axilla.

A

Infraclavicular
group

Lateral group

Central group

Anterior group

Axillary tail
of Spence
drained to
anterior
lymph node

Assessment	Normal Findings	Deviations From Normal
• Central axillary lymph nodes. Upper part of the humerus.		
• Subscapular lymph nodes. Anterior edge of the latissimus dorsi muscle along the posterior axillary line.		
• Subclavian lymph nodes. Upper and lower clavicular ridges (fingers hook over clavicle).		
• If nodes are palpable, note number, location, consistency, mobility, size, and shape. If node is present, ask client if it is tender.	• One or two small, soft, nontender nodes may be normal.	• Enlarged or tender lymph nodes.
• Palpate breast tissue with client supine and one arm behind the head (alternating with each breast).		

Assessment	Normal Findings	Deviations From Normal
• Have the client raise her hand and place it behind the neck. You may place a small pillow or towel under the shoulder blade to further position breast tissue. • During this portion of examination, review techniques for BSE carefully. • If client complains of a mass, begin with opposite breast for objective comparison. • Use the pads of the first three fingers to compress breast tissue gently against the chest wall, noting tissue consistency and presence of tenderness (Fig. 15-3).		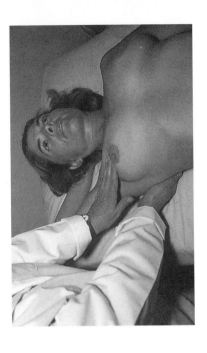 Fig. 15-3 Position of client and examiner for palpation of breast tissue against chest wall.

- Perform palpation systematically, covering the entire breast and tail in one of two ways:

  Clockwise or counterclockwise, forming small circles with the fingers along each quadrant and the tail.

  Back-and-forth technique with the fingers moving up and down across each quadrant.

- Breasts of a young client are dense, firm, and elastic. In an older client the tissue may feel stringy and nodular. The inframammary ridge at the lower edge of each breast may feel firm or hard but should not be confused with a tumor. The ridge may enlarge slightly during a menstrual period.

- During menstruation, there may be an increase in size and nodularity, and tenderness of the breasts may occur.

- A palpable, unilateral mass may suggest a malignancy.

Assessment	Normal Findings	Deviations From Normal
• While palpating breasts, take the client's fingertips and move them gently over breast tissue to help her learn to feel normal variations of her own breast.		• A single palpable mass that is hard, nontender, irregular in shape, fixed, and poorly delineated suggests a malignancy.
• Be sure she palpates the inframammary ridge, the lower edge of the breast that may feel firm and hard.		
• After light palpation, repeat the examination with deeper palpation.		
Examine any masses further for:	• Fibrocystic masses are usually multiple, bilateral, round, soft (lumpy) to firm in consistency, mobile, and tender, and are well delineated.	
• Quadrant location (e.g., upper outer, lower outer, tail).		
• Diameter.		
• Shape (round, discoid, irregular).		

- Consistency.
- Tenderness.
- Mobility.
- Discreteness (clear or unclear borders).
- Support large breasts with one hand and palpate breast tissue with the other against the supporting hand. Note consistency of tissues.
- Gently palpate the entire surface of the nipple and areola. Gently compress the nipple and note any discharge. If discharge appears, observe its color and attempt to determine the origin by massaging radially around the areola while watching for discharge through the ducts.
- If client has had a mastectomy, palpate unaffected breast in usual manner.

- During examination, the nipple may become erect and the areola wrinkled.
- No masses are present and no discharge should be produced.

- Galactorrhea (lactation not associated with childbearing) (Seidel et al, 1999).

Assessment	Normal Findings	Deviations From Normal
• Palpate affected area, paying particular attention to the surgical scar.		
• Palpate with two fingers for swelling, lumps, thickening, or tenderness, using small circular motion.		
Male Breast Assessment		
• Inspect breasts for size, symmetry, contour, skin color, texture, and venous patterns.	• Smooth and the color of neighboring skin.	• Same as seen in the female examination (see p. 365).
• Inspect nipple and areola for color and presence of nodules, edema, and ulceration.		
• Palpate breast for same characteristics as with female breasts. The examination can be done more quickly than for a female.	• Thin layer of fatty tissue overlying muscle is normal. Obese men have a thicker fatty layer.	• For males the same deviations may be present; the smaller amount of breast tissue in males presents lower risk of deviations.

UNEXPECTED ASSESSMENT FINDINGS—BREASTS

Assessment Findings	Significance	Next Step
• Peau d'orange appearance.	• Dimpling of the skin that gives it the appearance of the skin of an orange is caused by lymphedema. • Peau d'orange may begin in the nipples. • A sign of advanced breast cancer.	• Report to primary care provider. Client will need to be set up for a diagnostic mammogram as soon as possible. • Provide emotional support to client.
• Unilateral venous pattern.	• May be the result of increased blood flow to an underlying tumor.	• Complete careful breast examination. • Record and report findings to primary care provider. • Client will usually be sent for a diagnostic mammogram.
• Nipple retraction, discharge or bleeding.	• May be the result of an underlying tumor.	• If nipples are inverted, determine if new finding.

Assessment Findings	Significance	Next Step
	• Retraction or deviation of the nipple is caused by inward pulling from inflammation or a malignancy.	• Recent inversion or retraction can indicate malignancy. • Record and report findings.
• Galactorrhea.	• Lactation not associated with childbearing. Can be caused by drugs (e.g., estrogen, phenothiazines, tricyclic antidepressants).	• Review client's medications. • Record and report findings. • Report assessment finding to primary care provider.
• Gynecomastia (male breast enlargement).	• Caused by obesity, glandular enlargement, or chronic use of medication (e.g., digitalis).	• Review medication list. • Determine how long the client has experienced enlarged breasts. • Record and report findings.

Pediatric Considerations

- Breasts of infants of both sexes are often enlarged for a brief time after birth due to influence of maternal hormones during pregnancy.
- The right and left breasts of adolescent females may not develop at the same rate.
- Male adolescents may experience temporary unilateral or bilateral subareolar masses during puberty.

Gerontologic Considerations

- Chronic cystic disease diminishes after menopause.
- Adipose tissue increases, glandular tissue atrophies, suspensory ligaments relax, and breasts appear elongated or pendulous.
- Nipples become smaller and flatter.
- Gynecomastia in men after age 50 is usually unilateral. Causes include testicular or pituitary tumors, cirrhosis, estrogen therapy, and steroidal therapy (Lueckenotte, 2000).

Cultural Considerations

- The age-adjusted incidence of invasive breast cancer is highest among white, Hawaiian, and African-American women. The lowest rates occur in Korean, American Indian, and Vietnamese woman. White non-Hispanic woman have a rate four times higher than the women in the lowest rate group (Reis, 2000). White women are more likely to develop breast cancer than African-American women. African-American women are more likely to die of breast cancer than white women because of later detection and a more aggressive form of tumor.
- Recently, Japanese Americans have experienced an increased incidence of breast cancer, which may be related to diet and lifestyle (Giger, 1999). Between the ages of 55-69 years, white, Japanese and African-American woman have the highest incidence of in situ breast cancer.
- Non-Hispanic white and African-American women, age greater than 40 years, have similar follow-through in obtaining a mammogram at 68% and 67% respectively. Sixty-one

percent of Hispanic and Asian or Pacific Islander woman get a mammogram. American Indian and Alaskan Native women have the lowest percentage at 45% (USDHHS, 2001).

Client Teaching

- All women 20 years of age and older should perform a breast self-examination (BSE) monthly (Box 15-1). Always perform examinations around the last day of the menstrual period or the same day each month if the client has reached menopause or is on Depo provera for birth control.
- The American Cancer Society's recommendations (2000) for breast cancer detection in asymptomatic women include the following:
  - Age 20 to 39: Monthly BSE; clinical breast examination every 3 years;
  - Age 40 to 49: Monthly BSE; annual clinical breast examination; annual mammography.

- Over age 50: Monthly BSE; annual clinical breast examination; annual mammography.
- Some controversy exists among physicians regarding the efficacy of routine mammograms.
- African-American women tend to avoid regular mammograms more so than whites. Reinforce explanation of importance of regular examinations.
- Women with a family history of breast cancer should be examined annually by a primary care provider and have a baseline mammogram 10 years before the age the family member was diagnosed with breast cancer. For example, if the client's mother was diagnosed with breast cancer at the age of 45, all daughters should have a baseline mammogram by age 35 years.
- Discuss signs and symptoms of breast cancer. These include breast lump, thickening, swelling, distortion or tenderness, skin irritation or dimpling, and nipple pain, scaliness, or retraction (American Cancer Society, 2000).

BOX 15-1 Breast Self-Examination

Instruct client on breast self-examination. All women 20 years and older should perform this self-examination monthly using the following steps.

■ Stand before a mirror. Look at both breasts for anything unusual, such as discharge from the nipples, puckering, dimpling, or scaling of the skin.

■ To note changes in the shape of the breasts, perform the following measures (see the illustration).

■ Watch in the mirror while raising the arms above the head.

■ Press hands firmly on the hips and bow slightly toward the mirror when pulling the shoulders and elbows forward.

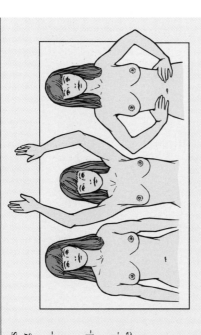

Continued

Illustrations from Payne WA, Hahn DB: *Understanding your health*, ed 2, St Louis, 1989, Mosby.

BOX 15-1 Breast Self-Examination—cont'd

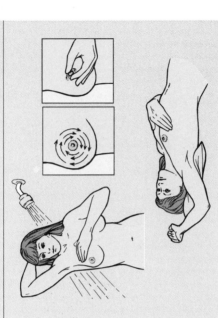

- In the shower or in front of the mirror, palpate each breast. Raise the right arm and use three or four fingers of the left hand to explore the breast carefully (see the illustration). Then start at the outer edge, pressing the flat part of the fingers in small circles, moving the circles slowly around the breast, gradually working toward the nipple (see the illustration). Pay close attention to the area between the breast and armpit and feel for unusual lumps or masses. Repeat the process for the left breast.

- Gently palpate each nipple, looking for discharge (see the illustration). Caution against pinching.

- Repeat the third and fourth steps lying down. Lie flat on the back with the right arm over the head and a small pillow under the right shoulder. Palpate the right breast (see the illustration). Repeat the process on the left breast.

- Call your physician if you find a lump.

Illustrations from Payne WA, Hahn DB: *Understanding your health*, ed 2, St Louis, 1989, Mosby.

Abdomen

Anatomy and Physiology

The abdominal cavity contains vital organs of numerous body systems. The peritoneum, a serous membrane, lines the cavity and protects many of the abdominal structures. The mesentery is a fold of peritoneum that covers most of the small intestine and anchors it to the posterior abdominal wall.

The stomach, a hollow organ, lies transversely in the upper left abdominal cavity under the costal margin. The small intestine is 21 feet long and coils through the abdominal cavity, from the pyloric orifice of the stomach to the ileocecal valve at the large intestine. The first 12 inches (30 cm) of the small intestine, the duodenum, forms a C-shaped curve around the head of the pancreas. The pancreatic and common bile ducts enter into the duodenum. The next 8 feet of intestine is the jejunum, which joins with the terminal section of the small intestine, the ileum. The small intestine completes digestion through the absorption of water and nutrients and secretion of substances to promote digestion and passage of contents.

The large intestine begins at the cecum, a 2- to 3-inch long pouch, in the lower right abdominal quadrant. The appendix extends from the base of the cecum. The ascending colon rises from the cecum along the right posterior abdominal wall to the undersurface of the liver. Once the colon turns toward the midline, it becomes the transverse colon. The transverse colon crosses the abdominal cavity toward the spleen and turns downward into the descending colon. This final segment of the large intestine travels along the left abdominal wall to the rim of the pelvis, where it turns into the S-shaped sigmoid colon. The rectum extends from the sigmoid to the muscles of the pelvic floor continuing as the anal canal and anus. The large intestine absorbs water, secretes mucus, and eliminates wastes as the material courses throughout the abdominal cavity.

The kidneys are located deep in the retroperitoneal space in both upper quadrants of the abdomen. Each kidney extends from the T12 to L3 vertebrae. The right kidney is usually lower than the left. These organs selectively filter, reabsorb, and secrete water and electrolytes delivered by means of the circulatory system to maintain fluid and electrolyte balance and eliminate wastes.

The bladder is a hollow, distensible organ that collects and eliminates urine formed by the kidneys. Normally the bladder lies below the symphysis pubis, but once it becomes distended it can become palpable just above the pubic bone.

The liver is located in the right upper quadrant just below the diaphragm. The liver's inferior surface touches the gall-bladder, stomach, duodenum, and hepatic curve of the large intestine. The hepatic artery transports blood directly to the liver from the aorta, and the portal vein carries blood from the digestive tract and spleen to the liver. The liver's functions include the formation of serum protein; production of bile; metabolism of fat, carbohydrate, and protein; detoxification of foreign substances; storage of vitamins and iron; production of antibodies; production of blood coagulation factors; and metabolism of bilirubin.

The gallbladder is a saclike organ about 4 inches (10 cm) long that is recessed in the inferior surface of the liver. The gallbladder concentrates and stores bile from the liver for the eventual emulsification of fats entering the small intestine. Contraction of the gallbladder moves bile through the common bile duct into the duodenum.

The pancreas lies behind and beneath the stomach, with its head along the curve of the duodenum and its tip almost touching the spleen. The organ is both an exocrine gland that secretes digestive enzymes and an endocrine gland that secretes insulin and glucagon.

The spleen is in the left upper quadrant, lying above the left kidney and just below the diaphragm. The organ consists of lymphoid tissue and functions to filter blood and manufacture lymphocytes and monocytes. In addition, the spleen contains a capillary and venous network that stores and releases blood.

The reproductive organs are located within the abdominal cavity. In the female, the vagina and uterus lie in the pelvic cavity between the bladder and rectum. The ovaries and fallopian tubes are located along the lateral pelvic wall at the level of the anterosuperior iliac spine. In the male, the spermatic cords, seminal vesicles, and prostate gland lie along the posterior wall and base of the bladder.

Muscles form and protect the abdominal cavity. In addition, tissues and bones outside the abdominal cavity (e.g., the spine) protect vital organs. These structures may be involved when clients complain of abdominal pain.

The abdominal aorta passes from the diaphragm through the abdominal cavity, just left of the midline. At the level of the umbilicus it branches into the two common iliac arteries.

Critical Thinking Application—Abdomen

Knowledge	Experience	Standards
• Apply your knowledge of the organs comprising the abdominal cavity and the location of each organ.	• Assessment of the abdomen is more difficult in obese clients. The extra fat layer covering the organs makes it difficult to detect abnormalities.	As you examine the abdomen apply the following principles: • Ensure the client is comfortable and has an empty bladder.

Knowledge	Experience	Standards
• Consider the function of the abdominal organs. Your ability to make an accurate assessment and diagnostic conclusions depends on your knowledge of the abdominal organs.	• Practice assessing the abdomen while visualizing the underlying organs. • If you are uncertain about any findings, have a more experienced practitioner confirm your assessment	• Auscultation is performed before palpation or percussion because manipulation of the abdominal organs can change the character of bowel sounds. • Be methodical in the order of auscultation, palpation, and percussion. • Localize findings according to the abdominal quadrants.

Abdominal Assessment

Equipment

- Stethoscope
- Adequate lighting
- Small centimeter ruler
- Tape measure
- Marking pencil
- Small pillow

Delegation Considerations

The abdominal examination requires critical thinking and knowledge application unique to a professional nurse. Delegation of the skill is inappropriate. Assistive personnel can learn to detect changes in abdominal size and client complaints of pain. Assistive personnel may first notice changes in bowel habits. Assistive personnel should be instructed to report any changes to you for verification.

Client Preparation

- The room should be warm, and the client's upper chest and legs should be draped.
- Expose the abdomen from just above the xiphoid process down to the symphysis pubis.
- Make sure lighting is good.
- The client lies supine with arms down at the side and knees slightly bent. A small pillow or rolled bath towel can be placed under the knees for support and relaxation of abdominal muscles. You may ask the client to place the soles of the feet on the examination table or bed to help relax the abdominal muscles.
- A small pillow may also be placed under the head to relax the abdominal muscles.
- Keep your hands and the stethoscope warm to help the client relax.

History

- If the client has abdominal or low back pain, assess the character of pain in detail (type, quality, location, severity, onset, frequency, aggravating factors, precipitating factors, and course). Ask the client what medications or positions alleviate the pain, if anything.
- Ask about the client's normal bowel habits and stool character. Ask whether the client uses laxatives or cathartics frequently and whether there have been recent changes.
- Ask whether the client has had abdominal surgery, trauma, or gastrointestinal (GI) diagnostic tests.
- Ask whether the client has had a recent weight change in the last week or intolerance to diet (e.g., nausea, vomiting, cramping), especially in the last 24 hours.
- Ask the client about any change in diet.
- Ask about belching, difficulty in swallowing, flatulence, bloody emesis (hematemesis), black or tarry stools (melena), heartburn, diarrhea, or constipation.
- Inquire about family history of cancer, kidney disease, alcoholism, hypertension, or heart disease.
- Determine if female client is pregnant; note last menstrual period.
- Assess client's usual intake of alcohol.
- Ask whether the client takes antiinflammatory medication, such as aspirin, ibuprofen, or steroids, or antibiotics that may cause GI upset or bleeding.

- Review client's history for the risk factors for hepatitis B virus (HBV) exposure
- Health care occupation
  - Hemodialysis
  - Intravenous drug user
  - Household or sexual contact with HBV carrier
  - Heterosexual person with more than one sex partner in previous 6 months
  - Sexually active homosexual or bisexual male
  - International traveler in area of high HBV infection rate

The abdominal examination primarily includes an assessment of structures of the lower GI tract in addition to the liver, stomach, kidneys, and bladder.

Abdominal pain is one of the most common symptoms clients will report when seeking medical care (Table 16-1). An accurate assessment requires matching data from the client's history with a careful assessment of the location of physical symptoms. Disturbances in a person's bowel elimination pattern can often be detected during an abdominal assessment. Because many factors influence bowel function (for example, dietary changes, medications, stress, surgery, fluid intake, activity), you can use assessment findings in caring for a variety of health problems. Your assessment of the abdomen determines the presence or absence of masses, tenderness, organ enlargement, and peristaltic activity.

Assessment of the abdomen involves examination of organs and tissues anteriorly and posteriorly (Fig. 16-1). When assessing the abdomen, use a system of landmarks to map out the abdominal region. The abdomen is divided into four equal quadrants, with the xiphoid process (tip of sternum) marking the upper boundary and the symphysis pubis delineating the lowermost boundary. Two imaginary lines cross at the umbilicus to form the quadrants. Assessment findings are recorded in relation to these four quadrants. For example, pain may be noted in the lower left quadrant (LLQ).

Table 16-1 Assessing Abdominal Pain

Abdominal pain can be assessed in a variety of ways to determine its significance:
- Clients may warn you to not touch a specific area; however, they may not have pain if their faces seem relaxed and unconcerned. When you touch they might recoil, but their expression remains unconnected.
- Clients with an organic cause for abdominal pain are usually not hungry.
- Ask the client to point to the location of the pain. If the finger goes to a fixed point (other than the navel), there is a likelihood that it has physical significance. If the finger goes to the navel and the client seems well, you should consider psychogenic causes.

Common Conditions Producing Abdominal Pain	Pain Characteristics
Appendicitis	Initially periumbilical or epigastric; colicky; later becomes localized to RLQ
Cholecystitis	Severe, unrelenting RUQ or epigastric pain; may be referred to right subscapular area
Pancreatitis	Dramatic, sudden, excruciating LUQ, epigastric or umbilical pain; may be present in one or both flanks; may be referred to left shoulder
Perforated gastric or duodenal ulcer	Abrupt RUQ; may be referred to shoulders
Intestinal obstruction	Abrupt, severe, spasmodic; referred to epigastrium, umbilicus
Leaking abdominal aneurysm	Steady throbbing midline over aneurysm; aneurysm may radiate to back, flank
Ectopic pregnancy	Lower quadrant; referred to shoulder with rupture is agonizing
Pelvic inflammatory disease	Lower quadrant increases with activity
Renal stones	Intense; flank, extending to groin and genitals; may be episodic

Modified from Seidel HM et al: *Mosby's guide to physical examination*, ed 4, St Louis, 1999, Mosby.

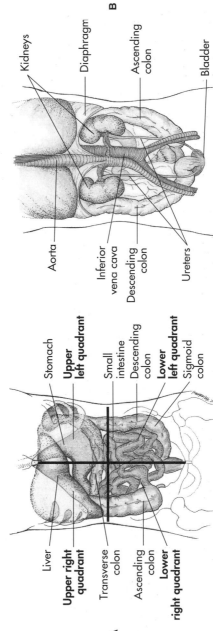

Fig. 16-1
Anterior (**A**) and posterior (**B**) views of the abdomen.

ASSESSMENT TECHNIQUES—ABDOMEN

Assessment	Normal Findings	Deviations From Normal
Inspection		
• Throughout the examination observe the client's movement and positioning.		• Lying still with knees drawn up, moving restlessly to find a comfortable position, splinting the abdomen, and lying on one side or sitting with knees drawn to chest are behaviors indicative of abdominal pain.
• Have client lie supine.	• Client is able to lie supine comfortably.	
• Ask client to locate any tender areas.	• Helps to focus the examination if abnormalities appear.	• Although this method is the traditional way to perform an assessment, room configuration or set up may necessitate examination from the client's left side.
• Assess tender areas last to minimize discomfort and anxiety.		
• Stand at client's right side.		
• Inspect the abdomen from above to detect abnormal shadows and movement.		

Assessment	Normal Findings	Deviations From Normal
• Sit down and inspect the abdomen from a lower position.		
• Observe the skin over abdomen for color, scars, venous patterns, and stretch marks (striae).	• Skin is the same color as the rest of body but may be pale if not exposed to the sun.	• Generalized color changes such as jaundice or cyanosis.
	• Venous patterns are normally faint except in thin, light-skinned clients.	
	• Striae (stretch marks) usually result from stretching of tissue. New stretch marks are pink or blue in color and turn silvery white over time.	• Striae may be the result of ascites, weight gain, or pregnancy.
		• Artificial openings may indicate an ostomy, ileoconduit, or drainage site from previous surgery.
		• Scars indicate past trauma or surgery.
		If a surgical scar is present, consider extent to which normal anatomy has been altered.

• To check prominent abdominal veins, compress a section of vein with two fingers next to each other; remove one finger and observe for filling.	• Blood fills from above to lower abdomen.	• Blood fills from lower to upper abdomen, indicating obstruction of inferior vena cava.
• Repeat procedure, removing other finger.		
• Look for evidence of lesions.	• Normal skin changes are present (see Chapter 7).	• Rash or nodules, abnormal skin changes.
• Note the position, shape, color, and presence of inflammation, discharge, or protruding masses from the umbilicus.	• Normal umbilicus is flat or concave midway between the xiphoid process and symphysis pubis. • Color is the same as surrounding skin. • No discharge is present.	• Discoloration, protruding or everted umbilicus.
• Inspect for contour, symmetry, and surface motion of the abdomen, noting any masses or bulging.	• A flat abdomen forms a horizontal plane from the xiphoid process to the symphysis pubis.	• Presence of a mass or asymmetry may indicate an underlying pathology.

Assessment	Normal Findings	Deviations From Normal
• After viewing from the seated position, move to a standing position behind the client's head to look at contralateral areas of the abdomen.	• A round abdomen is evenly convex, with maximum height at umbilicus. • A concave or scaphoid abdomen seems to sink into the muscular wall. The concave abdomen is common in thin adults.	
• Inspect for distention.	• Normal abdominal contour.	• Gas does not cause bulging of the flanks. • Do not confuse distention with obesity, which is marked by rolls of adipose tissue along the flanks and client denial of tightness
• While observing contour, ask client to take a deep breath and hold it.	• Contour remains smooth and symmetric.	• Enlarged organs in the upper abdominal area (e.g., liver, spleen) may descend below the rib cage to cause a bulge.

- Ask client to raise head (not shoulders).

- Abdominal musculature remains flat.

- Superficial wall masses, hernias, and muscle separations will become apparent during this maneuver.

- Inspect abdomen for normal respiratory movement.

- Males breathe more abdominally than costally. Females breathe more costally.

- Tightening of abdominal muscles during breathing with reduced ventilatory excursion may indicate guarding from abdominal pain.

- Smooth, even movement occurs with respiration.

- Note presence of peristaltic movement or aortic pulsation by looking across the abdomen from the side.

- Peristaltic movement may be visible in thin clients; otherwise no movement is present.

- Pronounced peristaltic wave is abnormal; may indicate an obstruction. Marked pulsation of aorta may indicate increased pressure or aneurysm.

- Aortic pulsations occur with each beat of systole and appear in the midline above the umbilicus.

Auscultation

If the client has a nasogastric tube to constant or intermittent suction, turn the suction off momentarily before auscultation.

Assessment	Normal Findings	Deviations From Normal
• Place the warmed diaphragm of the stethoscope first over the LLQ.		
• Apply very light pressure.		
• Ask the client not to speak.		
• To determine that bowel sounds are absent, you must listen continuously for 5 minutes (Seidel et al, 1999).		
• Listen for bowel sounds in all four quadrants.	• Bowel sounds are high-pitched, soft gurgling or clicking sounds that occur irregularly 5 to 35 times per minute (Seidel et al, 1999). Auscultate for at least 5 to 20 seconds to hear a bowel sound. Each bowel sound lasts about $\frac{1}{2}$ second to several seconds.	• Absent or hypoactive.
• Note their frequency and character.		

- Using the bell of the stethoscope, auscultate for bruits in the epigastric region and each of the four quadrants over the aortic, renal, iliac, and femoral arteries (Fig. 16-2) and the thoracic aorta.

- Normally there are no vascular sounds over the aortic, renal, iliac, or femoral arteries.

- Presence of a bruit indicates an aneurysm or narrowing of vessel.

  If bruits are heard, do not palpate the abdomen. Injury to an underlying aneurysm may result. Notify a physician immediately.

- Use the diaphragm of the stethoscope to auscultate over the liver and spleen for friction rubs.

- Normally no rubs are heard.

- A rub is a high-pitched rubbing sound that usually occurs on inspiration.

- Rubs indicate inflammation of serous tissue.

Percussion

The client who is ticklish presents a challenge to your abdominal examination. Have the client do the examination with your fingertips over his or her fingertips. After a time, you can let your fingers drift onto the abdomen while keeping your fingers primarily on the clients' fingers (Seidel et al, 1999).

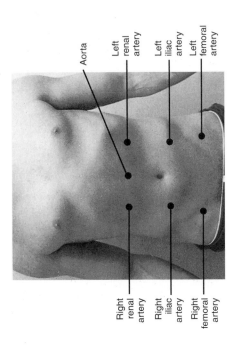

Fig. 16-2
Sites to auscultate for abdominal bruits.
(From Seidel HM et al: *Mosby's guide to physical examination*, ed 4, St Louis, 1999, Mosby.)

Assessment	Normal Findings	Deviations From Normal
• Systematically percuss over all four quadrants.	• Hollow organs such as the stomach, intestine, bladder, and aorta are tympanic.	• A dull note over an area not occupied by an organ may indicate a tumor.
• Note areas of tympany and dullness.	• A dull, medium- to high-pitched short sound can be heard over the liver, spleen, pancreas, kidneys, and a distended bladder.	
• Percuss potentially painful areas last.		
• Use percussion to locate borders of underlying organs.		
• Stand on client's right side and begin to percuss at the right iliac crest across from the umbilicus and upward along the right midclavicular line.	• Note changes from tympanic to dull once you percuss the liver's lower border (Fig. 16-3).	• A lower border can indicate organ enlargement or downward displacement of the organ by the diaphragm.
• Note when the percussion note changes from tympanic to dull.	• Usually the liver border is at the right costal margin or slightly below it.	
• Mark lower liver border with marking pen.		

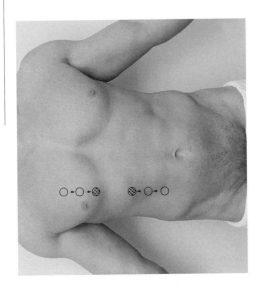

Fig. 16-3
Liver percussion route.
(From Seidel HM et al: *Mosby's guide to physical examination*, ed 4, St Louis, 1999, Mosby.)

Assessment	Normal Findings	Deviations From Normal
• Percuss the upper border by percussing down from the clavicle along the intercostal spaces at the midclavicular line.	• The liver's upper border is usually at the fifth, sixth, or seventh intercostal space.	• Diseases such as cirrhosis, cancer, and hepatitis cause liver enlargement.
• Note if sound changes from resonant to dull. Measure distance from upper to lower border.	• The distance between the upper and lower liver borders should be 6 to 12 cm (2 ½ to 5 inches).	
	• Liver span is usually greater in males and tall individuals than in females and short persons (Seidel et al, 1999).	
• Percuss over the lower left anterior rib cage and left epigastric region.	• The stomach's air bubble is tympanic and lower in pitch than tympany of the intestine.	
• With the client sitting or standing, use direct or indirect percussion to assess for kidney inflammation.	• Nontender.	• Inflamed kidney causes tenderness during percussion.

Assessment	Normal Findings	Deviations From Normal

- Use the ulnar surface of the partially closed fist and directly percuss posteriorly over the costovertebral angle at the scapular line.

Palpation

- Palpate the abdomen lightly over each of the four quadrants (Fig. 16-4).

- Initially avoid areas previously identified as problem spots.

- Lay palm of your hand lightly on abdomen, with fingers extended and approximated.

- Keep your palm and forearm horizontal.

- Placing the client's hand lightly over the examiner's hand can reduce tickling sensations.

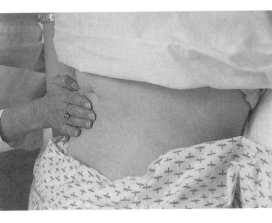

Fig. 16-4
Light palpation of the abdomen.
(From Potter PA, Perry AG: *Fundamentals of nursing,* ed 5, St Louis, 2001, Mosby.)

- With the pads of your fingertips, depress lightly ½ inch (1 cm) in a gentle dipping motion.

- Palpate to detect areas of muscular resistance, tenderness, abnormal distention, or superficial masses.

- During palpation observe client's face for any signs of discomfort.

- If you feel resistance, determine if it is voluntary or involuntary.

- Implement maneuvers to relax abdominal muscles. Have the client breath slowly through the mouth.

- Feel for relaxation of the abdominal muscles.

- Avoid quick jabs during palpation.

- Complete light palpation over those areas reported tender by the client.

- Abdomen is normally smooth with consistent softness and nontender without masses.

- A distended bladder may be felt just below the umbilicus and above the symphysis pubis.

- Muscles relax on expiration.

- Tightening or guarding by the client can occur with peritonitis, cholecystitis, and perforated ulcer.

- Tumors are palpable, especially in thin clients.

- Tenseness remains, likely because of an involuntary response to rigidity.

- Rigidity develops from peritoneal irritation.

Assessment	Normal Findings	Deviations From Normal
Note that if your hands are cold, the client is ticklish, or you palpate too deeply, the client may tense the abdominal muscles (guarding).	• Deep pressure may cause tenderness in the healthy client over the cecum, sigmoid colon, aorta, and midline near the xiphoid process (Seidel et al, 1999). No masses are felt.	• A deep mass can be a cyst or cancerous tumor.
• Use deep palpation to delineate abdominal organs and to detect less obvious masses.		
• Be sure your fingernails are short.		
• Depress your hands 1 to 3 inches (2.5 to 7.5 cm) into the clients' abdomen (Fig. 16-5).		
• Never use deep palpation over tender organs, areas of bruits, or a surgical incision.		
• Move the fingers back and forth over the abdominal contents.		

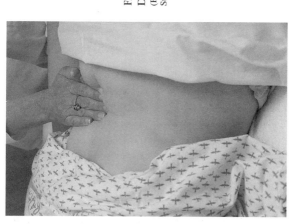

Fig. 16-5
Deep palpation of the abdomen.
(From Potter PA, Perry AG: *Fundamentals of nursing*, ed 5,
St Louis, 2001, Mosby.)

Assessment	Normal Findings	Deviations From Normal
• Note the characteristics of any deep mass, including size, location, shape, consistency, tenderness, pulsation, and mobility.		
• If tenderness is found, test for rebound tenderness: press the hand slowly and deeply into the involved area and then release quickly.	• No increase in pain.	• Pain elicited with release of the hand is a positive rebound test that can occur in clients with peritoneal inflammation or injury causing bile, blood, or enzymes to enter the peritoneal cavity.
• Have the client lift the head from the examining table, causing contraction of abdominal muscles.	• Masses in the abdominal wall will continue to be palpable.	
• Palpate around the umbilicus and umbilical ring.	• Area is free from bulges, nodules, and granulation.	• Bulges, nodules, inflammation, tenderness.
Palpate the liver's lower edge as follows:		
• Stand at the client's right side.		
• Place your left hand under the client's right posterior thorax at the eleventh and twelfth ribs. Apply upward pressure (Fig. 16-6).		

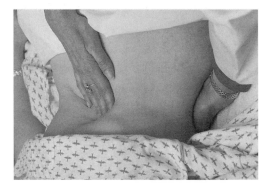

Fig. 16-6
Liver palpation.

Assessment	Normal Findings	Deviations From Normal
• With the fingers of the right hand pointing toward the right costal margin, place your hand on the RUQ well below the liver's lower border.	• The liver is usually difficult to palpate in a normal adult.	• Enlarged palpable liver.
• Press gently in and up with the right hand, while asking the client to inhale deeply.	• If palpable, the liver is firm, non-tender, and smooth and has a regular contour with a sharp edge.	
• Try to feel the liver's edge as it descends.		
• Palpate below the liver margin at the lateral border of the rectus muscle.	• Normal gallbladder is not palpable.	• Gallbladder is palpable and tender, indicating cholecystitis.
• If gallbladder disease is suspected, ask client to take a deep breath during palpation.		• Client will experience pain and quickly stop inspiration (Murphy's sign) as the inflamed gallbladder contacts your examining fingers.

- Palpate the spleen by reaching across the abdomen with your left hand. Place your hand beneath the client, over the left costovertebral angle.
- Press upward with your left hand.
- Place palm of your right hand with fingers extended on the abdomen below the left costal margin.
- Press fingertips inward toward the client's spleen while asking client to take a deep breath.
- Palpate edge of the spleen as it moves downward toward your fingers.
- To palpate for aortic pulsation, use the thumb and forefinger of one hand.
- Palpate slowly but deeply into the upper abdomen just left of the midline.

- A normal spleen is not palpable.

- A normal aortic pulsation is palpable.

- Spleen is enlarged and may be the result of portal hypertension or hemolytic anemia.

  Never vigorously palpate an enlarged spleen. Excessive manipulation can cause it to rupture.

- An aortic aneurysm causes pulsation to expand laterally.

Assessment	Normal Findings	Deviations From Normal
To assess for an ascitic fluid wave, ask the client or colleague for assistance (Seidel et al, 1999). See Fig. 16-7.		
• Have client lie supine.		
• Have client or another nurse press the edge of the hand and forearm firmly along the vertical midline of the abdomen.		
• Place your hands on each side of the abdomen and strike one side sharply with your fingertips.		
• Feel for the impulse of a fluid wave with the fingertips of your other hand.	• Absence of fluid wave.	• With ascites, a fluid wave is easily palpated.

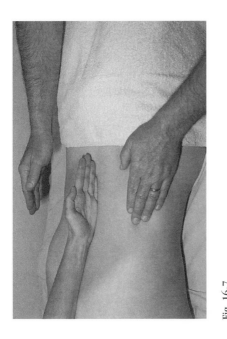

Fig. 16-7
Testing for fluid wave. Strike one side of the abdomen sharply with the fingertips. Feel for the impluse of a fluid wave with the other hand.

UNEXPECTED ASSESSMENT FINDINGS—ABDOMEN

Assessment Findings	Significance	Next Step
• Multiple abdominal bruises.	• May indicate accidental injury, physical abuse, or a type of bleeding disorder.	• Ask if client self-administers injections (e.g., insulin, heparin). • Review injection technique with client. • Record and report findings, including client's competency in self-administration of injections.
• Engorged, prominent veins.	• Can be caused by cirrhosis or abdominal malignancy.	• Review chart for history of abdominal malignancy or cirrhosis. • Record and report findings.
• Rash.	• Transient skin rash is common in hepatitis.	• Reassess presence of drug, food, or contact allergies.

Assessment/Finding	Rationale	Nursing Action
	Generalized pruritic, red, macular, and papular lesions that develop abruptly are likely caused by a drug reaction.	Record and report findings, describing the rash in detail (see Chapter 7).
Nodules.	May indicate intraabdominal lymphoma (Seidel et al, 1999).	Review chart for history of nodules.
		Record and report findings.
		If new finding, report to physician.
Generalized symmetric distention, resulting in the entire abdomen protruding.	Can be caused by a heavy meal, obesity, or gas.	If the abdomen appears distended, ask the client to roll onto side, and inspect for bulging flank.
	Distention from ascites causes flanks to bulge; when client rolls onto side, a protuberance forms on the dependent side.	Ask client whether abdomen feels unusually tight.
	An everted, pouched-out umbilicus can indicate distention.	Measure abdomen's girth by placing a tape measure around abdomen at umbilicus. Use a marking pencil to indicate where the tape measure was applied.
A bluish discoloration around the umbilicus (Cullen's sign).	Can indicate intraabdominal bleeding.	Monitor hemoglobin and hematocrit (H & H) and blood pressure.

Assessment Findings	Significance	Next Step
• Protruding umbilicus.	• May be caused by an underlying mass.	• Ask client if there is a history of abdominal trauma. • Record and report findings. • Notify physician if client exhibits signs of hypotension. • Clarify if client has known umbilical hernia.
• Absent bowel sounds.	• Indicates a cessation of GI motility that may be a result of bowel obstruction, paralytic ileus, or peritonitis.	• Be sure you auscultated for a full 5 minutes by the clock. • Determine when client had last bowel movement. • Assess for nausea, vomiting, ability to drink fluids. • Notify physician of abnormal findings. • Record and report findings.

- Hyperactive bowel sounds.

- Indicates increased GI motility from conditions such as inflammation, anxiety, diarrhea, bleeding, and excess ingestion of laxatives or certain foods.

- Ask clients if they have eaten any foods that increase bowel activity, (e.g., prunes, prune juice).
- Ask if client has taken any over-the-counter (OTC) laxatives or stool softeners.
- Ask client if bowel movements are soft, loose, or liquid.
- Ask if the client is experiencing any abdominal pain or cramping.
- Record and report findings.

- Palpable liver.

- Enlargement can be caused by hepatitis, cirrhosis, and cancer.
- In hepatitis the liver enlarges.
- In cirrhosis the liver has a firm, nontender border. Over time the liver becomes less palpable.

- Carefully note the liver borders.
- Report findings to primary care provider.
- Record and report assessment data.

Assessment Findings	Significance	Next Step
	• In carcinoma the liver becomes hard with nodules and an irregular border. The liver can be tender or nontender to palpation.	

Pediatric Considerations

- Distraction is important to help children relax when being assessed. Involve the child's parents. Do an abdominal examination first, especially if there is risk of the child becoming agitated.
- A child may confuse the pressure of palpation with pain. Children are also often ticklish.
- The abdomen of an infant or child should be rounded and dome shaped. Abdominal and chest movements are synchronous.

- Pulsations in the epigastric area are common in infants and children.
- Distended veins across the abdomen may indicate abdominal or vascular obstruction or abdominal distention.
- An umbilical hernia, which forms a visible and palpable bulge, is common in infants. A hernia will evert during coughing or sneezing.
- The umbilical stump should be dry and odorless.
- Visible peristaltic waves warrant careful evaluation and can indicate intestinal obstruction.

supine with knees slightly bent and head almost flat for most accurate measurement. With a nonstretchable tape measure, measure from the notch of pubis symphysis over the top of the fundus, without tipping the tape back. Measure in centimeters.

 Gerontologic Considerations

- Normally, older adults have reduced GI peristalsis and duller nerve sensations to the lower bowel, making constipation a common problem (Lueckenotte, 2000).
- The abdominal wall is thinner and less firm. Underlying organs are more easily palpated.
- The abdominal contour is often rounded as a result of loss of muscle tone.
- The older adult may experience impaired digestion and food intolerances caused by changes in bacterial flora of the intestine (Seidel et al, 1999).
- Liver size decreases after age 50. Hepatic blood flow is decreased as the cardiac output decreases. The ability of the liver to metabolize some medications decreases with age (Seidel et al, 1999).

- Bowel sounds are present within 1 to 2 hours of an infant's birth.
- An infant's abdomen may be more tympanic than an adult's, because the infant swallows air during feeding and crying.
- Organs palpable in children include the bladder, cecum, and sigmoid colon.
- Abdominal pain may be revealed by change in the pitch of crying, facial grimacing, and drawing the knees to the abdomen with palpation.
- Up until 4 or 5 years of age, a young child's abdomen takes on a potbellied appearance.
- Consider pregnancy in a young adolescent with a mass in the lower abdomen.

 Pregnancy Considerations

- Bowel sounds are diminished as a result of reduced peristalsis.
- Complaints of nausea and vomiting are common during the first trimester.
- Constipation is common.
- Assessment includes measurement of fundal height. Have the client empty her bladder. Then assist the client to lie

Cultural Considerations

- Native Americans have a high incidence of gallbladder disease (Seidel et al, 1999).
- The number of cancer deaths per 100,000 population caused by colon and rectal cancer is highest in the Czech Republic, Hungary, New Zealand, Singapore, Denmark, and Austria (American Cancer Society, 2000).
- The highest death rate per 100,000 population for stomach cancer occurs in Costa Rica, with the Russian Federation second (American Cancer Society, 2000).
- Cancer of the stomach, esophagus, and liver occurs more frequently among Japanese Americans than in whites which may be related to eating dry, salted fish (Giger, 1999).

Client Teaching

- Explain factors such as diet, regular exercise, limited use of OTC drugs causing constipation, establishment of regular elimination schedule, and a good fluid intake to promote normal bowel elimination.
- Caution the client about the dangers of excessive use of laxatives or enemas.
- If the client has chronic pain, explain measures for pain relief.
- If the client has acute pain, explain activities or positions to avoid.
- If the client is a health care worker or has contact with blood or body fluids of persons infected with hepatitis, encourage the client to receive the series of three vaccine doses.

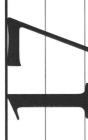

Genital-Urinary

Female Genital-Urinary Assessment

Examination of the female genitalia should be a part of all preventive health care examinations because of the high incidence of uterine and vaginal cancer. Deaths from uterine (cervix) cancer have declined over the last several decades because of regular checkups and use of the Papanicolaou (Pap) test (American Cancer Society, 2000). Ovarian cancer is the sixth leading cancer among women and the fifth leading cause of death among female reproductive cancers because of its silent nature (American Cancer Society, 2000). Women should have regular examinations to screen for cancer and sexually transmitted diseases (STDs). The average age of menarche among young girls has declined. Most

young girls are experiencing their first menstrual period between the ages of 9 to 12 years of age. The majority of male and female teenagers are sexually active by age 19 years, and some teenagers are sexually active by age 14 or 15 years (Wong, 1999).

Anatomy and Physiology

The female genitalia consist of external and internal genitalia. The external genitalia, referred to collectively as the *vulva*, include the mons pubis (veneris), labia majora, labia minora, clitoris, and vaginal opening (Fig. 17-1). The internal genitalia include the vagina, uterus, fallopian tubes, and ovaries (Fig. 17-2).

The labia have sensory receptors that are sensitive to touch, pressure, pain, and temperature. The two labia minora, which are just inside the labia majora, are thin folds of pigmented skin that extend upward to form the clitoral hood. These inner folds possess many blood vessels and have many sensory nerve endings.

When the clitoral hood is pulled back, the glans of the clitoris is revealed. The clitoris looks like a smooth, shiny pea. The clitoris has many nerve endings and is very sensitive to touch, pressure, and temperature.

The vaginal opening, or introitus, is between the urethra and the anus. The hymen is a membranous fold of tissue that partially covers the introitus. The hymen has no known function and usually remains intact until the first intercourse or use of tampons.

The Bartholin's glands are two small ducts that open on the inner surface of the labia minora next to the vaginal opening. The glands secrete a small amount of lubricating fluid.

The vagina is a thin-walled, muscular organ that tilts upward at a 45-degree angle toward the small of the back. The walls of the vagina consist of a thin outer serosa; a middle layer of smooth, involuntary muscle that is continuous with

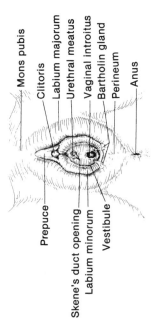

Fig. 17-1
External female genitalia.
(From Seidel et al: *Mosby's guide to physical examination*, ed 4, St Louis, 1999, Mosby.)

Labels:
- Prepuce
- Skene's duct opening
- Labium minorum
- Vestibule
- Mons pubis
- Clitoris
- Labium majorum
- Urethral meatus
- Vaginal introitus
- Bartholin gland
- Perineum
- Anus

The mons pubis is a layer of fatty tissue that covers the pubic bone and is covered by pubic hair in the postpubescent female. The two labia majora are fatty folds of skin whose outer surfaces are covered with pubic hair and whose inner surfaces are smooth and hairless. The labia majora extend down from the mons veneris and form the outer boundaries of the vulva.

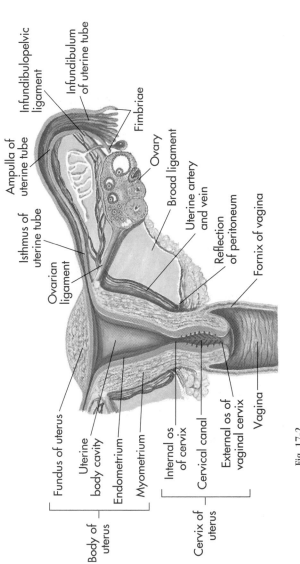

Fig. 17-2
Cross-sectional view of internal female genitalia and pelvic contents.

the muscle of the uterus; and an inner layer of moist mucous membrane called *mucosa*. The vagina serves as a passageway for menstrual flow and childbirth.

The uterus is a thick-walled muscular organ located between the urinary bladder and rectum. The uterus is about 3 inches (7.5 cm) long and looks like a small, upside-down pear. The wide upper part of the uterus is known as the *body*. The bottom part, called the *cervix*, protrudes into the vagina. The inner lining of the cervix contains many glands that secrete varying amounts of mucus that plug the opening to the uterus during pregnancy.

The two fallopian tubes begin at the uterus and end in long, fingerlike fimbriae near the ovaries. The chief function of the fallopian tubes is a conduit for the passage of both egg and sperm for fertilization.

The two walnut-size ovaries, one on each side of the uterus, have two functions. The ovaries produce eggs that are released into the fallopian tubes, and they secrete female hormones and small amounts of androgen directly into the bloodstream.

Critical Thinking Application—Female Genital-Urinary Assessment

Knowledge	Experience	Standards
• Consider the knowledge you have regarding communication techniques, human sexuality, and cultural diversity.	• Use your experience in determining a convenient time for conducting examination of the external genitalia. The external portion of the examination can be performed during hygiene	During the examination of the female genitalia apply the following principles: • Always use a relaxed approach, keeping the client as comfortable as possible.

- A complete and detailed history will help guide the examination. Complete the history before the examination.

- The examination of genitalia is intrusive. The client expects you to perform professionally and efficiently. The procedure is embarrassing and can be a source of great anxiety for the client.

- Consider the knowledge you have regarding GU function. Signs and symptoms identified during the gynecological examination may reflect problems involving the urinary system.

care, toileting, and during care of an indwelling urinary catheter.

- In the outpatient setting, the genitalia are examined during the annual "Well Woman" examination.

- Through experience, you will learn where the exam is placed in the overall physical examination.

- The female genital examination can be done last or after the abdominal examination, when the client is already supine.

- If you are a male care provider, offer the client the option of having a second provider in the room during the examination. Many older female clients are uncomfortable having a male perform the genitourinary (GU) examination.

- Adolescents may prefer to have a parent in attendance during the examination. Give the client and parent a choice.

- If you suspect sexual abuse, interview and examine the client in private to make her feel comfortable to report any problems. Presence of a spouse or sexual partner will usually discourage honest reporting.

A health care provider has a legal obligation to maintain a client's confidentiality (e.g., in the case of an STD) unless required by law to report those who pose a risk to the health or lives of innocent parties.

Female Genital-Urinary Assessment

Equipment

- Examination table with stirrups
- Disposable or metal vaginal speculum of correct size.
- Adjustable lamp
- Sink
- Water-soluble lubricant
- Clean disposable gloves
- Glass microscope slides
- Sponge forceps or swabs
- Plastic spatulas and/or cytobrush
- Fixative spray
- Collection device for obtaining gonococcal (GC)/chlamydia samples; viral swab for swabbing suspected herpes lesions
- Special collection swabs (usually Dacron tipped) and lab-specific collection devices if obtaining rectal swabs for STD (Check with the laboratory that will be processing the specimen.)
- Hemocult card with developer

Delegation Considerations

The examination of the genitalia requires critical thinking and knowledge application unique to a professional nurse. Delegate of the examination to assistive personnel is inappropriate. Assistive personnel will perform perineal hygiene and care for indwelling catheters. Ensure that assistive personnel know to report problems (e.g., unusual discharge; client complaint of genital tenderness or pain; presence of lesions, masses, or bleeding) and avoid any attempt to manipulate or inspect the client's genitalia other than that required for hygiene. A female colleague usually accompanies male care providers during the female examination.

Client Preparation

- Have the client empty her bladder before the examination so that a urine specimen may be obtained.
- Because the client may be embarrassed by the lithotomy position, use a calm, reassuring, and attentive approach; position and drape the client carefully, explain each part of the examination in advance, and avoid any delays or interruptions during assessment.

- Maintain eye contact with the client, both before and during the examination as much as possible. Ask if this is the client's first pelvic examination.
- Assist the client to the lithotomy position, in bed or on the examining table for an external genitalia assessment only.
- Assist client into the stirrups if the speculum examination is to be performed. Have the woman stabilize each foot in a stirrup and then have her slide the buttocks down to the edge of the examining table. Place your hand at the edge of the table, and instruct her to move down until touching your hand.
- If the client has pain or deformity of the joints, paralysis, spasticity, or muscle weakness, an alternative position may be necessary to perform the examination. One option is to have only one leg abducted, or the client can assume a side-lying position on the left side with her right thigh and knee drawn up to her chest. Offer a pillow for the client's head. Drape the client so that one corner of the drape covers the perineal area until the examination begins. Other options include the following:
  - a diamond-shaped position (woman lies on back with knees bent so that both legs are spread flat and the heels meet at the foot of the table; insert speculum with handle up),

- M-shaped position (woman lies on back, knees bent and apart, feet resting on the examination table close to the buttocks; insert speculum handle up), or
- the V-shaped position (woman lies on back with straightened legs spread out to either side of table; inserted speculum handle up) (Seidel et al, 1999).

History

If client arrives at the emergency room with emotional or physical manifestations of shock, hysteria, crying, anger, reduced level of consciousness, reported pain in the genital area, and signs of physical trauma, expect rape. Suspected sexual abuse or rape requires immediate medical management. Assess for physical injuries before beginning the history. Gather a history of the assault (who, what, where, when, why) and follow agency protocol to ensure a complete medical and legal review (Lewis et al, 2000).

- Has the client had previous illness (e.g., STD) or surgery involving reproductive organs?
- Assess normal urinary elimination pattern: frequency of voiding; history of nocturia; character and volume of urine; daily fluid intake; symptoms of burning, urgency, and fre-

quency; involuntary loss of urine, or stress incontinence and hematuria.

- Review menstrual history, including:
  - age at menarche (first menstrual period)
  - frequency and duration of menstrual cycle
  - character of flow (that is, amount, number of pads or tampons used in 24 hours, presence of clots)
  - presence of dysmenorrhea (painful menstruation)
  - pelvic pain
  - date of last menstrual period (first day of last cycle)
  - premenstrual symptoms, such as headaches, weight gain, edema, mood changes, relief measures
- Ask the client to describe obstetric history, including each pregnancy, history of abortions, and any miscarriages. Have the client describe current and past contraceptive practices and problems encountered. Discuss risks of STDs, such as chlamydia, syphilis, human papillomavirus (HPV) and human immunodeficiency virus (HIV) infection.
- Determine if client has signs and symptoms indicating an STD:
  - vaginal discharge
  - painful or swollen perianal tissues
  - genital lesions
  - rectal discharge
  - dysuria
  - urinary frequency
  - pelvic lymphadenopathy
  - malaise
  - headache
  - arthralgia
  - abdominal pain
- Ask if client has had signs of bleeding or pain outside of normal menstrual period or after menopause or has had unusual vaginal discharge (signs of cervical cancer and endometrial cancer).
- Assess if client has history of condyloma acuminatum infection (genital warts), herpes simplex, or cervical dysplasia; has multiple sex partners; smokes; has had multiple pregnancies; or was young at first intercourse (risk factors for cervical cancer).
- Assess if client has history of ovarian dysfunction, cancer of the breast or endometrium, irradiation of pelvic organs, endometriosis, family history of ovarian or breast cancer, or history of infertility or nulliparity (risk factors for ovarian cancer).

- Assess if client is postmenopausal, obese, or infertile; had early menarche (before age 12); had late menopause (after age 50); has history of hypertension, diabetes, or liver disease; or has family history of endometrial, breast, or colon cancer (risk factors for endometrial cancer).

- Does the client have symptoms of genitourinary problems such as dysuria, frequency, urgency, nocturia, hematuria, incontinence, or stress incontinence?

- Assess client's attitudes or feelings about sexual partners and sexual lifestyle.

- For pregnant women, determine expected date of delivery or weeks of gestation, involuntary passage of fluid, presence of bleeding, and associated symptoms.

- Consider factors in general survey that rule out risks for sexual abuse (see Chapter 6).

Assessment Techniques—Female Genital-Urinary

Assessment of the female genitalia consists of examination of external genitalia and speculum examination of internal geni-talia, described separately in the following sections. Nurse practitioners, midwives, and physicians typically perform speculum examinations. However, it is important for you to understand the procedure because a primary care provider will need your assistance.

The speculum examination is performed to assess the internal genitalia for cancerous lesions and other abnormalities and to collect specimens for a Pap smear to test for cervical and vaginal cancer. Women who are, or have been, sexually active or who have reached age 18 years should have annual Pap smears until three or more tests are negative. Thereafter the Pap test may be performed less frequently at the physician's discretion (American Cancer Society, 2000). Women age 40 years and over should have an annual pelvic examination by a health professional. Women at high risk of developing endometrial cancer should have an endometrial tissue sample evaluated at menopause. Pap smear tests are highly effective in detecting cervical cancer early. The test is less effective in detecting endometrial cancer and only rarely uncovers ovarian cancer.

ASSESSMENT TECHNIQUES—FEMALE GENITAL-URINARY

Assessment	Normal Findings	Deviations From Normal
Female External Genitalia		
⊙ *Standard Precautions Alert* *Glove both hands.*		
• Sit at the end of the examination table or bed. **Do not touch the perineal area without warning the client. Touch one thigh first and advance to the perineum.**		
• Inspect quantity and distribution of hair growth; look for presence of lice or nits.	• Preadolescent has no pubic hair except for fine body hair. During adolescence, hair grows along the labia, becoming darker, coarser, and curlier as it spreads over the pubic symphysis. In an adult, hair grows in a triangle over the perineum and along the medial surfaces of the thighs. Hair is free of lice or nits.	• Unusual growth or distribution of hair can indicate hormonal problems. See Chapter 6 for description of lice. • Client may shave pubic area.

- Inspect the surface characteristics of the labia majora.

- Explain that the next phase of the examination is to inspect deeper perineal structures.

- With nondominant hand, gently place thumb and index finger inside labia minora and retract tissues outward. Be sure to maintain a firm hold during retraction.

- Inspect characteristics of labia minora and mucous membranes between labia majora and minora.

- Note any inflammation, edema, lesions, or lacerations.

- The perineal skin is smooth, clean, and slightly darker than other skin.

- The labia majora may be gaping or closed, appear dry or moist, and are usually symmetric.

- After menopause, the labia majora become thinner.

- After childbirth, the labia majora are separated and the labia minora are more prominent.

- Mucous membranes appear dark pink and moist. The labia minora are normally thinner than the labia majora, and one side may be larger.

- Inner surface should be moist and dark pink.

- In virgins, the labia minora lie together.

- After childbirth or intercourse, the labia tend to gape or fall to the side.

- Unusual change in skin color or pigmentation is one sign of sexual abuse. White, chalky, malodorous discharge within labial folds can indicate poor hygiene habits.

- Scarring in genital area can indicate sexual abuse.

- Vesicular lesions, moist ulcerations, and crusting of erosions are progressive signs of herpes simplex virus, type 2.

- The perineal area can be inflamed. Discrete single or multiple papillary growths that are white to gray appearing on the vulva are manifestations of condylomata acuminata (Lewis et al, 2000).

Assessment	Normal Findings	Deviations From Normal
• Use other hand to palpate the labia minora between your thumb and second finger.	• Tissue should feel soft without tenderness.	
• Inspect the clitoris for size, shape, and color. Look for inflammation, irritation, or discharge in tissue folds.	• The size of the clitoris is variable, but the clitoris normally does not exceed 2 cm in length and 0.5 cm in diameter.	• Enlargement of the clitoris may indicate a masculinizing condition (Seidel et al, 1999).
		• An inflamed clitoris appears bright cherry red. The clitoris is a common site for syphilitic lesions, which appear as small, open ulcers that drain serous material.
• Observe urethral orifice carefully for color and position; note any discharge, polyps, or fistulas.	• Urethral orifice is normally intact without inflammation.	• Inflammation and reported irritation are signs of repeated urinary tract infections (UTI) or insertion of foreign objects.
	• The urethral meatus is anterior to the vaginal orifice and is pink, often appearing as an irregular slit or opening in the midline.	• Dysuria, hematuria, enuresis, and frequent UTIs are signs and symptoms of sexual abuse.

- If inflammation is suspected, check for urethral discharge by placing index finger inside vaginal orifice and gently milking the urethra from inside outward.

- If urethral drainage is present, change to a clean pair of gloves afterwards.

- Note the condition of the hymen.

- Inspect appearance of vaginal introitus; look for inflammation, edema, discoloration, discharge, fistulas, and lesions.

- Absence of urethral discharge.

- In virgins the hymen may restrict the opening of the vagina. Only remnants of the hymen remain after sexual intercourse or use of tampons.

- Vaginal introitus is usually a thin vertical slit or a large orifice. Tissue is moist.

- Women who have had multiple vaginal child births often have an opening that extends upward, interfering with the view of the urethra.

- Urethral discharge is a sign of STD.

- Discoloration of tissues with vaginal odor and pain can indicate sexual abuse.

- Vulvar trauma with erythema and extension of injury to anal area are signs of rape.

- Foul-smelling discharge can be symptomatic of vaginal infection.

Assessment	Normal Findings	Deviations From Normal
		• *Candida*, a common yeast infection, causes white, curdlike discharge with mild to severe itching and erythema of the labia.
		• *Trichomonas vaginalis* causes a copious, frothy, gray/green discharge and foul odor, with severe itching with or without erythema of the vulva.
• With the labia still retracted, examine Skene's and Bartholin's glands.		
• Inform client you are going to insert one finger in her vagina and that she will feel pressure.		
• With the palm facing upward, insert index finger of examining hand into vagina as far as second joint.	• Normally no discharge or tenderness is present.	• Discharge appears, indicating infection.

- Exert upward pressure, milking Skene's glands by moving the finger outward.

- Look for discharge and note any tenderness. Repeat on other side.

- Note the color, odor, and consistency of any discharge present.

- If inflammation and edema are found near the posterior end of the introitus, suspect infection of Bartholin's glands.

- Palpate the glands one side at a time with thumb and index finger between labia majora and introitus.

- Note swelling, tenderness, masses, or discharge.

- Inspection and palpation of the perineum and anal area (see Chapter 18) may be done at this time. Change gloves before proceeding.

Protocol may require collection of urethral discharge for a culture analysis.

- Painful swelling, hot to touch indicate abscess of the gland.

- A nontender mass suggests a Bartholin cyst (Seidel et al, 1999).

- The Bartholin's gland normally cannot be palpated.

- Surface is smooth.

- Tissue will feel thick and smooth in nulliparous women and thinner and rigid in multiparous women.

- Presence of external hemorrhoids, venereal warts, lesions, or fissure.

Assessment	Normal Findings	Deviations From Normal

Speculum Examination

- Be sure client is comfortable in stirrups and/or in lithotomy position.

- Select the proper size speculum. (A small speculum will fit women less sexually active, a medium size is best for sexually active women, and a large size works well for women who have delivered children vaginally.)

- Warm the speculum by placing it under running water.

- If you plan to obtain a cytology specimen, do not use lubricant. Lubricant can interfere with Pap smear studies and other swabs used to obtain samples for suspected STDs.

- Water-soluble lubricant can be used for all other examinations.

- Connect light source to plastic disposable speculum.

- If using a metal, nondisposable speculum, adjust light source over your shoulder to the examination site. Explain to the client what you are doing during the examination.

- Have the client breath slowly to relax.

Insert speculum:

- Hold the speculum in your dominant hand.

- If the client has never had a speculum examination, take time to show the client the speculum. Have the client handle it and feel it against her inner thigh. Show the client how the speculum will be adjusted, especially the noise made by opening the plastic, disposable speculum.

Assessment	Normal Findings	Deviations From Normal

- Then, insert two fingers of nondominant hand gently just inside the vaginal introitus. Feel for any abnormalities.

- With the same two fingers, press down on the perineal body just inside the introitus.

- After checking to be sure that the speculum blades are closed, introduce the closed speculum obliquely (rotated 50 degrees counterclockwise from the vertical position) past the fingers (Fig. 17-3, A).

- Client may feel some discomfort as vaginal opening is stretched.

Be especially sensitive to young women who have not had sexual intercourse. Go slowly. Give the client time to relax.

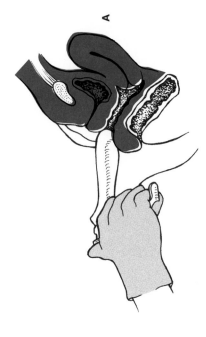

A

Fig. 17-3

Speculum insertion. **A,** Insert into vaginal opening.

Continued

- The speculum is inserted downward at a 45-degree angle toward the examination table to avoid trauma to the urethra. (This maneuver corresponds with the normal downward slope of the vaginal canal.)

- Do not pull pubic hair or pinch the labia.

- After the wide portions of the blades have passed the introitus, remove your fingers and rotate the speculum so that the blades are horizontal (Fig. 17-3, *B*).

- Insert the speculum the length of the vaginal canal.

- Open the blades slowly after full insertion and move the speculum to visualize the cervix (Fig. 17-3, *C*).

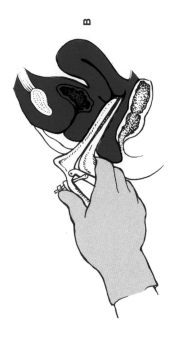

B

Fig. 17-3, cont'd
Speculum insertion. **B,** Gently insert until you reach the cervix.
Continued

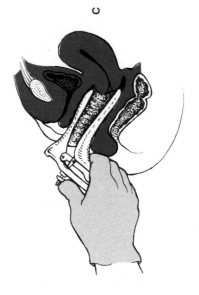

C

Fig. 17-3, cont'd
Speculum insertion. C, Gently open speculum to visualize
cervix.

Assessment	Normal Findings	Deviations From Normal
• When the cervix is in full view, the blades are locked in the open position by pressing on the thumbpiece or tightening the thumbscrew.		
• Inspect the cervix for color, appearance of the cervical os, or opening, size, surface characteristics, discharge, and symmetry.	• Cervix is glistening pink, smooth, and round. • Diameter is about 1 inch (2.5 to 3 cm) in a young woman and smaller in an older adult. • Cervix is midline without lesions. • The cervix becomes bluish during pregnancy.	• A pale cervix indicates anemia. • An enlarged cervix may indicate an infection. • Presence of friable tissue, red patchy areas, granular areas, and white patches can indicate inflammation, infection (e.g., STD), or carcinoma (Seidel et al, 1999).
• If discharge is present, note the color, odor, amount, and consistency.		
• Describe any irregularities or lesions as being in a 12 o'clock position, 6 o'clock position, and so forth around the cervix.	• The cervical os is usually small and closed in women who have not had children, or is larger and slightly curved after childbirth.	

Assessment	Normal Findings	Deviations From Normal
• Pay careful attention to the position of the cervix.	• In multiparous women the cervical os may have gaps.	• A cervix pointing anteriorly indicates a retroverted uterus.
	• Cervix in the horizontal position indicates a uterus in midposition.	• A cervix pointing posteriorly indicates an anteverted uterus.
		• A pelvic mass or pregnancy, or adhesions can cause deviation to the right or left.
		• See Table 17-2 for classification of cytologic findings of Pap tests.
• Label Pap slide in pencil with the client's name, birth date, and the specimen source (vaginal, endocervical, ectocervical).	• Normal results on the Pap smear are negative.	
• Collect Pap smear specimens from two sites (Table 17-1): ectocervix (outer cervix) and endocervix.		

Table 17-1 Methods for Obtaining Pap Smears

Location		Technique
Outer cervix (ectocervix)		Use plastic spatula. Place tip of longer arm in os. Rotate spatula 360 degrees, scraping outer surface of cervix. Apply cells to glass slide. Apply fixative solution and label slide.
Endocervix		Use cervical brush (cytobrush). WARNING: Do *not* use on pregnant clients. Gently insert brush through os. Rotate brush 180 to 360 degrees. Apply cells by rolling and twisting brush on glass slide. Apply fixative solution and label slide.

Table 17-2	Classification of Cytologic Findings of Pap Tests		
Papanicolaou Class	Dysplasia	CIN	Bethesda System
Class I			
Normal smear	Negative	Negative	Within normal limits
Class II			
Atypical cells, no dysplasia	Reactive atypia	Koilocytosis or HPV	Regeneration, repair
	Koilocytosis or HPV	CIN 1	Inflammation
	Mild dysplasia		Low-grade squamous intraepithelial lesion
Class III			
Abnormal cells consistent with dysplasia	Moderate dysplasia	CIN 2	
Class IV			
Abnormal cells consistent with CIS	Severe dysplasia, CIS	CIN 2	High-grade squamous intraepithelial lesion
		CIN 3	
Class V			
Abnormal cells consistent with invasive or squamous cell origin	Squamous cell carcinoma	Squamous cell carcinoma	Squamous cell carcinoma

From Stenchever MA: *Office gynecology*, St Louis, 1992, Mosby.

CIN, Cervical intraepithelial neoplasia; *CIS*, carcinoma in situ; *HPV*, human papilloma virus.

Assessment	Normal Findings	Deviations From Normal
• Ensure spatula and cytobrush are rotated completely around the cervix.		
• Apply cells and secretions to glass microscope slides, apply fixative solution, and send to laboratory.		
• If using Thin Prep Pap, label jar with client's name, birth date, and source of specimen.		
• Using Thin Prep brush, insert broom into the cervical os and rotate fully for 5 rotations.		
• Then place broom in solution and rotate 10 times, knocking on sides of container to help release cells.		
• Inspect the vaginal walls while withdrawing the speculum.	• Vaginal walls are normally pink throughout and free from discharge and lesions.	• White, yellow, gray, or greenish discharge indicates infection.

Assessment	Normal Findings	Deviations From Normal
• Inspect the vaginal wall's color, surface characteristics, and secretions. • Be careful not to pinch the vaginal wall when closing the speculum. • Rotate it slowly during withdrawal.	• Surface is moist, smooth, or rugated. • Secretions are thin, clear or cloudy, and odorless.	• Bleeding may occur in a variety of conditions (e.g., midcycle spotting, delayed menstruation with excessive bleeding, frequent bleeding, intermenstrual or irregular bleeding, postmenopausal bleeding). • Ovulatory alterations, polyps, intrauterine devices, contraceptive use, hormonal disturbances, and uterine or cervical cancer (Thompson, 2001) may cause these conditions.
• As the speculum is withdrawn, the blades tend to close themselves. • Avoid pinching the mucosa and maintain downward pressure to avoid trauma to the urethra. • Deposit speculum in proper biohazard waste container.		

Standard Precautions Alert If drainage is present, change gloves.

- With a gloved index and middle finger in the vaginal orifice, ask the client to squeeze inward over your fingers to check for muscle strength.

- To check for prolapsed bladder (cystocele) or rectum (rectocele), ask the client to push or bear down as if having a bowel movement.

- Then ask the client to bear down while watching for urinary incontinence.

- Some nulliparous women can squeeze fairly tightly.

- Multiparous women may have less muscular control.

- No bulging of tissue through the vaginal orifice should occur while straining.

- No incontinence noted.

- Vaginal walls bulge, blocking the introitus.

- A portion of the vaginal wall and bladder may prolapse or fall into the orifice anteriorly; this is a cystocele.

- Bulging of the posterior wall may be caused by prolapse of the rectum (rectocele).

Any unexpected prolapse should be reported to a physician immediately.

- Vaginal walls bulge, blocking the introitus.

- A portion of the vaginal wall and bladder may prolapse or fall into the orifice anteriorly; this is a cystocele.

Assessment	Normal Findings	Deviations From Normal
• Inspection and palpation of the perineum and anal area (see Chapter 18) may be done at this time.	• Surface is smooth.	**Any expected prolapse should be reported to a physician immediately.**
• Complete the examination by performing a digital rectal examination for all women over the age of 40 years and for those with problems of rectal bleeding (see Chapter 18).	• Tissue will feel thick and smooth in nulliparous women and thinner and rigid in multiparous women.	
• Complete the examination by providing a warm wash cloth or premoistened towel for the client to cleanse the perineum and anal area.		

- Advanced practitioners will proceed to a bimanual examination and rectovaginal examination to complete the annual pelvic examination.

UNEXPECTED ASSESSMENT FINDINGS—FEMALE GENITAL-URINARY

Assessment Findings	Significance	Next Step
• Hematuria.	• May be the result of a UTI, kidney stone, or pyleonephritis.	• Assess vital signs for fever. • Observe urine for frank blood. • Complete urine dipstick if ordered. • Ask client if she is experiencing any flank or low back pain.

Assessment Findings	Significance	Next Step
		• Assess for costovertebral angle (CVA) tenderness.
		• Record and report findings.
		• Notify physician of findings.
• Vesicular lesions, moist ulcerations, and crusting erosions (herpes simplex virus, [HSVI or HSVII]).	• Sexually transmitted disease.	• Ask client about sexual practices, recent sexual contacts, knowledge of lesions, and any history of previous lesions.
		• Notify primary care provider.
		• Be prepared to obtain viral culture.
		• Record and report findings.
• Candidaisis (a white, curdlike discharge with mild to severe itching and erythema of the labia).	• Indicates a vaginal yeast infection.	• Discuss signs and symptoms with client.
	• May be caused by recent antibiotic treatment, persistently elevated glucose, or suppressed immune system.	• Determine onset of infection.
		• Be prepared to obtain slides for potassium hydroxide (KOH) and wet prep.

- *Trichomonas vaginalis* (a copious, frothy, gray/green discharge with foul odor, with severe itching with or without erythema of the vulva).

- Sexually transmitted disease.

- Record and report findings.

- Discuss current sexual partners.

- Both the client and partner will need to be treated.

- Record and report findings.

Refer to p. 472 for sexually transmitted diseases common to both men and women.

🌸 Pediatric Considerations

- To examine the genitalia of the newborn, hold infant's legs in a frog position. Labia majora completely cover the clitoris and labia minora at full term.

- Any swelling of the labia majora and minora usually disappears in a few weeks.

- Newborns may have a mucoid, whitish vaginal discharge up to 4 weeks after birth caused by passive hormonal transfer from mother to infant (Seidel et al, 1999).

- With children and presexual female adolescents, assessment is of the external genitalia only. To examine the external genitalia of a young child, position child in parent's lap or on examination table in frog position, knees flexed and drawn up.

- A speculum examination is performed only when the child is experiencing bleeding, discharge, trauma, or when sexual abuse is suspected.

- Sources of perineal irritation in children include bubble baths, soaps, detergents, and urinary tract infection. A foul odor may be the result of a foreign body.

- Swelling of vulvar tissue should alert the examiner to sexual abuse. Further evidence includes scarring of genital, anal, and perianal areas; unusual changes in skin color; anorectal itching, bleeding, or pain; and genitourinary problems such as rash or sores, vaginal odor, bleeding, and discharge (Seidel et al, 1999).

Pregnancy Considerations

- Examination follows the same procedure as for nonpregnant adult women.
- The cervix gradually becomes soft, and the vulva acquires a bluish color from increased vascularity. Vaginal secretions also increase. The fundus flexes easily on the cervix.
- Estimation of the bony pelvis size is made.

Gerontologic Considerations

- Older women may need more time to assume the lithotomy position and assistance to hold the legs in place.
- Labia become atrophied with advancing age, thus appearing flatter and smaller.
- Pubic hair is gray and sparse.
- Cervix is smaller and paler.
- Vaginal epithelium is thinner, drier, and less vascular, and the cervix and uterus become smaller.
- Dry, scaly, nodular lesions may be malignant changes.

Cultural Considerations

- Female Mexican Americans have a strong social value that women do not expose their bodies to men or even other women. During a pelvic examination, a female Mexican-American client may express "feeling hot" because of embarrassment (Giger, 1999).
- Chinese Americans may view the examination of genitalia as being offensive (Giger, 1999). You must provide thorough explanations regarding the reason for the procedures used in the examination.
- Until the early 1900s, traditional practitioners were not allowed to touch the bodies of Vietnamese female clients except to take their pulse. Figurines were used for the female client to indicate where she was having problems. Today, many Vietnamese persons still place an emphasis on virginity at the time of marriage and continue to have strong feelings about unmarried young women having pelvic examinations (Giger, 1999).
- Japanese Americans place a high value on the family system. Family name and honor are important. Be cognizant of the issue of confidentiality and respect. Information should

not be shared even with extended family members who appear close to a client (Giger, 1999).

■ Russian Americans generally accept health examination of the genitalia without argument if adequate information and justification are provided and permission has been requested (Giger, 1999).

■ Young, virginal Bosnian women may refuse a speculum examination. Virginity until married is important in the culture. Breaking the hymen on the wedding night and bleeding on the wedding night sheets assures the man his new wife was a virgin.

Client Teaching

■ Instruct the client about purpose and recommended frequency of Pap smears and gynecological examinations.

■ Counsel client with STD about diagnosis and treatment.

■ Instruct client on how to perform genital self-examination (GSE):
  ■ Use a mirror.
  ■ Position self to see the area covered by the pubic hair.
  ■ Spread pubic hair apart, looking for bumps, sores, or blisters.

■ Look for any genital warts, which may appear as small, bumpy spots and then enlarge to fleshy, cauliflower-like lesions.
  ■ Spread outer vaginal lips apart and look at the clitoris for bumps, blisters, sores, or warts.
  ■ Look at both sides of the inner vaginal lips.
  ■ Finally, look at the area around the urinary and vaginal opening for bumps, blisters, sores, or warts.

■ Explain warning signs of STD: pain or burning on urination, pain in pelvic area, bleeding between menstruation, an itchy rash around vagina and vaginal discharge that is different from usual.

■ Teach ways to prevent STD: preventive measures (e.g., male partner's use of condoms, restricting number of sexual partners, avoiding sex with persons who have several other partners, perineal hygiene measures).

■ Explain risk factors for cervical, endometrial, and ovarian cancer (see history section).

■ Tell clients with STDs that they must inform sexual partners of the need for an examination.

■ Reinforce the importance of perineal hygiene.

■ Discuss with clients alternate sources of sexual satisfaction.

■ Discuss options for birth control.

Male Genital-Urinary Examination

The genitalia should be assessed routinely during health promotion examinations. Although testicular tumors make up about 0.7% of all forms of cancer in men, it is important for men to know how to perform testicular self-examinations (Table 17-3).

Anatomy and Physiology

The external male genitalia are the penis and scrotum. The male internal genitalia include the testicles, which produce hormones and sperm; the epididymis and vas deferens, a system of ducts that transport sperm; and the prostate gland, seminal vesicles, and Cowper's glands. These secretions become part of the ejaculated semen (Fig. 17-4).

The penis consists of the shaft, which is composed primarily of erectile tissue, and the glans, which has both erectile and sensory tissue. The penile shaft is comprised of three parallel tubes: two corpora cavernosa, which lie side by side, and beneath them a single corpus spongiosum, which surrounds the urethra.

The anterior end of the corpus spongiosum fits over the corpora cavernosa and is called the *glans*. The glans resembles an acorn. The area where the glans arises abruptly from the shaft is called the *corona*, meaning crown. If the male is uncircumcised, the skin of the shaft continues forward and forms a loose-fitting hood over the glans. This hood is called the *foreskin* or *prepuce*. On the undersurface the glans is attached to the prepuce by a thin fold of skin called the *frenulum*.

The scrotum is a thin, loose sac of skin that protects the two testicles. The scrotum is located at the base of the penis. The scrotum is divided into two compartments, each containing a testis, epididymis, and part of the vas deferens. The testes, epididymis, and parts of the vas deferens located in the scrotum are considered internal organs even though located outside the body cavity.

The left testicle usually hangs lower than the right testicle. The testicles have two main functions: to produce sperm and to produce hormones. The sperm drain into the epididymis, a duct that lies just outside the testicle. The vas deferens is a long tube from each testicle that goes up and out of the scrotum. The vas deferens curves around the urinary bladder and then turns downward and opens into an enlargement 4 inches (10 cm) long called the *ampulla*. The ampulla is a reservoir

Table 17-3   Male Genital Self-Examination

All men 15 years and older should perform this examination monthly using the following steps:

Genital Examination

Perform the examination after a warm bath or shower when the scrotal sac is relaxed.

Stand naked in front of a mirror and hold the penis in your hand and examine the head. Pull back the foreskin if uncircumcised.

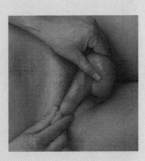

Testicular Self-Examination

Look for swelling or lumps in the skin of the scrotum while looking in the mirror.

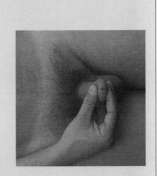

Continued

Table 17-3 Male Genital Self-Examination—cont'd

All men 15 years and older should perform this examination monthly using the following steps:

Genital Examination—cont'd

Inspect and palpate the entire head of the penis in a clockwise motion, looking carefully for any bumps, sores, or blisters.

Look also for any bumpy warts (see the illustration).

Look at the opening at the end of the penis for discharge.

Look along the entire shaft of the penis for the same signs.

Be sure to separate pubic hair at the base of the penis and carefully examine the skin underneath.

Testicular Self-Examination—cont'd

Use both hands, placing the index and middle fingers under the testicles and the thumb on top (see the illustration).

Gently roll the testicle, feeling for lumps, thickening, or a change in consistency (hardening).

Find the epididymis (a cordlike structure on the top and back of the testicle; it is not a lump).

Feel for small, pea-sized bumps on the front and side of the testicle. The lumps are usually painless and are abnormal.

Call your physician if you find a lump.

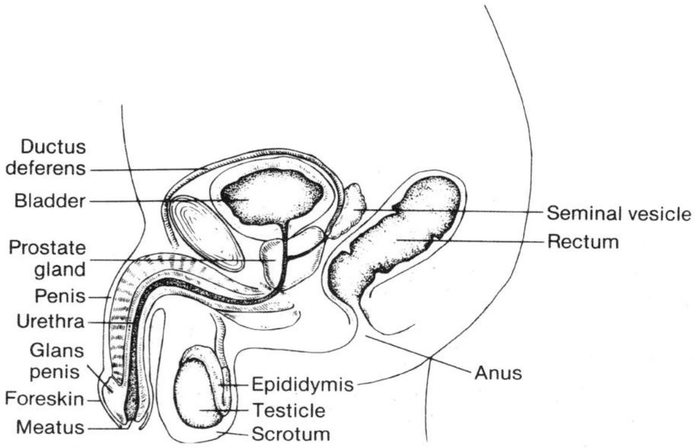

for the sperm before it is discharged into the ejaculatory duct. This duct carries them through the prostate into the posterior urethra. The urethra extends from the bladder to the penis tip and carries urine or semen.

The prostate is about the size of a chestnut and surrounds the urethra at the bladder neck. It produces the major volume of ejaculatory fluid. The ejaculatory ducts and a portion of the urethra pass through the prostate.

Fig. 17-4
Male sex organs.

Critical Thinking Application—Male Genital-Urinary

Knowledge	Experience	Standards
• Refer to the knowledge you have regarding communication techniques, human sexuality, and cultural diversity.	• Use your experience to find a convenient time during hygienic care or catheter care to perform the male genitalia examination.	During the examination of the male genitalia apply the following principles:
• The examination may cause the male client considerable embarrassment. The client will expect you to be professional and efficient.		• Always use a relaxed approach, keeping the client as comfortable as possible.
• Refer to the knowledge you have regarding normal genitourinary function.		• If you are a female provider, offer the client the option of having a second provider in the room during the examination.
		• Adolescents may prefer to have parents in attendance during the examination. Give the client and parent a choice.
		• If you suspect sexual abuse, interview and examine the client in private to

make him feel comfortable. The presence of a spouse or sexual partner will usually discourage honest reporting.

• A health care provider has a legal obligation to maintain a client's confidentiality (e.g., in the case of an STD) unless required by law to report those who pose a risk to the health or lives of innocent parties.

Assistive personnel usually provide routine hygiene and catheter care to clients. Ask assistive personnel to observe for unusual discharge, color change, presence of lesions, and the client's report of genital pain. Any changes should be reported to you. Instruct staff not to manipulate the genitalia more than is required for routine hygiene.

Client Preparation

■ Ask client whether he needs to empty his bladder.
■ Make sure the room is warm.
■ Have the client lie supine, with the chest, abdomen, and

Male Genital-Urinary Assessment

Equipment

■ Disposable gloves
■ Cotton swab applicator
■ Tongue blade

Delegation Considerations

The examination of the male genitalia requires critical thinking and knowledge application unique to a professional nurse.

- Assess client's sexual history and use of safe sex habits (e.g., use of condoms, number of sexual partners). Are there concerns about sexual partner or sexual lifestyle?
- Does client have difficulty achieving erection or ejaculation?
- Determine whether the client has had previous surgery or illness involving urinary or reproductive organs, including STD.
- Has client noted penile pain or swelling, lesions of genitalia, or urethral discharge (signs and symptoms of STD)?
- Has client noted heaviness or painless enlargement of testes or irregular lumps (signs and symptoms of testicular cancer)?
- Review medications that might influence sexual performance: diuretics, sedatives, antihypertensive agents, tranquilizers.
- Assess client's knowledge of testicular self-examination.
- Does the client conduct a self-examination routinely?
- Ask client for date(s) of the most recent prostate specific antigen (PSA) test and digital rectal examination.

lower legs draped. The client may also stand during the examination.

- Examine the genitalia carefully and completely but also briskly.
- Adolescents and men are fearful of having an erection during the examination.
- Because the client may feel anxious during the examination, particularly with a female nurse, help him relax, and explain each step of the examination. Have a second nurse in attendance to assure the client that you, as the examiner, will perform in an ethical manner. Legally, this protects you against any unfounded complaints regarding sexual harassment or abuse.

History

- Assess normal urinary elimination pattern: frequency of voiding; history of nocturia; character and volume of urine; daily fluid intake; symptoms of burning, urgency, and frequency; difficulty starting stream; and hematuria.

ASSESSMENT TECHNIQUES—MALE GENITAL-URINARY

Assessment	Normal Findings	Deviations From Normal
⊙ *Standard Precautions Alert* *Apply disposable gloves.*		
• Assess the sexual maturity of the client.	• First sign of puberty, an increase in genital and pubic hair development, is variable but usually starts around 9 to 10 years of age.	• Slow development of sexual maturity may indicate hormonal imbalance or may be familial.
• Note character and distribution of pubic hair, size of penis, and size and condition of scrotal tissues.	• During preadolescence there is no pubic hair except for fine body hair.	
	• By puberty, pubic hair extends from the base of the penis over the symphysis pubis and becomes coarse and curly.	
	• No hair covers the penis.	
	• The penis slowly lengthens, reaching to at least the bottom of the scrotum.	

Assessment	Normal Findings	Deviations From Normal
• Inspect the skin covering the genitalia for lice, nits, rashes, excoriations, or lesions.	• Skin is clear, without lesions.	• *Pediculus pubis* (lice) is spread by sexual contact. The infestation causes intense itching from biting lice. Scratching may cause secondary infection.
• If lice are present, dispose of gloves and reapply another pair. **Lice are highly contagious.**	• The scrotal skin becomes wrinkled and darker than surrounding skin.	
• Explain that the next portion of examination involves manipulation of the genitalia.		
• Manipulate the genitalia gently to avoid discomfort.		
• Inspect structures of the penis. Begin by inspecting the dorsal vein.	• Normally apparent along shaft.	
• In uncircumcised males, retract the foreskin to reveal the glans and urethral meatus.	• In uncircumcised males, foreskin retracts easily.	• Phimosis is a tightening of the foreskin, causing difficulty in retracting the tissue. Phimosis is the result of infection and congenital abnormality.
	• A bit of white, cheesy smegma may be seen over the glans.	

Note position of meatus and observe for discharge, lesions, edema, and inflammation.	If client is circumcised, glans is exposed and no smegma will be present. Glans and meatus are without inflammation. The meatus is slitlike and normally positioned just millimeters from the tip of the glans.	In some congenital conditions the meatus is displaced along the penile shaft. In hypospadias the meatus is located on the ventral surface of the glans or penile shaft. Syphilitic chancres usually occur on the glans and are painless lesions with indurated borders and a clear base.
Inspect the glans around its entire circumference for signs of lesions. Look carefully along dorsal side.	Glans is smooth and pink without lesions.	Herpetic lesions appear as superficial vesicles on the glans, foreskin, scrotum, or penile shaft. Lesions are often painful. Herpetic lesions rupture to form shallow, moist ulcerations. Herpetic lesions usually heal without a scar.

Assessment	Normal Findings	Deviations From Normal
• Palpate any lesion gently to note tenderness, size, consistency, and shape.		• Condyloma acuminatum (genital warts) are soft, reddish or gray lesions that develop on the foreskin, glans penis, penile shaft, and scrotum. • Penile cancer is rare but may be mistaken for condyloma acuminatum.
• Compress the glans gently between the thumb and index finger. • Observe the opening of the urethral meatus and note the color and any discharge. (Client can be asked to perform this measure for you.)	• Opening is glistening and pink. • No discharge.	• Bright erythema or discharge indicates inflammation or STD.
• Inspect the dorsal and urethra surfaces of the penis for any lesions, scars, or areas of edema.	• No lesions or edema.	• A client who has lain in bed for a prolonged time may develop dependent edema in the penile shaft. Lesions resulting from STD can be found on penile shaft.

- Gently palpate the shaft between thumb and first two fingers to note any localized areas of hardness or tenderness.

- If abnormal discharge from meatus is present, obtain specimen by gently milking penis from base to urethra.

- Brush culture swab across meatus. (Client again may assist with this procedure.)

- Pull retracted foreskin down to its original position at this point in the examination.

- Be particularly gentle when touching the scrotum. Inspect the scrotum's size, color, shape, and symmetry, and observe for lesions and edema.

- Penis should be soft and free of nodules.

- Hardened area, mass or nodule.

- Discharge may indicate a sexually transmitted infection.

- Scrotum hangs freely from perineum behind penis.

- The left testis may normally be lower than the right.

- The skin of the scrotum is normally loose; surface may be coarse.

- Sebaceous cysts (Seidel et al, 1999) commonly cause lumps in scrotal skin.

- Edema of scrotum may be from fluid retention caused by cardiac, hepatic, or renal disease.

Assessment	Normal Findings	Deviations From Normal
• Gently lift scrotum to view posterior surface.	• There are no lesions observed. • The skin color is often more deeply pigmented than body skin. The scrotum normally contracts in cold temperatures and relaxes in warm temperatures.	
• While the client retracts the penis upward, gently palpate the testes between thumb and first two fingers and note size, shape, and consistency; ask client whether palpation reveals any unusual tenderness. Continue palpation of epididymis, a cordlike structure along posterolateral surface of testicle.	• Testes should be sensitive to gentle compression but not tender. The testes are normally oval and approximately ½ to 1 inch (1 to 2.5 cm) in diameter. The testes feel smooth, rubbery, and free from nodules; the epididymides feel smooth, nontender, and resilient.	• An infection, tumor, or cyst may cause changes in texture or size of testes. Infection will cause tenderness. • Palpable, painless, pea-size lumps involving testis may indicate testicular tumor. • In diabetic neuropathy the testes are insensitive to painful stimuli (Seidel et al, 1999).
• Have client palpate testes at this time to become familiar with consistency of normal tissue.		

- Continue the examination by palpating the vas deferens separately as it forms the spermatic cord toward the inguinal ring.

- Assess cremasteric reflex by stroking the inner thigh with the end of a tongue blade or your finger.

- Ask client to stand for assessment of the inguinal ring and canal.

- During inspection, ask the client to bear down as if having a bowel movement.

- Inspect both inguinal areas for signs of obvious bulging.

- Vas deferens feels smooth and discrete, without nodules or swelling.

- Testicle and scrotum rise on the stroked side.

- Abdominal muscles tighten and scrotum lowers as client bears down.

- No bulging or protrusion is observed in scrotal sac or inguinal area.

- Lumpiness may be caused by changes from diabetes.

- Lack of reflex.

- Indirect inguinal hernia (most common) appears as soft swelling in area of internal ring with pain on straining.

- Direct inguinal hernia forms bulge that is usually painless.

Assessment	Normal Findings	Deviations From Normal
• Palpate the inguinal ring and canal to be sure a hernia is not present.		
• Have client relax and take a deep breath.		
• Begin by gently inserting the examining finger into the lower scrotal sac and carry it upward along the vas deferens into the inguinal canal (Fig. 17-5).		
• Follow the spermatic cord up to the inguinal ring.		
• Do not force finger into inguinal canal.		
• When the finger reaches the farthest point along the canal, ask client to cough and strain down.		

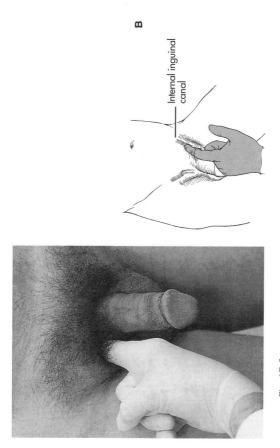

Fig. 17-5

A, Right inguinal hernia check. **B,** Left inguinal hernia check.

Internal inguinal canal

A

B

Assessment	Normal Findings	Deviations From Normal
• Repeat on left side.	• As client strains, no bulging pressure will be felt against fingertips; a tightening around the finger is normal.	• Indirect inguinal hernia comes down inguinal canal and touches fingertip on examination. Direct inguinal hernia pushes against side of finger on examination.
• Palpate the prostate gland during rectal examination (see Chapter 18).		

UNEXPECTED ASSESSMENT FINDINGS—MALE GENITAL-URINARY

Assessment Findings	Significance	Next Step
• Hematuria.	• May be the result of a urinary tract infection (UTI), kidney stone, or pyelonephritis.	• Assess vital signs for fever. • Observe urine for frank blood. • Complete urine dipstick if ordered.

- Difficulty starting stream of urine, decreased force of stream, or interrupted stream of urine.

- Usually caused by an enlarged prostate.
- May indicate prostatitis.

- Ask client if he is experiencing any flank or low back pain.
- Assess for costovertebral angle (CVA) tenderness.
- Record and report findings.
- Notify physician of findings.
- Perform a direct rectal examination (DRE) to assess size of prostate.
- Obtain urine sample.
- Assess for infection (e.g., elevated temperature, malaise, malodorous urine).
- Notify physician of findings.
- Record and report findings.

Assessment Findings	Significance	Next Step
• *Pediculus pubis*.	• A form of lice that attach their eggs to pubic hair. Spread by sexual contact, the infestation results in the lice biting, which causes intense itching. Scratching may cause secondary infection.	• Isolate a single louse with transparent tape, or remove a single pubic hair and attach to transparent tape and then to a microscope slide. • Review under microscope with physician. • Discuss sexual contacts with client. (See Chapter 7 for laundry instructions.) • Record and report findings.
• Condyloma acuminatum.	• Sexually transmitted disease.	• Discuss sexual partners with client. • Record and report location, size, and number of lesions. • Be prepared to assist the physician with chemical removal. • Record and report findings.

- Syphilitic chancres.

- Swollen, tender testicle.

- Sexually transmitted disease.

- May indicate an inflammation or infection.

- Discuss sexual partners with client.

- Report findings to physician for validation and verification.

- Counsel the client about safe sexual practices.

- Record and report findings.

- Be prepared to obtain urine specimen and gonococcal/chlamydia culture.

- Instruct client to elevate swollen testicle with bath towel and apply ice.

- Notify primary care provider.

- Record and report findings.

Pediatric Considerations

- Examine newborns for congenital anomalies; note size of penis, placement of urethral opening, and other anomalies.
- The foreskin in an uncircumcised infant is usually tight. The foreskin should retract enough to permit a good urinary stream. Uncircumcised infants (2 to 3 months of age) should not have foreskin retracted too far to inspect the urethra because foreskin retracted too far is at risk of tearing membrane. The foreskin becomes fully retractable by 3 or 4 years of age (Seidel et al, 1999).
- Undescended testes are common in premature infants.
- The scrotum in infants often appears large in relation to the rest of the genitalia.
- If either testis is not palpable, check to see if in inguinal canal. Alert physician.
- In children the testes should be about 1 cm (½ inch) in size.
- With adolescents, genital examination may be left until last because adolescents are more likely to be embarrassed. The examiner should proceed calmly as with all other segments of the examination. Note degree of maturation.

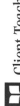

Gerontologic Considerations

- The size and firmness of the testes generally decrease with age.
- Scrotum becomes more pendulous because of loss of muscular tone.

Cultural Considerations

- Testicular cancer occurs most frequently among whites and is rare in African Americans.

 Client Teaching

- If the client expresses interest or concern about STDs, contraceptive techniques, physiological functioning, and other matters of human sexuality, you may choose to provide information after the examination. Measures to prevent STDs include the following:
  Use of condoms.
- Avoiding sex with partner who becomes infected.
- Restricting number of sexual partners.
- Avoiding sex with persons who have multiple partners.
- Instruct client to practice routine genital and testicular self-examination (Table 17-3).

18

Rectum and Anus

For both male and female clients, assessment of the rectum and anus can generally best be performed immediately after assessment of the genitalia. For males, rectal assessment includes assessment of the prostate gland.

Anatomy and Physiology

The rectum is the terminal portion of the lower gastrointestinal (GI) tract. The GI tract is a hollow tube, 4 to 6 inches (10 to 15 cm) in length containing folds of mucus-lined tissue. The rectum extends from the sigmoid colon to the muscles of the pelvic floor, where it continues as the anal canal. The anal canal is 1 to 1 ½ inches (2.5 to 4 cm) in length and is normally kept closed by the internal and external sphincters. The canal extends in a line toward the umbilicus before turning into the mucus-lined rectum. The anus contains a rich supply of sensory nerve fibers. At the junction of the anal canal and rectum, the rectum balloons out and turns posteriorly into the hollow of the coccyx and sacrum.

The urge to defecate occurs when the rectum fills with feces, causing reflex stimulation that relaxes the internal sphincter. Defecation occurs as the external sphincter, under voluntary control, relaxes. Defecation ensures the elimination of solid wastes.

In males the prostate gland is located at the base of the bladder. The gland surrounds the urethra and is palpable, because its posterior surface comes in contact with the anterior rectal wall.

Critical Thinking Application—Rectum and Anus

Knowledge	Experience	Standards
• Use your knowledge of the anatomy of the anus and rectum during your examination.	• Assessment of the anus, rectum, and prostate takes practice.	• Apply the following principles during the rectal and anal examination:
• Recall your knowledge of risk factors for colorectal and prostate cancer.	• As you perform digital rectal examinations, you will learn the feel of the anal sphincter.	• Maintain the client's comfort and privacy.
• Use communication techniques to help the client who may be uneasy about the examination.	• Experience with palpation of prostate will allow you to accurately assess changes in the size and texture.	• The examination can be uncomfortable and embarrassing for some clients.
	• Whenever you detect abnormalities, have an experienced practitioner confirm your findings until you are competent in prostate examination.	

Rectal and Anal Assessment

Equipment

- Disposable gloves
- Lubricant
- Examination light

Delegation Considerations

Examination of the rectum and anus requires critical thinking and knowledge application unique to a professional nurse. Delegation of the examination to assistive personnel is inappropriate. Ensure assistive personnel are instructed to report problems such as blood in the stool, difficulty starting urinary stream (in males), and change in clients' bowel habits.

Client Preparation

- Use a calm, gentle approach. Explain what will happen, step by step, before beginning the examination.
- Drape client so that only anal area is exposed.
- The female client is assessed in the lithotomy position if rectal assessment follows vaginal examination. Otherwise the female should assume a side-lying or Sims' position.
- The male client is asked to stand and bend forward with hips flexed, knees slightly bent, and upper body resting across the examination table.
- Nonambulatory male clients may be assessed in the Sims' position.

History

- Has the client experienced bleeding from the rectum, black or tarry stools (melena), rectal pain, or change in bowel habits (constipation or diarrhea)?
- Determine whether the client has personal history of colorectal cancer, polyps, or inflammatory bowel disease. Note if client is over 40 years of age.
- Assess dietary habits for high fat intake or deficient fiber content that may be linked to bowel cancer.
- Has the client ever undergone screening for colorectal cancer (digital rectal exam, fecal occult blood, sigmoidoscopy, colonoscopy)?
- Assess medication history for use of laxatives or cathartics, codeine, or iron preparations, which can alter elimination patterns.
- Ask if male client has experienced weak or interrupted urine flow, inability to urinate, difficulty in starting or

stopping urine stream, polyuria, nocturia, hematuria, or dysuria. The answers to these questions will give you information about the size of the prostate.

■ Assess client's family history: colon cancer (Box 18-1), familial polyposis, Gardner's syndrome, Peutz-Jeghers syndrome.

BOX 18-1 Signs and Symptoms of Colorectal Cancer

- Change in bowel habits.
- Diarrhea, constipation or feeling the bowel does not completely empty.
- Bright red or very dark blood in the stool.
- General abdominal discomfort, e.g., frequent gas pains, bloating, fullness, cramps.
- Unexpected or known weight loss.
- Constant fatigue.
- Vomiting.

(American Cancer Society: *2001 Cancer facts and figures*, Atlanta, 2001, The Society.)

ASSESSMENT TECHNIQUES—RECTUM AND ANUS

The primary purpose of the rectal examination is to determine the presence of masses or irregularities of the rectal walls. The integrity of the external anal sphincter can also be assessed. The examination includes screening for rectal cancer. Incidence rates for colon and rectal cancer have fallen in recent years (American Cancer Society, 2000). In males the rectal examination provides access to the condition of the prostate gland. The incidence of prostate cancer in the United States is on the rise because of improved detection methods. Prostate cancer is the second leading cause of death in men (American Cancer Society, *2001 cancer facts and figures*, Atlanta, 2001, The Society).

Assessment	Normal Findings	Deviations From Normal
◉ **Standard Precautions Alert** *Apply disposable gloves.*		
Rectal Examination		
• Inspect the perianal tissues and sacrococcygeal areas. Look for lumps, rashes, inflammation, excoriation, and scars.	• Skin is smooth and uninterrupted.	• Fungal infection can cause perianal irritation.
• Palpate surrounding tissue.	• Area is nontender.	• Area is tender to palpation.
• With nondominant hand, retract client's buttocks to inspect the anal area for skin characteristics, lesions, external hemorrhoids, fissures and fistulas, inflammation, rashes, or excoriations.	• Anal tissues are moist and hairless compared with perianal skin.	• External hemorrhoids appear as dilated veins that look like reddened protrusions.
	• Tissue is coarser and more darkly pigmented.	

Assessment	Normal Findings	Deviations From Normal
	• The anus is held closed.	• Pilonidal cysts are located in the midline, superficial to the coccyx and lower sacrum, and look like dimples with a sinus tract opening.
		• Perianal abscesses appear as areas of swelling with erythema of the anus, internally and externally.
		• Abscesses are extremely painful and tender.
• Ask client to bear down as if having a bowel movement. (Note presence of internal hemorrhoids or fissures.)	• No protrusion of tissue.	• Hemorrhoids may protrude.
• Use clock referents (e.g., 12 o'clock and 6 o'clock) to describe location of findings.		• Rectal mucosa may prolapse through the anal ring as the client strains.
• Apply lubricant to gloved index finger of nondominant hand.		• A prolapse is pink and looks like a doughnut or rosette (Seidel et al, 1999).

Some institutions do not permit nurses to perform digital examinations. Be sure that nails are trimmed short. Providers with long, artificial nails put the client at risk for rectal tears and injury.

- Press finger pad against the anal opening (Fig. 18-1).

- Ask client to bear down as though having a bowel movement.

- As the anal sphincter relaxes, insert fingertip gently into the anal canal directed toward the umbilicus.

- Explain that client may have sensation of need to have a bowel movement while your finger is inserted.

To avoid mucosal tissue injury, never force digital insertion.

- Have client tighten the external sphincter around the finger and note the tone of the anal sphincter.

- Muscles close snugly and evenly around finger, without discomfort to client.

- Weakened sphincter indicates a neurological problem.

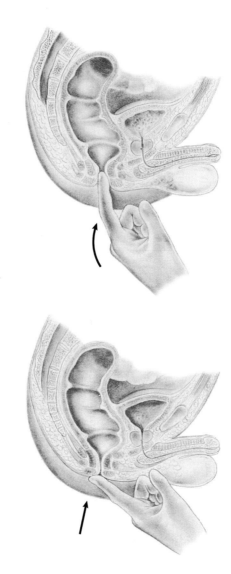

Fig. 18-1
Palpation of rectum.
(From Seidel HM et al: *Mosby's guide to physical examination*, ed 4, St Louis, 1999, Mosby.)

Assessment	Normal Findings	Deviations From Normal
• Continue examination, being aware of the course of the anal canal.	• Anal ring should feel smooth.	• Anal ring is tender or ragged.
• Rotate examination finger to palpate the muscular anal ring. Feel for any tissue irregularities.		
• Beyond the anal canal, palpate each side of the rectal wall for tenderness, irregularities, polyps, masses, or nodules.	• Rectal wall feels even and smooth. Stool is commonly found in rectum.	• Masses can be benign or malignant.
• Once the finger is advanced fully, have the client bear down again. This maneuver will cause any high lesions to descend against your fingertip.	• No lesions or masses are palpable.	• Palpation of a mass or nodule could indicate an internal hemorrhoid, a polyp, or a metastatic lesion.
• In male clients, turn the hand so that the finger palpates the anterior rectal wall.	• Gland is firm, without bogginess, tenderness, or nodules.	• Prostate enlargement is classified by amount of projection into the rectum.
• Warn the client that he may feel the urge to urinate, but will not.		• Grade I is 1- to 2-cm protrusion; grade II, 2- to 3-cm; grade III, 3- to 4-cm; grade IV, more than 4-cm protrusion (Seidel et al, 1999).

Assessment	Normal Findings	Deviations From Normal
• Palpate prostate gland to determine size, shape, firmness, tenderness, or lesions (Fig. 18-2). • The cervix may be palpable during rectal palpation through the anterior rectal wall. • Do not mistake the cervix or an inserted tampon for a rectal tumor.	• Male prostate is palpable anteriorly as a rounded, heart-shaped structure, 1 to 1 ½ inches (2.5 to 4 cm) in diameter, divided into two lobes by a small groove. It is normally firm, and non-tender. The prostate is often described as feeling like a pencil eraser. • Normally less than 1-cm protrusion into the rectum is found.	

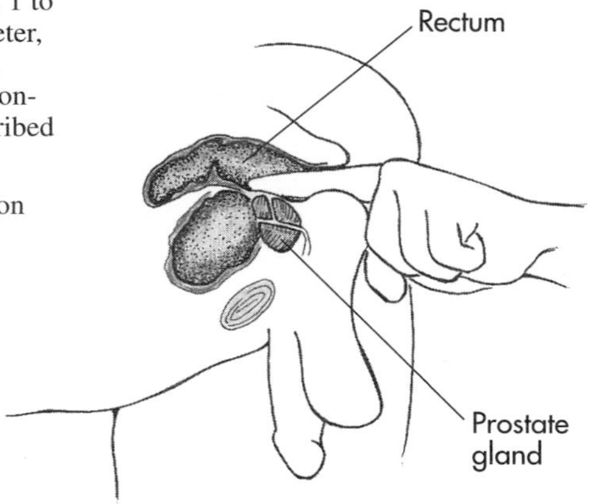

Fig. 18-2
Palpation of prostate.

- Gently withdraw finger and examine for fecal material.
- Complete the examination by offering the client a warm wash cloth or prepared wipe, or assisting with cleansing the anal and perineal area.

- Stool should be soft and brown.

- Blood or pus is abnormal.
- Test stool on gloved finger for occult blood.
- Stool characteristics can indicate disease.

UNEXPECTED ASSESSMENT FINDINGS—RECTUM AND ANUS

Assessment Findings	Significance	Next Step
• Acute rectal pain.	• May be caused by fissures, inflamed hemorrhoids, or hard, constipated stool.	• Inspect rectum for fissure or hemorrhoid. • Ask client about constipation or difficult stools. • Record and report findings. • If hemorrhoid or fissure is large, inflamed, or bleeding, notify the physician.

Assessment Findings	Significance	Next Step
• Rectal mass is palpable.	• A cancerous tumor is usually felt as a polypoid mass with nodular raised edges. The consistency is stony and contour is irregular (Seidel et al, 1999).	**Report any masses to the physician**
• Hardness or nodules on prostate.	• May indicate presence of a cancerous lesion.	• Report finding to physician. • Note if new finding. • Physician may repeat examination and order prostate specific antigen (PSA) for confirmation.
• Blood in feces.	• Reasons include ingestion of iron, steroids, and aspirin-containing medications; anal fissures; coagulation disorders; peptic ulcers; swallowed blood; foreign body trauma; and hemorrhoids	• Record and report finding. • The physician may order fecal occult blood (FOB) times three to determine if the finding is a single episode or occurs with each stool.
• Intermittent pencil-shaped stools.	• Caused by spasmodic rectal contractions.	• Record and report findings. • Determine from client how long the change in stool pattern has been noticed.

• Persistent pencil-shaped stools.	• Indicates permanent stenosis or con-stricture from a malignancy (Seidel et al, 1999).	• Record and report findings. • Determine from client how long the change in stool pattern has been noticed.
• Fatty stools (float in the toilet bowel, may be light brown or chalky colored).	• Seen in pancreatic disorders and malabsorption syndromes.	• Record and report findings. • Determine from client how long the change in stool pattern has been noticed.
• Mucus in fecal matter.	• Characteristic of intestinal inflammation and mucous colitis (Seidel et al, 1999).	• Record and report findings. • Determine from client how long the change in stool pattern has been noticed.
• Pipestem and ribbon stools.	• Indicates lower rectal stricture (Seidel et al, 1999).	• Record and report findings. • Determine from client how long the change in stool pattern has been noticed.

Pediatric Considerations

- In the neonate, passage of meconium stool within the first 48 hours of life indicates anal patency.
- Rectal examinations are deferred in infants and children unless an abnormality is suspected.
- Routinely inspect the anal region and perineum, examining buttocks for redness, masses, and evidence of change in firmness. Pinworms, *Candida*, or other diaper irritants often cause perirectal redness and irritation.
- Asymmetric creases in the buttocks may indicate congenital hip dislocation.
- Parents should be assured that toilet training is individualized for children and cannot begin until the child has mature neurological and muscular development.

 Gerontologic Considerations

- Older clients may only be able to assume left lateral side-lying position.
- Anal sphincter tone may be reduced.
- Older men have some degree of benign prostatic hyperplasia (BPH). The gland will feel smooth, rubbery, and symmetric. An annual examination is recommended to monitor recurrent urinary tract infections and to ensure that carcinoma does not exist.

 Cultural Considerations

- Performance of the rectal examination is an invasive procedure. Review the cultural considerations regarding touch on p. 27. Be respectful of the clients' wishes. It may be necessary to have a family member or other health care provider in the room before performing the examination.

Client Teaching

- Teach client common signs and symptoms of colorectal cancer (see Box 18-1, p. 478).
- Discuss risk factors for colorectal cancer (Box 18-2).
- Discuss the American Cancer Society's guidelines for early detection of colorectal cancer (Box 18-3).
- Discuss diet plan to reduce fat and increase fiber content.
- Warn client about problems caused by overuse of laxatives, cathartics, codeine, and enemas.
- Discuss risk factors for prostate cancer with male client (Box 18-4).
- Review signs and symptoms of prostate enlargement and possible prostate cancer (Box 18-5).
- Review the American Cancer Society's guidelines for early detection of prostate cancer (Box 18-6).

BOX 18-2 Risk Factors for Colorectal Cancer

- Age greater than 50 years.
- Diets high in beef, animal fat, and calories and low in fiber.
- History of colon polyps, Crohn's disease.
- History of ovarian, uterine, breast, or colorectal cancer.
- First-degree relative with colorectal cancer.
- History of ulcerative colitis greater than 10 years' duration.
- Familial polyposis, Gardner's syndrome, Peutz-Jeghers syndrome.

(From National Cancer Institute: *What you need to know about cancer of the colon and rectum*. U.S. Department of Health and Human services, Public Health Service, National Cancer Institute, NIH Publication No. 97-1552, Bethesda, Maryland, 1999; Seidel et al, *Mosby's guide to physical examination*, St Louis, 1999, Mosby.)

BOX 18-3   Recommendations for Early Detection of Colorectal Cancer

After 40 years of age:
• Digital rectal examinations (DRE) annually.

After 50 years of age:
• Fecal occult blood test (FOB) (guaiac test) performed yearly.
• Flexible sigmoidoscopy, involving visual inspection of the rectum and lower colon with a flexible, hollow, lighted tube and performed by a physician.
• If flexible sigmoidoscopy is normal and annual FOB is normal, then a repeat flexible sigmoidoscopy is performed every 5 years.

Or

• Colonoscopy. If colonoscopy is normal and annual FOB is normal, repeat colonoscopy every 10 years.

Or

• Double contrast barium enema. If normal, repeat every 5-10 years.

(American Cancer Society, *2001 Cancer facts and figures*, Atlanta, 2001, The Society.)

BOX 18-4   Risk Factors for Prostate Cancer

• Age greater than 65 years.
• African-American descent.
• Family history of prostate cancer.
• Diet high in animal fat.
• Live in North America and Northwestern Europe.

(From American Cancer Society, *2001 Cancer facts and figures*, Atlanta, 2001, The Society.)

BOX 18-5 Signs and Symptoms of Prostate Enlargement or Cancer

- Weak or interrupted urine flow.
- Difficulty starting or stopping urinary stream.
- Inability to urinate.
- Frequency, especially at night.
- Hematuria.
- Pain or burning on urination.
- Constant pain in the lower back, pelvis or upper thighs.

(From American Cancer Society, *2001 Cancer facts and figures*, Atlanta, 2001, The Society.)

BOX 18-6 Recommendations for Early Detection of Prostate Cancer

- Digital rectal examination performed annually after age 40.
- Prostate specific antigen (PSA) blood test performed annually after age 50.

If either test result is suspicious, a prostate ultrasound examination should be performed.

(From American Cancer Society, *2001 Cancer facts and figures*, Atlanta, 2001, The Society.)

Musculoskeletal System

19

Musculoskeletal assessment can be conducted as a separate examination or integrated appropriately with other parts of the total physical examination. You can also integrate this assessment as the client moves about or performs physical activity.

Anatomy and Physiology

The musculoskeletal system is the body's main line of defense against external forces. Physical performance requires bones, muscles, and joints that function smoothly and effortlessly. The musculoskeletal system is a bony structure with its joints held together by ligaments, attached to muscles by tendons, and cushioned by cartilage. The musculoskeletal system provides support, protection, body movement, hematopoiesis, heat production, and mineral storage.

The skeleton consists of four types of bones: long bones (e.g., humerus, femur), short bones (e.g., phalanx), flat bones (e.g., scapula), and irregular bones (e.g., vertebra) (Thibodeau and Patton, 2000). Bones serve differing needs such as bearing weight and offering protection to underlying structures. Bones differ not only in size and shape but also in the types of bone tissue that comprises them. Compact bone is dense and solid in appearance, whereas cancellous bone is spongy. Bone is anatomically organized so that its great strength and minimal weight result from the interrelationships of its structural components (Thibodeau and Patton, 2000).

An articulation or joint is a point of contact between bones. Although most joints (e.g., diarthrodial) allow considerable movement, others are completely immovable or allow limited motion. The existence of movable joints permits us to perform complex, highly coordinated, and purposeful movements. Most joints are diarthrodial; that is, freely moving articulations that are enclosed by a capsule of fibrous articular cartilage, ligaments, and cartilage covering opposing bones. Each articular cavity is lined with a synovial membrane that secretes synovial fluid. Bursae develop in the spaces of connective tissue between tendons, ligaments, and bones to promote motion and reduce friction. Table 19-1 describes the classification of joints.

Bones and joints cannot move themselves. Skeletal muscle tissue attaches to the skeleton and is responsible for voluntary body movement. Skeletal muscle cells have several characteristics that permit them to function: excitability (capable of responding to nerve signals), contractility (capable of contracting to produce movement), and extensibility (capable of extending or stretching to allow muscles to return to resting length). Muscles perform a function that is often overlooked. Muscle cells, like all cells, produce body heat through catabolism. Because of the highly active nature of muscle cells, skeletal muscle contractions produce a major share of total body heat.

Table 19-1 Classification of Joints

Type of Joint	Example	Description
Synarthrosis		No movement is permitted
Suture	Cranial sutures	United by thin layer of fibrous tissue
Synchondrosis	Joint between the epiphysis and diaphysis of long bones	A temporary joint in which the cartilage is replaced by bone later in life
Amphiarthrosis		Slightly movable joint
Symphysis	Symphysis pubis	Bones are connected by a fibrocartilage disk
Syndesmosis	Radius-ulna articulation	Bones are connected by ligaments
Diarthrosis (synovial)		Freely movable; enclosed by joint capsule, lined with synovial membrane
Ball and socket	Hip	Widest range of motion, movement in all planes
Hinge	Elbow	Motion limited to flexion and extension in a single plane
Pivot	Atlantoaxis	Motion limited to rotation
Condyloid	Wrist between radius and carpals	Motion in two planes at right angles to each other, but no radial rotation
Saddle	Thumb at carpal-metacarpal joint	Motion in two planes at right angles to each other, but no axial rotation
Gliding	Intervertebral	Motion limited to gliding

From Seidel HM et al: *Mosby's guide to physical examination*, ed 4, St Louis, 1999, Mosby.

Critical Thinking Application—Musculoskeletal System

Knowledge	Experience	Standards
• Refer to your knowledge of anatomy and physiology of the skeletal and muscular system. A detailed understanding will help you recognize alterations and anticipate how changes in other body systems affect muscular and skeletal function.	• Learn how to combine elements of the musculoskeletal examination with other body system examinations. For example, when examining the head and neck, it would be easy to assess range of motion (ROM) and muscle strength for major joints and muscle groups.	During examination of the musculoskeletal system, apply the following principles: • Know the normal ROM for each joint. • Never move or force a joint beyond the client's current ROM. • Use caution when examining a sports injury.
• Refer to your knowledge of changes in musculoskeletal function as a result of aging. Age-related changes can significantly affect an older client's mobility and make an examination challenging. The older adult will require special consideration in your examination.	• Most people have experienced some type of injury to their musculoskeletal system, such as a sprained ankle, bruised hand, or injured finger. Remember that pain is associated with such an injury and requires you to carefully support and examine the affected area.	• Support the full length of the body part being examined. • Consider the client's level of fatigue or the existence of symptoms such as shortness of breath in determining how extensive an examination can be performed.

Musculoskeletal Assessment

The integrity of the musculoskeletal system is vital for persons to move about freely and care for themselves. Disorders of the musculoskeletal system can range from alterations causing minor discomfort, such as sprained ligaments, to life-threatening conditions, such as muscular dystrophy. The musculoskeletal system is complex in that it is influenced by endocrine and neurological function. Your examination includes assessment of the bones; supportive tissues, such as cartilage, tendons, and fasciae; muscles; and joints. Give particular attention to areas of limited or absent movement to determine the level and extent of a client's disability. The client may exhibit problems resulting from disease of bones or joints, trauma, endocrine imbalance affecting muscle function, or disorders of the nerves that innervate the musculoskeletal system.

Equipment

- Goniometer (usually available from physical therapy department; used to measure degrees of flexion and extension)
- Tape measure

Delegation Considerations

Physical examination of the musculoskeletal function requires critical thinking and knowledge application unique to a professional nurse. Delegation of this assessment to assistive personnel is inappropriate. Assistive personnel often assist clients with ambulation, transfer, and positioning, and should be trained in recognizing problems with gait and ROM. Inform assistive personnel about the following:

- Clients at risk for gait problems.
- The importance of never moving or forcing a joint beyond the client's current ROM.
- Clients with muscular weakness, who require special assistance with transfer and ambulation.
- The need to report any problems noted in ROM, appearance of joint, or muscle strength to you.

Client Preparation

- Depending on the muscle groups assessed, the client sits, lies supine, or stands.
- Be sure the client's muscles and joints are fully exposed and free to move.
- Keep client warm and comfortable.

History

- Ask if client is involved in competitive sports, particularly any involving collision and contact. Does the client warm up adequately?
- Is the client in good physical condition?
- Has the client had a rapid growth spurt (adolescents)?
- Does the client wear protective equipment?
- Review client history for heavy alcohol use, cigarette smoking, constant dieting, calcium intake less than 500 mg daily, thin and light body frame, nulliparous state, occurrence of menopause before age 45 years, postmenopausal state, bilateral oophorectomy, and family history of osteoporosis (risk factors for osteoporosis) (Box 19-1).
- Ask the client to describe history of problems in bone, muscle, or joint function, including history of recent falls, trauma, lifting heavy objects, and bone or joint disease with sudden or gradual onset. Have client point out the locations of alterations.
- Assess the nature and extent of any stiffness or pain, including location; duration; severity; type of pain; and predisposing, aggravating, and relieving factors.

BOX 19-1 Risk Factors for Osteoporosis

- Asian, Native American, or Caucasian
- Northwestern European descent
- Blonde or red hair
- Thin, light body frame
- Family history
- Nulliparous
- Postmenopausal
- Menopause before age 45 years
- Calcium intake <500 mg/day
- Frequent dieting
- Scoliosis or rheumatoid arthritis
- Diabetes, hypercortisolism, or hyperthyroid
- Use of steroids, thyroxine, or heparin
- Poor dentition
- History of previous fractures
- Cigarette smoker
- Heavy alcohol use
- Heavy use of soda or pop

(Modified from Seidel HM et al: *Mosby's guide to physical examination,* ed 4, St Louis, 1999, Mosby).

- Ask whether the client has noticed a change in ability to perform self-care tasks such as bathing, feeding, dressing, toileting, and ambulating or social functions such as household chores, work, recreation, and sexual activities (Table 19-2).

- For women over age 50 years, assess height decrease to predict osteoporosis. Subtract current height from maximum adult height.

Table 19-2   Functional Assessment: Musculoskeletal Assessment

Activity to Observe	Indicators of Weakened Muscle Groups
Rising from lying to sitting position	Rolling to one side and pushing with arms to raise to elbows; grabbing a siderail or table to pull to sitting
Rising from chair to standing	Pushing with arms to supplement weak leg muscles; upper torso thrusts forward before body rises
Walking	Lifting leg farther off floor with each step: shortened swing phase; foot may fall or slide forward; arms held out for balance or move in rowing motion
Climbing steps	Holding handrail for balance; pulling body up and forward with arms; uses stronger leg
Descending steps	Lowering weakened leg first; often descends sideways holding rail with both hands; may watch feet

Picking up item from floor	Leaning on furniture for support; bending over at waist to avoid bending knees; uses one hand on thigh to assist with lowering and raising torso
Tying shoes	Using footstool to decrease spinal flexion
Putting on and pulling up trousers or stockings	Difficulty may indicate decreased shoulder and upper arm strength; these activities often performed in sitting position until clothing is pulled up
Putting on sweater	Putting sleeve on weaker arm or shoulder first; uses internal or external shoulder rotation to get remaining arm in sleeve
Zipping dress in back	Difficulty with this indicates weakened shoulder rotation
Combing hair	Difficulty indicates problems with grasp, wrist flexion, pronation and supination of forearm, and elbow rotation
Pushing chair away from table while seated	Standing and easing chair back with torso; difficulty indicates problems with upper arm, shoulder, lower arm strength, and wrist motion
Buttoning button or writing name	Difficulty indicates problem with manual dexterity and finger-thumb opposition

From Seidel HM et al: *Mosby's guide to physical examination*, ed 4, St Louis, 1999, Mosby.

ASSESSMENT TECHNIQUES—MUSCULOSKELETAL SYSTEM

Assessment	Normal Findings	Deviations From Normal
• Inspect gait as client walks into examination room and stands.	• Gait is normal, with arms swinging freely at sides.	• Dragging of the foot, shuffling, or unsteady gait may indicate neurological problem (see Chapter 20).
• Observe for foot dragging, shuffling or limping, balance, presence of obvious deformity in lower extremities, and position of the trunk in relation to the legs.	• Head and face lead body, and balance is good. • Toes should point straight ahead. • **Posture is erect.**	• Localized injury or deformity might also cause dragging of the foot. • Posture is stooped, angled to the side, which may indicate posturing to minimize pain.
• Stand behind client and observe postural alignment (position of hips relative to shoulders).	• Head is held erect, with hips and shoulders aligned in parallel.	• *Lordosis* is an abnormal posturing with a swayback or increased curvature of the lumbar spine.
• Look at client's ability to stand erect and note symmetry of body parts.	• There is an even contour of shoulder, level scapulae, and iliac crests, and alignment of head over gluteal folds is normal.	• *Kyphosis*, or hunchback, is an exaggeration of the posterior curvature of the thoracic spine.
• Look sideways at cervical, thoracic, and lumbar curves (Fig. 19-1).	• Normal cervical, thoracic, and lumbar curves are present.	• *Scoliosis* is lateral spinal curvature.

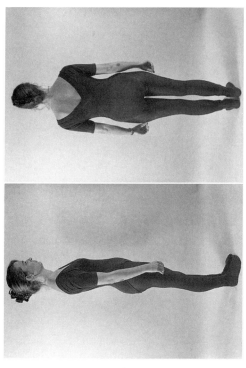

Fig. 19-1
Postural positions. **A**, Side view. **B**, Posterior view.

Assessment	Normal Findings	Deviations From Normal
• Note client's base of support and weight-bearing stability. If you detect a problem or wish to inspect gait more closely, refer to neurological examination (see Chapter 20).	• Weight is evenly distributed. • The client stands on right and left heels and toes. • Pregnant woman's base of support is shifted forward with a compensatory lordosis and forward cervical flexion.	
• Make a general observation of the extremities. • Look at overall size, gross deformity, bony enlargement, alignment, and symmetry.	• Bilateral symmetry exists in length, circumference, alignment, and the position and number of skin folds.	• Asymmetry may indicate trauma, previous surgery, or skeletal deformity.
• Conduct gross examination of muscles. • Note size and presence of fasciculations or spasms.	• Muscle size is approximately symmetric bilaterally. Dominant forearm may be larger in laborers or athletes. • No atrophy or hypertrophy seen.	• Swelling, hemorrhage, pain, loss of function, muscular atrophy, contraction, or spasm.

- Inspect the skin and subcutaneous tissues overlying muscles, bones, and joints for discoloration, swelling, or masses.

  - Bluish or black discoloration of tissue; swelling, pain on movement, and erythema; or swelling and enlargement of soft tissue involving diarthrodial joints (e.g., fingers, feet) (Fig. 19-2).

- Gently palpate all bones, joints, and surrounding muscles in a complete examination (e.g., client with arthritis or other systemic problem).

  - Tissue tends to conform to shape of body part, without swelling or masses.

- Note any heat, tenderness, edema, crepitus, or resistance to pressure.

  - Muscle tone is firm.

  - No discomfort occurs when pressure is applied.

  - No deformities or crepitus.

  - A fracture is indicated by edema, pain, loss of function, color changes, and paresthesias.

In a focused assessment, palpate only an involved area.

Palpate any inflamed joints last.

Range of Joint Motion and Muscle Tone and Strength

When client has obvious traumatic injury to the bone or joint, do not assess ROM. A physician or qualified practitioner will fully assess the extent of injury.

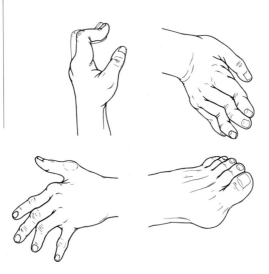

Fig. 19-2
Typical deformities of rheumatoid arthritis.
(From Lewis SM et al: *Medical-surgical nursing*, ed 5, St Louis, 2000, Mosby.)

Assessment	Normal Findings	Deviations From Normal
• Assist client in putting each major joint through its full ROM (Table 19-3, Figures 19-3 through 19-6).		
• Observe equality of motion in same body parts.		
• Give client adequate space to move each muscle group.		
• *Active motion:* Instruct client in moving each joint through its normal range independently.	• Full active ROM is present in all joints with good muscle tone.	
• *Passive motion:* Have client relax. Support the extremity at the joint while you move the joint passively until the end of the range is felt.	• ROM is equal between contralateral joints.	
Do not force any joint through its ROM.		

Table 19-3   Terminology for Normal Range of Motion Positions

Term	Range of Motion	Examples of Joints
Flexion	Movement decreasing angle between two adjoining bones; bending of limb	Elbow, fingers, knee
Extension	Movement increasing angle between two adjoining bones	Elbow, knee, fingers
Hyperextension	Movement of body part beyond its normal resting extended position	Head
Pronation	Movement of body part so that frontal or ventral surface faces downward	Hand, forearm
Supination	Movement of body part so that the front or ventral surface faces upward	Hand, forearm
Abduction	Movement of extremity away from midline of body	Leg, arm, fingers
Adduction	Movement of extremity toward midline of body	Leg, arm, fingers
Internal rotation	Rotation of joint inward	Knee, hip
External rotation	Rotation of joint outward	Knee, hip
Eversion	Turning of body part away from midline	Foot
Inversion	Turning of body part toward midline	Foot
Dorsiflexion	Flexion of toes and foot upward	Foot
Plantar flexion	Bending of toes and foot downward	Foot

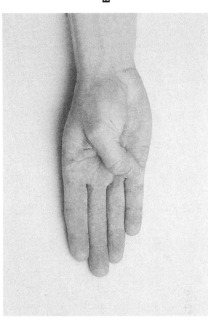

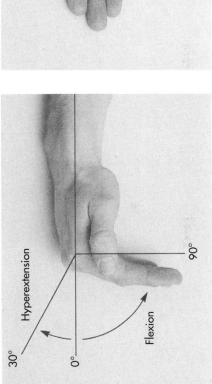

Fig. 19-3

Range of motion of the hand and wrist. **A,** Metacarpophalangeal flexion and hyperextension. **B,** Finger flexion; thumb to each fingertip and to the base of the little finger.

(From Seidel HM et al: *Mosby's guide to physical examination,* ed 4, St Louis, 1999, Mosby.)

Continued

D

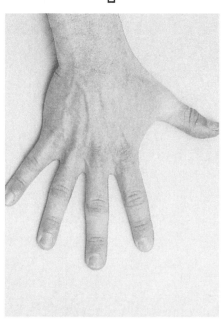

C

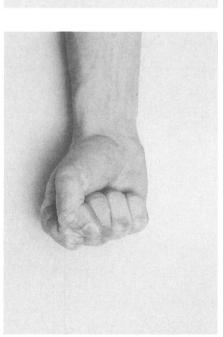

Fig. 19-3, cont'd
C, Finger flexion; fist formation. **D,** Finger abduction.
(From Seidel HM et al: *Mosby's guide to physical examination,* ed 4, St Louis, 1999, Mosby.)

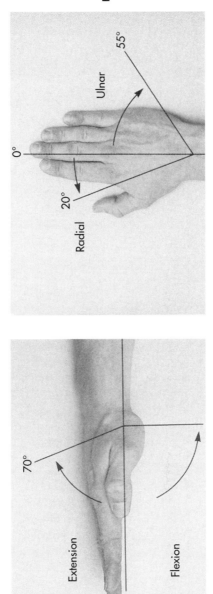

Fig. 19-3, cont'd
E, Wrist flexion and hyperextension. **F,** Wrist radial and ulnar movement.
(From Seidel HM et al: *Mosby's guide to physical examination,* ed 4, St Louis, 1999, Mosby.)

Fig. 19-4
Range of motion of the hip. **A,** Hip flexion, leg extended.
B, Hip hyperextension, knee extended.
(From Seidel HM et al: *Mosby's guide to physical examination*, ed 4, St Louis,
1999, Mosby.)

Continued

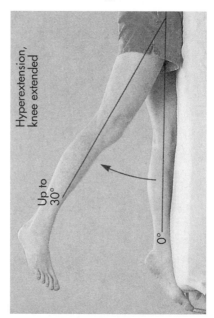

B

Hyperextension,
knee extended

Up to
30°

0°

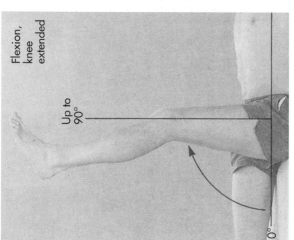

Flexion,
knee
extended

Up to 90°

0°

A

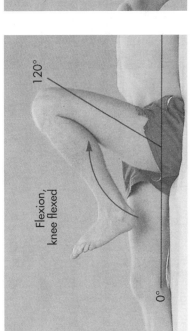

Fig. 19-4, cont'd

C, Hip flexion, knee flexed. **D,** Abduction.

(From Seidel HM et al: *Mosby's guide to physical examination,* ed 4, St Louis, 1999, Mosby.) *Continued*

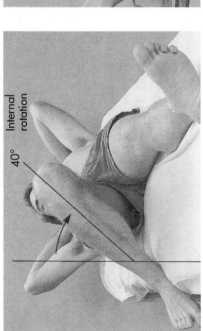

Fig. 19-4, cont'd
E, Internal rotation. **F,** External rotation.
(From Seidel HM et al: *Mosby's guide to physical examination,* ed 4, St Louis, 1999, Mosby.)

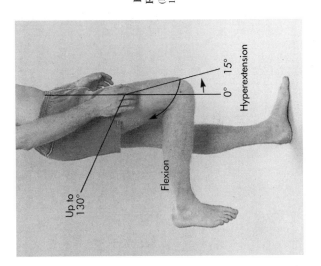

Fig. 19-5
Range of motion of the knee: flexion and extension.
(From Seidel HM et al: *Mosby's guide to physical examination*, ed 4, St Louis, 1999, Mosby.)

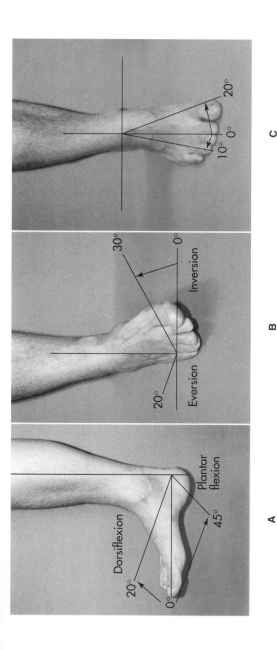

A

B

C

Fig. 19-6
Range of motion of the foot and ankle. **A**, Dorsiflexion and plantar flexion. **B**, Inversion and eversion. **C**, Abduction and adduction.
(From Seidel HM et al: *Mosby's guide to physical examination*, ed 4, St Louis, 1999, Mosby.)

Assessment	Normal Findings	Deviations From Normal
• If a joint appears to have increased or limited ROM, measure precise degree of motion with goniometer:		
• Position center of protractor at center of joint being measured.		
• Extend each arm of goniometer along body parts extending from joint.		
• Measure joint angle before moving joint.		
• Move the joint through its full ROM, and measure angle again (Fig. 19-7).	• ROM angle is full for measured joint.	• Decreased ROM.
• Compare reading with normal degree of joint movement.		

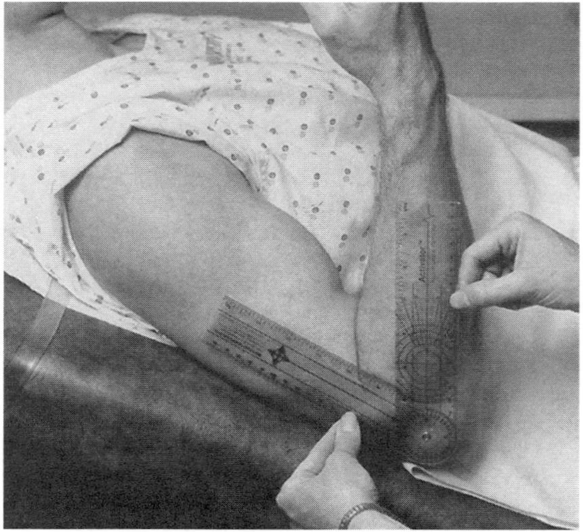

Fig. 19-7
Measuring ROM with goniometer.

Assessment	Normal Findings	Deviations From Normal
• While measuring ROM, note any instability of joint:		
• Palpate for unusual movement of joint during its movement. Note any deformity.		
• Palpate joint for swelling, stiffness, tenderness, and heat; note any redness.	• No discomfort should occur when applying pressure to bones and joints. • No nodules or evidence of swelling is seen.	• Swelling, stiffness, tenderness, heat, redness.
• While assessing ROM, ask client to allow extremity to relax or hang limp. • Support extremity and move limb through ROM to detect muscular resistance (Fig. 19-8).	• Normal tone causes mild, even resistance to movement through entire ROM.	• Hypertonicity (increased tone) occurs with sudden movement of joint, causing considerable resistance. • Hypotonic (decreased tone) muscle moves without resistance; muscle feels flabby.

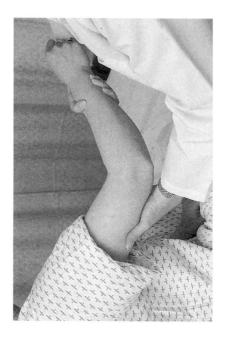

Fig. 19-8
Nurse assesses muscle tone.
(From Potter PA, Perry AG: *Fundamentals of nursing*, ed 5, St Louis, 2001, Mosby.)

Assessment	Normal Findings	Deviations From Normal

- Assess muscle strength.

- Be sure client is in a stable position, one that will allow active contraction of muscle groups.

- Assess muscle strength by gradually applying increasing pressure to muscle group.

- Have client resist pressure applied by trying to move against resistance (e.g., flex elbow).

- Have client maintain resistance until told to stop.

- Compare symmetric groups.

- For example: Place hand on side of client's face (Fig. 19-9) as client turns head laterally against resistance (neck muscles).

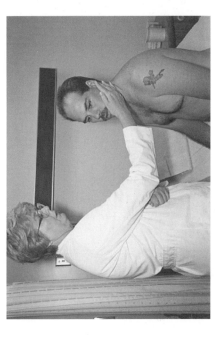

Fig. 19-9
Testing muscle strength.

Assessment	Normal Findings	Deviations From Normal
• Place one hand over each of the client's deltoid muscles. Have the client abduct arm to 90 degrees; have client hold position against resistance (deltoid muscle).	• Muscle strength is bilaterally symmetric with resistance to opposition.	
• Place one hand on dorsal surface of client's neutrally positioned foot as client tries to bend foot up (ankle and foot).	• Dominant arm may be slightly stronger than nondominant arm.	
Client's position should not be one that would easily cause a loss of balance or a fall.		
Rate muscle strength on a scale of 0 to 5:		
• **0** = No voluntary contraction		
• **1** = Slight contractility, no movement		
• **2** = Full ROM, passive		
• **3** = Full ROM, active		

- **4** = Full ROM against gravity, some resistance
- **5** = Full ROM against gravity, full resistance
- If muscle weakness is noted, measure muscle size by placing a tape measure around muscle body's circumference and compare with opposite side.

- Circumference is symmetric bilaterally.
- Dominant side of upper or lower extremity may be larger in athletes or laborers.

- Reduced circumference indicates muscle atrophy.
- A muscle that is atrophied or reduced in size may feel soft and boggy on palpation.

UNEXPECTED ASSESSMENT FINDINGS—MUSCULOSKELETAL SYSTEM

Assessment Findings	Significance	Next Step
Marked swelling, hematoma, ecchymosis, bruising, pain, and loss of function of extremity or joint.	Serious muscle sprain.	• Immobilize the extremity or joint, elevate, and apply ice. • Notify physician of finding. • Assess level of pain, weight bearing, and use.

Assessment Findings	Significance	Next Step
• Muscular atrophy.	• Can be the result of disuse from paralysis.	• Perform appropriate neurological assessment (see Chapter 20). • Record and report findings. • Assess ROM and determine limits. • Provide appropriate support (e.g., splint, brace, and sling).
• A fracture of the bone.	• Can cause muscle contractions and spasms leading to shortening of tissue around the bone.	• In acute injury, immobilize the extremity, elevate, evaluate severity of pain, notify physician, and apply ice. • Assess for weight bearing, compound fracture and neurological deficit (see Chapter 20). • Record and report findings.
• Bluish or black discoloration of tissues.	• Indicates hematoma or bruising.	• Assess for recent injury. • Apply ice, elevate, and limit use. • Record and report findings.

- Swelling, pain on movement, and erythema of major joint.
- Bursitis is an inflamed bursa.

  - Have client reduce weight bearing and use of involved joint.
  - Evaluate for neurological deficit (see Chapter 20).
  - Record and report findings.

- Swelling and enlargement of soft tissue involving diarthrodial joints (e.g., fingers, feet) (Fig. 19-2).
- Rheumatoid arthritis.
- Rheumatoid arthritis causes joints to sometimes feel warm to the touch.

  - Report finding to physician.
  - Administer nonsteroidal anti-inflammatory (NSAID) medications as ordered.
  - Record medication and assessment.

- Decreased ROM.
- Can be the result of chronic contracture or deformity (painless) or from painful conditions such as muscle strain, sprain, or fracture.

  - Assess for limitations of movement.
  - If acute injury, reduce weight bearing, apply ice, and elevate affected area.
  - If chronic contracture or deformity, ask client how to position extremity for maximal comfort.
  - Record and report findings.

Assessment Findings	Significance	Next Step
• Joint swelling.	• Can indicate cyst, bony overgrowth, arthritic changes, hematoma, or fracture.	• Evaluate for range of motion, crepitus, tenderness, and heat for palpable mass. • Notify physician of new findings. • Be prepared for neurological examination (see Chapter 20) and possible order for X-ray examination of involved joint or extremity. • Record and report findings.

Pediatric Considerations

■ Fully undress an infant and observe the posture and spontaneous generalized movements.

■ In the neonate the spine is gently rounded rather than the characteristic S shape. Hyperflexibility of the joints is characteristic of Down syndrome.

■ Arms and legs should flex symmetrically in infants. The axillary, gluteal, femoral, and popliteal creases should also be symmetric, and the limbs should move freely (Seidel et al, 1999).

■ Newborns have some resistance to full extension of the elbows, hips, and knees.

■ A newborn's hands should open periodically with the fingers fully extended. When the hand is fisted, the thumb is positioned inside the fingers.

- Infants should be checked for hip dislocation throughout the first 12 months of life. (This maneuver requires a special examination technique.)
- An infant has a bowlegged pattern until 18 to 24 months of age. Young children have a lumbar curvature of the spine and a protuberant abdomen.
- Toddlers usually have a wide-based gait until 2 years of age.
- Watch children during play to assess musculoskeletal function.

 Gerontologic Considerations

- The older adult fatigues easily; has a slower reaction time as a result of a decrease in nerve conduction and muscle tone; and may not display smooth, coordinated movement. Allow clients in this age-group adequate time for rest during the physical examination.
- Older adults have a decrease in muscle mass, tone, and strength as a result of a decrease in muscle cell decreases. The elasticity of the ligaments, tendons, and muscles also decrease (Lueckenotte, 2000).
- Older adult men take smaller steps and have a wider base of support. Women become bowlegged, with a narrow base of support, causing a waddling gait (Lueckenotte, 2000).

- Older clients lose height because intervertebral space narrows as a result of water loss. The curve of the back flattens, resulting in a decrease in the flexion and extension of the lower back (Lueckenotte, 2000).
- The client's posture may display increased dorsal kyphosis, with flexion of the hips and knees. Extremities may appear long if the trunk has diminished in length.
- It is especially important to assess an older adult's functional abilities (Table 19-3).
- Fractures are common in the older adult. Care should be taken to reduce the older adult's risk for falls.
- Older adults are at greater risk for osteoporosis and stress fractures, osteopenia, osteoarthritis, rheumatoid arthritis, and polymyalgia rheumatica.

 Cultural Considerations

- Motor development of African-American infants is often advanced over that of whites; thus African-American children under 3 years of age may reach developmental milestones earlier. White children start to catch up by 3 years of age (Seidel et al, 1999).

- There is a high prevalence of arthritis, including rheumatoid arthritis, among selected American Indians (Giger, 1999).
- Osteoporosis is less prevalent in African-American women than in white women.
- Eskimos and Native Americans are more likely to have 25 vertebrae than other races (Seidel et al, 1999).
- Femurs of Native Americans are often quite convex anteriorly, while African Americans usually have straight femurs (Seidel et al, 1999).
- Elongated second tarsal is seen most often in Melanesians, Vietnamese and Caucasians. African Americans have the lowest incidence (Lueckenotte, 2000).

Client Teaching

- Instruct the client about correct posture. Consult with a physical therapist about exercises to improve the client's posture.
- Explain to clients with low back pain that they can benefit from modification of worker risk factors (e.g., lifting heavy weights, use of protective equipment), regular aerobic exercise, exercises that strengthen the back and increase trunk flexibility, and learning how to lift properly.

- Instruct the client on a proper exercise program to promote good bone health, such as walking three or more times a week. Instruct on risk factors for osteoporosis (Box 19-1). Encourage calcium intake of 1000 to 1500 mg per day.
- Postmenopausal women need 1500 mg of calcium per day. Increased vitamin D will aid calcium absorption and is especially important in the older adult who has decreased vitamin D absorption from the sun.
- For clients with osteoporosis, instruct on proper body mechanics and ROM (e.g., swimming) and moderate weight-bearing exercises (e.g., walking, light weight lifting) to minimize trauma and subsequent bone fractures.
- Instruct older adults on the use of assistive devices such as zippers on clothing instead of buttons, elevated chairs to minimize bending of hips and knees, and use of crutches and walkers.
- Instruct older adults to pace activities to compensate for loss in muscle strength.
- Discuss pain-relief measures such as relaxation, massage, distraction, and heat applications.
- For clients with an unstable gait, discuss safety precautions in the home such as removal of throw rugs and installation of grab bars alongside stairs.

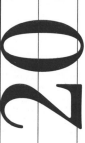

20

Neurological System

The neurological system assessment includes the following: mental and emotional status, behavior and appearance, language function, intellectual function, cranial nerve function, sensory function, motor function, and reflexes. Assessment of neurological functions can be complex because of the factors that influence function, such as oxygenation, metabolic balance, and circulatory status. The examination can be time consuming, but neurological measurements can be integrated with other parts of the physical examination. For example, mental and emotional status can be observed while taking the nursing history. Reflexes can be measured during the musculoskeletal system examination. Your judgment is necessary in determining the extent of a neurological examination.

Anatomy and Physiology

The central nervous system (CNS) is composed of the brain and spinal cord. The CNS coordinates and controls body functions through the reception, storage, processing, and transmission of information.

The peripheral nervous system (PNS) is composed of motor (efferent) and sensory (afferent) nerves that carry information to and from the CNS. The motor division has two subdivisions: the somatic, or voluntary, nervous system and the autonomic, or involuntary, nervous system. Sympathetic and parasympathetic branches of the autonomic nervous system regulate nervous activity. The neurological system is responsible for initiation and coordination of movement, reception and perception of sensory stimuli, organization of thought processes, control of cognitive and voluntary behaviors such as speech, and storage of memory. The neurological system is closely integrated with all other body systems, particularly the endocrine system.

The brain is composed of the cerebrum, cerebellum, and brainstem and continues with the spinal cord, which extends from the foramen magnum to the lower border of the first lumbar vertebra. The two cerebral hemispheres comprise the greatest mass of the cerebrum. The outer layer, or cortex, integrates sensory and motor function and enables one to conduct higher-level functions dealing with behavior, learning, and language. The brain is divided into five lobes, each with a specific function (Box 20-1).

The cerebellum functions with the cerebrum in the integration of voluntary movement. By processing nerve impulses from the eyes, ears, touch receptors, and musculoskeleton, the cerebellum integrates with the vestibular system sensory data for muscle tone, equilibrium, and posture.

The brainstem consists of the midbrain, pons, and medulla and lies as a pathway between the brain and spinal cord. Nuclei from the 12 cranial nerves arise from the brainstem. The brainstem controls important vital functions such as respiratory, circulatory, and vasomotor activities; controls reflexes such as swallowing, coughing, pupillary response, and vomiting; and acts as a relay center for ascending and descending spinal tracts.

Fibers, grouped into tracts, run through the spinal cord carrying sensory, motor, and autonomic impulses between higher centers in the brain and the body. Myelinated fibers of the spinal cord contain the ascending (sensory) and descending (motor) tracts. The gray matter contains the nerve cell bodies, comprising the anterior and posterior horns of the spinal cord. The ascending tracts mediate various sensations by transmitting precise information about the type of stimulus and its location. The posterior (dorsal) column spinal tract carries the nerve fibers for discriminatory sensations, such as touch, joint position, two-point discrimination, deep pressure, and vibration. The spinothalamic tracts carry nerve fibers for sensations of light and crude touch, pressure, temperature, and pain. The descending tracts originate in the brain and carry impulses to various muscle groups with inhibitory or facilitatory actions. The tracts also send impulses for the control of muscle tone and posture.

Thirty-one pairs of spinal nerves arise from the spinal cord and exit at each intervertebral foramen (Fig. 20-1). The sensory and motor fibers of each spinal nerve supply and receive information in a specific part of the body called a *dermatome* (Fig. 20-2). Within the spinal cord, each spinal nerve separates into a ventral and dorsal root. Motor fibers of the ventral root carry impulses from the spinal cord to the muscles and glands. The sensory fibers of the dorsal root carry impulses from sensory receptors of the body to the spinal cord.

BOX 20-1   Functions of the Lobes of the Brain

Frontal Lobe

Voluntary skeletal movement
Speech formation
Emotions, affect, and drive
Self-awareness, appropriateness

Parietal Lobe

Processes and interprets temperature, pressure, pain, size, shape, texture, and two-point discrimination
Visual, gustatory, olfactory, and auditory sensations
Comprehension of written words and awareness of body position (proprioception)

Temporal Lobe

Perception and interpretation of sounds
Determination of source of sounds

Comprehension of the spoken word and written language
Integrates taste, smell, and balance
Integrates behavior, emotion, and personality

Occipital Lobe

Contains primary vision center

Limbic System

Responsible for behavior that determines survival, such as aggression, affection, fear, and mating

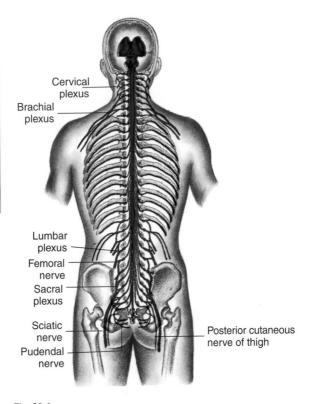

Cervical plexus

Brachial plexus

Lumbar plexus

Femoral nerve

Sacral plexus

Sciatic nerve

Pudendal nerve

Posterior cutaneous nerve of thigh

Fig. 20-1
Posterior view of exiting spinal nerves in relation to vertebrae.

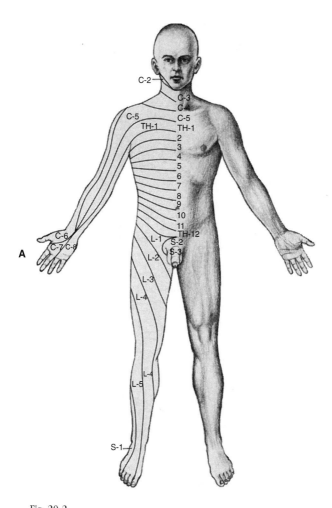

Fig. 20-2

A, Anterior view of sensory dermatomes.

(From Thompson JM et al: *Mosby's clinical nursing,* ed 5, St Louis, 2001, Mosby.)

Continued

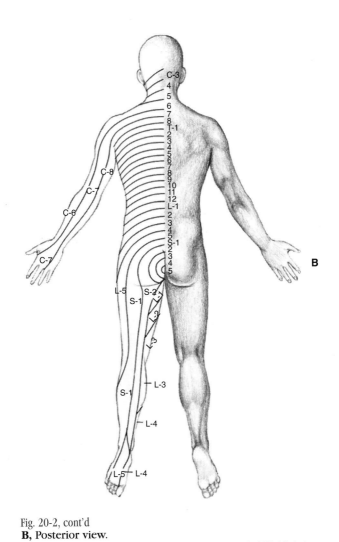

Fig. 20-2, cont'd
B, Posterior view.
(From Thompson JM et al: *Mosby's clinical nursing,* ed 5, St Louis, 2001, Mosby.)

Critical Thinking Application—Neurological System

Knowledge	Experience	Standards
• Refer to your knowledge of neurological anatomy and physiology. Clinical signs and symptoms can help localize any type of neurological pathology.	• Because the neurological system is so complicated, combining different aspects of the examination during a review of other body systems is used in practice. For example, examination of the cranial nerves can occur while examining the eyes, ears, pharynx, and head and neck; certain motor functions can be assessed while examining the musculoskeletal system.	• Because neuropathways cross within either the brain or spinal cord, remember that physical signs on one side of the body generally indicate a problem on the opposite side.
• Refer to your knowledge of communication techniques. Clients with neurological alterations may have visual, auditory, cognitive, and speech impairments, all of which can affect their ability to communicate.		• When testing neurological function, be sure the client is aroused to the highest level of consciousness possible.
• Refer to your knowledge of psychology and normal behavior. Neurological problems can create subtle and sometimes obvious behavioral changes.		• When clients have a reduced level of consciousness, it is unnecessary to raise your voice. Speak in a clear and normal tone of voice.

Knowledge	Experience	Standards
		• When testing motor function, be sure to demonstrate the maneuver you wish the client to attempt. Poor performance can result from lack of understanding the maneuver rather than neurological impairment.
		• To ensure an objective assessment, consider the client's cultural and educational background, values, beliefs, previous experiences, and current level of coping. Such factors influence a client's response to questions.

Neurological Assessment

Your assessment will focus on a client's sensory, motor, affective, and intellectual capacities. Disturbances in any of these functions can cause serious physical and psychological compromise and may make clients incapable of caring for themselves. Neurological disorders often place a client at significant risk for injury. Neurological deficits can have an effect on a client's self-concept and create a significant threat to the lifestyle of clients and their family members.

Equipment

- Reading material
- Vials containing aromatic substances (e.g., vanilla, coffee)
- Familiar objects (e.g., coin, paper clip)
- Tongue blades (2)
- Snellen chart
- Penlight
- Vials containing sugar or salt
- Two test tubes, one filled with hot water and one filled with cold water
- Cotton balls or cotton-tipped applicators
- Tuning fork
- Reflex hammer

Delegation Considerations

The neurological examination requires critical thinking and knowledge application unique to a professional nurse. Delegation of the neurological examination to assistive personnel is inappropriate. Assistive personnel should know to inform you of any changes in a client's behavior or level of consciousness. When caring for clients with motor or sensory limitations, inform care providers of the safety precautions and position requirements needed to prevent injury to the client.

Client Preparation

- During the mental and emotional assessment, a client may assume a comfortable sitting or lying position.
- A client sits during cranial nerve assessment.
- Assessment of sensory, motor, and reflex function can require the client to assume various positions.

- Discuss with the client's spouse, family members, or friends any recent changes in the client's behavior (for example, increased irritability, mood swings, memory loss).
- Assess client for history of changes in vision, hearing, smell, taste, and touch.
- If an older adult client displays sudden acute confusion (delirium), review history for drug toxicity (anticholinergics, diuretics, digoxin, cimetidine, sedatives, antihypertensives, antidysrhythmics), serious infections, metabolic disturbances, heart failure, and severe anemia.
- Has the client had a history of head or spinal cord trauma, meningitis, congenital anomalies, neurological disease, or psychiatric counseling?
- If client exhibits behavioral changes, screen for evidence of depression (for example, troubling thoughts or feelings, change in outlook on life, feeling hopeless, reduced energy level, change in eating habits, spends more time sleeping, talks about hurting self).

History

- Determine if the client is taking prescribed analgesics, sedatives, hypnotics, antipsychotics, antidepressants, or nervous system stimulants such as medications or caffeine. Also determine if the client uses illicit street drugs.
- Assess specifically the client's use of alcohol or sedative-hypnotics, which can cause tremors, ataxia, and changes in peripheral nerve function.
- Determine if client has recent history of seizures or convulsions. Clarify sequence of events that occur during a seizure (aura, fall to ground, motor activity, loss of consciousness); character of any symptoms; and relationship of seizure to time of day, fatigue, or emotional stress.
- Screen the client for headaches (including migraines), tremors, dizziness, vertigo, numbness or tingling of a body part, visual changes, weakness, pain, or changes in speech (combinations of these symptoms can indicate neurological pathology). Determine onset, duration, precipitating factors, and other concomitant symptoms.

ASSESSMENT TECHNIQUES—NEUROLOGICAL SYSTEM

Assessment	Normal Findings	Deviations From Normal
• Perform a focused neurological assessment when client has no neurological illness, symptoms, or recent history of head or spinal cord injury or disease.		
• A focused neurological assessment includes mental status; level of consciousness; orientation to person, place and time; pupillary reflexes; movement of extremities; sensation; and deep tendon reflexes.		
Mental and Emotional Status		
• While interacting with the client throughout the examination, pose questions and observe the appropriateness of emotions and thoughts expressed.		

Assessment	Normal Findings	Deviations From Normal
• For client who is alert and conscious, conduct a mental status examination. Folstein's Mini-Mental State (MMS) is a good tool (see Chapter 6).	• Client demonstrates immediate recall of past events; is able to perform cognitive exercises. Maximum score on MMS is 30.	• Depressed clients without dementia usually score between 24 and 30. A score of 21 or less is found in clients with dementia, delirium, schizophrenia, or an affective disorder (Lueckenotte, 2000; Seidel et al, 1999).
• For client in whom alertness is questioned, assess level of consciousness and orientation by directing questions and giving instructions that require a response.		
• Be sure client is fully awake before testing.		
• Note appropriateness of emotions, responses, and ideas expressed.		
• Use the Glasgow Coma Scale (GCS) to measure consciousness objectively (Table 20-1).	• GCS score is 13 or higher.	• Client shows confusion or reduced level of consciousness.

Table 20-1	Glasgow Coma Scale	
Action	Response	Score
Eyes open	Spontaneously	④
	To speech	3
	To pain	2
	None	1
Best verbal response	Oriented	⑤
	Confused	4
	Inappropriate words	3
	Incomprehensible sounds	2
	None	1
Best motor response	Obeys commands	⑥
	Localized pain	5
	Flexion withdrawal	4
	Abnormal flexion	3
	Abnormal extension	1
	Flaccid	1
	Total Score	⑮

Assessment	Normal Findings	Deviations From Normal
The GCS can be misleading in clients with sensory losses. Clients are responsive but unable to sense painful stimuli over certain areas of the body.		
• Rephrase or ask similar question if uncertain whether client understands.		
• For client whose responses are inappropriate, ask short, to-the-point questions regarding information the client knows (e.g., "Tell me your name," "Tell me where you live," "What is the name of this place?").	• Client is able to respond to questions correctly with little hesitancy.	• Client is slow to respond and difficult to arouse, fails to answer all questions correctly, or is unable to respond.
• For client who is unable to respond to questions of orientation, offer simple commands (e.g., "Squeeze my fingers," "Move your toes").	• Client responds appropriately to command.	• Client fails to respond to command. Inability to move extremity (especially on one side) indicates motor deficit rather than change in level of consciousness.

- Client fails to respond to command. Test response to painful stimuli by applying firm pressure with thumb over root of client's fingernail.

Do not pinch skin; it can cause bruising.

Behavior and Appearance

- During initial general survey (see Chapter 6) and throughout the examination, observe the client's mannerisms and actions, noting verbal and nonverbal behaviors.

- Does the client respond appropriately to directions?

- What type of mood is displayed?

- Does the client cooperate with the examination?

- Client withdraws hand from painful stimulus.

- The client should behave in a manner expressing concern and interest in the examination.

- Client should make eye contact with you. Client normally is anxious or concerned about findings.

- No response to pain, indicating severe lowering of consciousness.

- Euphoria or lack of concern is exhibited.

Assessment	Normal Findings	Deviations From Normal
• Observe client's appearance: personal hygiene, cleanliness, choice of clothing and appropriateness to setting and type of weather, and use and appropriateness of makeup.	• Client is well-groomed and shows appropriate dress for weather.	• Appearance is unkempt, choice of clothing is inappropriate for weather, and makeup is excessive. May be result of emotional problem, psychiatric disturbance, or organic brain syndrome. **Variations in appearance may result from cultural preference, inability to attend to or perform self-care, inability to keep clothing clean, or poor self-image.**
Language • Observe manner of client's speech. • Note voice inflection, tone, and volume. When apparent communication with a client is unclear (e.g., misuse of	• The client's voice should have inflections, be clear and strong, and increase in volume appropriately. • Speech should be fluent and articulate.	• Speech is slow and slurred.

words, hesitations, creation of new words), assess the following:

- Ask the client to name familiar objects to which you point.

- Ask the client to respond to simple verbal and written commands such as "Stand up" or "Sit down."

- Ask the client to read simple sentences out loud.

Intellectual Function

- Use an approach that does not threaten or make the client feel uncomfortable.

- Ask questions about concepts or ideas with which the client is familiar.

- Client names objects correctly.

- Client can follow commands.

- Client reads sentences correctly.

- Client is unable to name objects appropriately.

- Client is unable to follow commands.

- Inability of client to understand spoken or written words may indicate a form of aphasia (expressive, receptive, or global).

Assessment	Normal Findings	Deviations From Normal
• Ask client to repeat a short series of numbers forward and then backward (e.g., 7, 3, 1 and 1, 3, 7). Gradually increase the number of digits until client fails to repeat digits correctly.	• Immediate recall: client is able to repeat series of five to eight digits forward and four to six backward.	• Immediate recall is impaired; associated possibly with depression or diffuse brain disease.
• Refer to MMS examination for test of short-term memory, registration, and recall (see Chapter 6).	• Client is able to name three objects and recall them later during the examination.	• Client is unable to recall objects.
• Have client recall verifiable events occurring during the same day, such as what was eaten for breakfast or form of transport used to arrive at clinic or hospital.	• Client recalls events.	• Impairment can be related to various neurological or psychiatric disorders.
• Ask client to recall previous medical history or family history of illness; ask date of client's birthday or a special day in history.		• Loss of immediate and recent memory with retention of remote memory suggests dementia (Seidel et al, 1999).

- Ask open-ended questions rather than simple "Yes" or "No" questions.

- Confirm the client's answers with family or friends if necessary.

- Have client follow a series of commands (e.g., tap your head, smile, raise one finger) or repeat a short story you relate.

- Client's attention span is normal.

Ask client to identify analogies or associations between terms or simple concepts. Go from simple to complex:

- What is similar about these objects: a plane and a bird, a tree and a rose, a river and a lake?

- Complete the following comparison: A dog is to a beagle as a cat is to a _____.

- Fatigue, anxiety, or medication effects may cause easy distraction, confusion, or impaired memory.

Assessment	Normal Findings	Deviations From Normal
• What is the difference between these two objects: a computer and a typewriter, a doctor and a nurse?	• Client makes correct analogy or association.	• Inability to describe similarities or differences can be caused by pathology of the cerebral cortex or by lower intelligence.
• Ask the client (without paper and pencil) to perform simple arithmetic calculations: Subtract 6 from 40 and 6 from that answer, etc. Add 9 to 60 and 9 to that, etc.	• Calculations should be completed within a minute, with few errors.	• Impairment of arithmetic skills can be associated with depression and diffuse brain disease.
• Ask client a series of questions designed to measure judgment and reasoning: Ask what client knows about reason for hospitalization, plans for the future, or how the client would react if he or she suddenly became ill at home.	• Client exhibits clear reasoning; evaluates situation, and offers appropriate response.	• Explanations are incongruent; judgment is impaired.
• Have client explain meaning of simple proverb (e.g., "A stitch in time saves nine," "Don't count your chickens before they're hatched"). Note if	• Abstract reasoning is intact, as evidenced by adequate interpretation of phrase.	• Abstract reasoning can be impaired by organic brain syndrome, brain damage, or lack of intelligence.

the client's explanation is relevant and concrete.

Cranial Nerve Function

- Assess the function of each of the 12 cranial nerves (Table 20-2).

- Many of the tests can be integrated during earlier portions of the physical examination.

Sensory Function

- Perform all sensory testing with client's eyes closed and be sure not to give client cues as to correct response (e.g., pattern in which body part is stimulated).

- All cranial nerves are intact.

The client's ability to perform intellectual functions has implications for the remainder of the neurological examination. You may have to skip or delay parts of the examination that require feedback if the client is confused or irritable.

- Inability to perform as expected.

Table 20-2 Cranial Nerve Function and Assessment

Number	Name	Type	Function	Method
I	Olfactory	Sensory	Sense of smell	Ask client to identify different nonirritating aromas such as coffee and vanilla.
II	Optic	Sensory	Visual acuity	Use Snellen chart or ask client to read printed material while wearing glasses.
III	Oculomotor	Motor	Extraocular eye movement	Assess directions of gaze.
IV	Trochlear	Motor	Pupil constriction and dilation	Measure pupil reaction to light reflex and accommodation.
			Upward and downward movement of eyeball	Assess directions of gaze.
V	Trigeminal	Sensory and motor	Sensory nerve to skin of face	Lightly touch cornea with wisp of cotton. Assess corneal reflex. Measure sensation of light pain and touch across skin of face.
			Motor nerve to muscles of jaw	Palpate temples as client clenches teeth.
VI	Abducens	Motor	Lateral movement of eyeballs	Assess directions of gaze.

Continued

Table 20-2	Cranial Nerve Function and Assessment—cont'd			
Number	Name	Type	Function	Method
VII	Facial	Sensory and motor	Facial expression	As client smiles, frowns, puffs out cheeks, and raises and lowers eyebrows, look for asymmetry.
			Taste	Have client identify salty or sweet taste on front of tongue.
VIII	Auditory	Sensory	Hearing	Assess ability to hear spoken word.
IX	Glossopharyngeal	Sensory and motor	Taste	Ask client to identify sour or sweet taste on back of tongue.
X	Vagus	Sensory and motor	Sensation of pharynx	Ask client to say "Ah." Observe palate and pharynx movement.
			Movement of vocal cords	Assess speech for hoarseness.
XI	Spinal accessory	Motor	Movement of head and shoulders	Ask client to shrug shoulders and turn head against passive resistance.
XII	Hypoglossal	Motor	Position of tongue	Ask client to stick out tongue to midline and move it from side to side.

Assessment	Normal Findings	Deviations From Normal
• Ask client to say when a particular stimulus is perceived. Be sure to test sensation bilaterally.		
Perform the following tests on the client's hands, lower arms, feet, and lower legs:		
(If impairment is found, describe by the distribution of major peripheral nerves or dermatomes.) (See Fig. 20-2.)		
• *Light touch:* Apply light wisp of cotton to sensitive points along the skin's surface (face, neck, top of hands). Ask client to voice when sensation is felt.		
It is always important to show the client what you will be using to test sensation. Then have client close eyes to test sensation, e.g., "Tell me where you feel being touched."		

- *Pain Sensation:* Break one end of a tongue blade. Alternately apply the sharp and blunt ends of the tongue blade to the skin's surface. Note areas of numbness or increased sensitivity by asking if client feels a "sharp" or "dull" sensation.

- *Vibratory Sensation:* Apply stem of vibrating tuning fork to the distal interphalangeal joint of fingers and interphalangeal joint of great toe, elbow, and wrist. Ask client to indicate when vibration is first felt and when vibration stops. Ensure client feels vibration and not just pressure.

- *Position Sense:* Grasp finger or toe, holding it by its sides with thumb and index finger. Alternate moving finger or toe up and down. Ask client to state when finger (or toe) is up or down. Perform on both sides and with fingers and toes.

Assessment	Normal Findings	Deviations From Normal
• *Temperature:* Touch skin with test tube filled with hot or cold water. Ask client if sensation of hot or cold is felt. (Omit if pain sensation is normal.)		• Impaired sensory reception can be the result of local peripheral nerve injury, spinal cord injury, or disturbance in sensory cortex.
• *Two-point discrimination:* Using two 10-gauge wires, lightly apply one or both simultaneously to skin's surface. Ask client if one or two pricks are felt. Find distance at which client can no longer distinguish two points.	• Sensation for touch, pain, vibration, and position is intact. • Client can discriminate two points as close as 2 to 8 mm (fingertips), 8 to 12 mm (palms), 40 mm (forearms), and 75 mm (upper arms and thighs) (Barkauskas, 1998).	
Test the client's cognitive ability to interpret sensations:		
• *Stereognosis:* Place a coin or paper clip in client's hand and ask client to identify object.	• Client is cognitively able to interpret sensation and identify object (stereognosis).	• Client incorrectly identifies object.

- *Graphesthesia:* Draw a letter or number with the end of a tongue blade on the client's palm. Have the client identify the figure.

- Client is able to readily recognize figure or letter drawn on palm.

- Letter or number cannot be identified. Inability to perform these tests may indicate lesion of the sensory cortex or posterior columns of spinal cord (Seidel et al, 1999).

Motor Function
Gait

- Assess gait, stance, gross muscle movement, involuntary muscle movement, and muscle strength and tone following procedures described in musculoskeletal assessment (see Chapter 19).

- To further assess gait, ask client to walk a straight line with eyes open, then turn and walk back with eyes closed. Note gait sequence, arm movements, and degree of steadiness. **Stand near client with your arms extended, but not touching client.**

- Client walks with first heel striking the floor and then moving to full contact with the floor.

- Second heel pushes off, leaving the ground.

- Body weight transfers from first heel to the ball of its foot.

- Client shuffles, staggers, reels, has leg lag, or has foot flop. Gait abnormalities may be caused by alterations such as pinched sciatic nerve (foot flop), hemiparesis (dragging or circling stiffly), cerebellar ataxia (wide based and staggering), or sensory

Assessment	Normal Findings	Deviations From Normal
		ataxia (wide based, feet thrown forward and out, client watches ground).
	• Leg swing accelerates as weight is removed from second foot.	
	• Second foot is lifted and travels ahead of the weight-bearing first foot, swinging through.	
	• Second foot slows in preparation for heel strike. Balance is steady.	
Test client's coordination and fine motor skills. For each of the following tests, demonstrate the maneuver first, then have the client repeat the maneuver, noting smoothness, rhythm, and speed:		
• *Romberg's Test:* Client stands with feet close together, arms at the sides, eyes closed. Note presence of swaying. (Stand close to client with arms outstretched to catch client in case of fall.)	• Slight swaying is expected but should not cause risk of falling.	• Loss of balance (positive Romberg's test) indicates cerebellar ataxia or vestibular (CN VIII) dysfunction.

- *Rapid Alternating Movement:* Ask client to sit. Demonstrate for client the method for rapidly striking thigh with palm of hand, evenly, without hesitation. Have client repeat.

  Next demonstrate and have client alternately strike thigh with hand supinated and then pronated.

- *Finger to Finger Test:* Stand in front of client, holding your index finger stationary 2 feet away from client's face.

- *Finger to Nose Test:* Ask client to touch your finger with index finger and then to touch own nose alternately.

- Test lower extremities for coordination by asking the client to lie supine.

- Place your hand at ball of client's foot. Ask client to tap hand with foot as quickly as possible. Note speed and smoothness of movement.

- Client performs all maneuvers smoothly, rhythmically, and with increasing speed.

- Taps foot evenly and quickly without hesitation.

- Stiff, slow, or nonrhythmic movement can indicate proprioception or cerebellar dysfunction.

- Tremors of hand may appear.

Assessment	Normal Findings	Deviations From Normal
Reflexes • Assess deep tendon reflexes (Table 20-3). • Reflexes are graded 0 to 4. 0> No response. 1 = Low normal with slight muscle contraction. 2 = Normal, visible muscle twitch and movement of arm/leg. 3 = Brisker than normal but may not indicate disease. 4 = Hyperactive, very brisk; spinal cord disorder suspected.	• Reflexes are symmetrical.	• Absent or hyperactive reflexes.

Table 20-3 Common Reflexes

Type	Procedure	Normal Reflex
Deep Tendon Reflexes		
Biceps	Flex the client's arm up to 45 degrees at the elbow with palms down; place your thumb in the antecubital fossa at the base of the biceps tendon and your fingers over the biceps muscle; strike the thumb with the reflex hammer	Flexion of arm at elbow
Triceps	Flex the client's arm at the elbow up to 90 degrees, holding the arm across the chest, or hold the upper arm horizontally and allow the lower arm to go limp; strike the triceps tendon, just above the elbow	Extension at elbow
Patellar	Have the client sit with legs hanging freely over the side of the table or chair or have the client lie supine and support knee in a flexed 90-degree position; briskly tap the patellar tendon just below the patella	Extension of lower leg
Achilles'	Have the client assume the same position as for patellar reflex; slightly dorsiflex the client's ankle by grasping the toes in the palm of your hand; strike Achilles' tendon just above the heel at the ankle malleoli	Plantar flexion of foot
Plantar (Babinski)	Have the client lie supine with legs straight and feet relaxed; take the handle end of the reflex hammer and stroke the lateral aspect of the sole from the heel to the ball of the foot, curving across the ball to the medial side	Bending of the toes downward

Continued

Table 20-3 Common Reflexes—cont'd

Type	Procedure	Normal Reflex
Cutaneous Reflexes		
Guteal	Have the client assume a side-lying position; spread apart the client's buttocks and lightly stimulate the perineal area with a cotton-tipped applicator	Contraction of anal sphincter
Abdominal	Have the client stand or lie supine; stroke the abdominal skin with the base of a cotton-tipped applicator over the lateral borders of the rectus abdominal muscles toward the midline; repeat the test in each abdominal quadrant	Rectus abdominal muscles contract with pulling of umbilicus toward the stimulated side
Cremasteric	Stroke the inner upper thigh of the male client, using a cotton-tipped applicator	Scrotum elevates on stimulated side

Assessment	Normal Findings	Deviations From Normal
• Have client relax extremity to be tested and avoid voluntary movement.		
• Position limb to slightly stretch the muscle being tested.		
• Palpate each tendon to locate correct point for stimulation.		
• Hold reflex hammer loosely so it can swing freely between thumb and fingers.		
• Tap tendon briskly (Fig. 20-3).		
• Compare symmetry of reflex from one side of body to the other.		

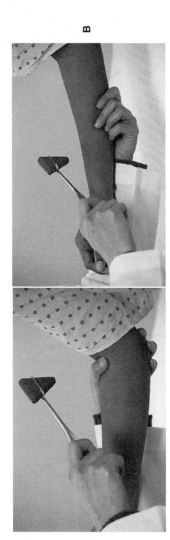

B

A

Fig. 20-3

Checking reflexes. **A,** Biceps. **B,** Brachioradial.
(From Seidel HM et al: *Mosby's guide to physical examination,* ed 4, St Louis, 1999, Mosby.)

Continued

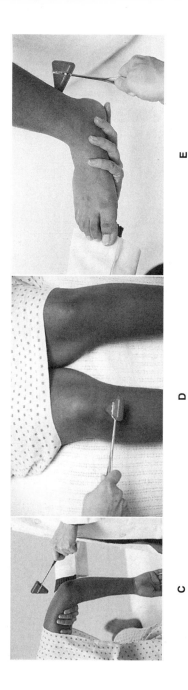

Fig. 20-3, cont'd

C, Triceps. **D,** Patellar. **E,** Achilles'.

(From Seidel HM et al: *Mosby's guide to physical examination,* ed 4 St Louis, 1999, Mosby.)

Assessment	Normal Findings	Deviations From Normal
• If necessary, distract client during testing to increase reflex response by asking the client to clench teeth while testing upper extremities or asking the client to interlock hands and pull outward during testing of lower extremities.		

UNEXPECTED ASSESSMENT FINDINGS—NEUROLOGICAL SYSTEM

Assessment Findings	Significance	Next Step
• Confusion or reduced responsiveness. • Alterations in level of consciousness (in order of increasing alteration): • Irritability, short attenion span, or dulled perception of environment.	• May result from pain, fever, substance abuse, electrolyte imbalance, side effects, or toxic effects of medications, circulatory shock, severe anemia, hypoxia, diabetic coma, or liver failure.	• Evaluate possible causes of change in mental status. • Record and report findings. **Any sudden change in level of consciousness requires immediate**

- Disorientation.
- Inability to recall name or time of day.
- Inability to follow even simple commands such as "Move your toes."
- Responsive only to painful stimuli.
- Completely unresponsive to verbal and painful stimuli (comatose).

- May represent acute confusion in the older adult, worsening cerebral edema in the client with head injury, metabolic or oxygenation problem, or acute neurological event, such as a stroke or transient ischemic attack.
- Be alert for a slowly deteriorating mental status.

assessment and notification of the physician.

- Abnormal cranial nerve responses:

- Inability to identify aroma or agnosia.

- Cranial nerve I.

- Reduced visual acuity.

- Cranial nerve II.

- Correlate with other assessment findings.
- If new finding or related to recent trauma, notify physician as soon as possible.

Assessment Findings	Significance	Next Step
• Abnormal direction of gaze, pupil reacts slowly to light or is nonreactive.	• Cranial nerve III.	• Complete neurological examination to elicit other abnormalities.
• Abnormal direction of gaze in upward and downward diagonals.	• Cranial nerve IV.	• Record and report findings.
• Absent corneal reflex, absent sensation of light touch across skin of face, client unable to clench teeth.	• Cranial nerve V.	
• Abnormal direction of gaze laterally.	• Cranial nerve VI.	• Correlate with other assessment findings.
• Inability to smile symmetrically, absent or one-sided blinking and raising of eyebrows, irregular or unequal facial movement, inability to identify taste on front of tongue.	• Cranial nerve VII.	• If new finding or related to recent trauma, notify physician as soon as possible.
• Inability to hear spoken word.	• Cranial nerve VIII.	• Complete neurological examination to elicit other abnormalities.

Finding	Interpretation	Nursing Action
Inability to identify taste on back of tongue, absent gag reflex.	Cranial nerve IX.	• Record and report findings. • Correlate with other assessment findings.
Unequal or absent rise of uvula and soft palate as client says "Ah," absent gag reflex.	Cranial nerve X.	• If new finding or related to recent trauma, notify physician as soon as possible.
Inability to shrug shoulders against resistance.	Cranial nerve XI.	• Complete neurological examination to elicit other abnormalities.
Tongue deviates to side.	Cranial nerve XII.	• Record and report findings.
Absent reflexes.	May indicate neuropathy or lower motor neuron disease.	• Correlate with other assessment findings, such as low back pain or pain in the cervical thoracic area for upper extremity findings.
Hyperactive reflexes.	Suggests an upper motor neuron disorder.	• Record and report findings. • Notify physician if new finding.

- Observe children at play, noting gait and fine motor coordination. The child can hop or do the heel-to-toe test in an improvised game.
- Young children have a wide-based gait. The school-age child walks with feet closer together.

A number of reflexes to assess an infant's developmental status exist, including the following:

- *Rooting reflex:* Infant turns head toward side of face stroked (disappears at 3 to 12 months of age).
- *Grasp reflex:* Infant flexes the hand or toes when light touch is applied to the palm of the hand or the sole of the foot (disappears at 3 months of age).
- *Moro's reflex:* Sudden jarring of infant while lying down causes infant to suddenly extend and abduct extremities. Crying also is elicited (disappears at 3 to 4 months of age).
- *Stepping reflex:* Infant is held upright so that the feet touch a flat surface to stimulate walking movement (disappears at 3 to 4 weeks of age).

Pediatric Considerations

- Parents should act as resources for information regarding any recent change in child's behavior, attention span, or school performance.
- Memory testing may begin at about 4 years of age. The number of words or numbers a child can repeat in order varies by age.
- Use of the Denver Developmental Screening Test (DDST) can determine whether the child is developing language and personal-social skills as expected.
- Use a Snellen, "E," or picture chart to test child's visual acuity.
- To assess cranial nerves, often games must be played to elicit response, such as imitating the examiner puffing out the checks or making facial expressions.
- Observe child eating a cookie or cracker to assess jaw strength.
- In sensory testing, children can point to areas touched. Superficial pain is usually not tested because of child's fear of sharp objects.

Gerontologic Considerations

- The older adult may need additional time to respond to questions requiring the use of memory, judgment, or other cognitive functions.

- Commonly, older clients show symptoms of forgetfulness resulting from normal neurological changes. Sudden confusion, however, is usually unrelated to age. The older client is at greater risk of confusion from acute conditions such as dehydration, infection, drug toxicity, hyponatremia, and hypoglycemia.

- Delirium is an acute disturbance of consciousness that is accompanied by a change in cognition. Delirium cannot be accounted for by a preexisting or evolving dementia. Delirium develops over a short period of time, usually hours to days, and tends to fluctuate during the course of the day. Usually delirium is a direct physiological consequence of a general medical condition. Client has reduced clarity of awareness of environment, client's ability to focus or shift attention is impaired, person is easily distracted, there is an accompanying change in cognition (recent memory impaired, disorientation to time and place, language distur-

bance), and the client has perceptual alterations (e.g., illusions, hallucinations).

- Deterioration of intellectual function should not be found unless the client has a disease of the CNS.

- Some problem-solving skills deteriorate with aging, but this may be related to disuse. Recent memory deteriorates before remote memory.

- See Chapters 8 and 9 regarding the older adult's limitations resulting from visual and hearing impairment.

- Atrophy of the taste buds is normal in older clients.

- Conduction velocity in peripheral nerves declines with age.

- The tactile and vibratory senses are blunted, and therefore more strong stimuli are required to test this sense.

- Proprioception in the older adult becomes increasingly less functional with age.

- Older clients have reduced pain sensation bilaterally.

- A normally slow reaction time may cause coordination testing to be less rhythmic in older adults.

- Slight swaying when the client stands with feet together and eyes closed is normal for an older client.

- Reflexes are normally less brisk or even absent in older clients.

- Reflex response diminishes in the lower extremities before the upper extremities are affected (Seidel et al, 1999).

- For clients with sensory or motor impairments, explain measures to ensure the client's safety; for example, use of ambulation aids, using caution when applying ice packs or heating pads.
- Teach older clients to observe skin surfaces for areas of trauma.
- See Chapters 8 and 9 regarding instructions for clients with hearing and vision loss.
- If client has reduced corneal reflex, advise on use of ophthalmic drops to keep cornea moistened.
- If a client has difficulty swallowing, instruct family on ways to properly prepare food or assist client with feeding.
- Teach older adult to plan enough time to complete tasks, because reaction time is slowed.
- Gait is characterized by short, uncertain steps. Shuffling may also occur.

Cultural Considerations

- Many Mexican Americans believe that health represents a state of equilibrium in the universe wherein the forces of "hot," "cold," "wet," and "dry" must be balanced. Headaches may have a causative agent thought to have a hot or cold quality. If a headache is seen to be caused by a "hot" factor, cold herbs may be placed on the temples to absorb the heat. Paralysis is thought to be caused when cold air enters the body (Giger, 1999).
- Cerebrovascular disease mortality is the highest for Japanese living in Japan, intermediate for Japanese living in Hawaii, and lowest for Japanese living on the U.S. mainland.

Client Teaching

- Explain to the client's family and friends the implications of any behavioral or mental impairment shown by the client.

Nutrition

21

A nutritional assessment includes physical measurements and anthropometry, laboratory tests, dietary history and health history, and clinical observations.

You are in an excellent position to recognize signs of poor nutrition and to take steps to initiate change. Close daily contact with clients and families enables you to make observations about clients' physical status, food intake, weight gain or loss, and responses to therapy. A nutritional assessment is designed to identify clients' nutritional deficiencies that adversely affect health, to assist in planning and delivering nutritional care, and to evaluate the efficacy of nutritional care.

Critical Thinking Application—Nutrition

Knowledge	Experience	Standards
• Refer to your knowledge regarding principles of nutrition and the function of the gastrointestinal (GI) system.	• Consider the factors that influence your own appetite and selection of foods. This personal experience will help you in identifying a client's food preferences, dietary habits, and problems that result when nutrition is inadequate.	• When performing a nutritional assessment apply the following principles:
• Clients will exhibit alterations that involve either a change in dietary intake or a change in the physiological systems that influence food.		• Collaborate closely with a clinical dietitian if one is available.
• Be aware of developmental variables influencing normal nutritional needs, as well as the influence of culture on dietary preferences.	• Assessment can be very effective if performed while a client is eating or preparing food in the home.	• When assessing a client's typical diet history, assess not only the foods eaten but also how they are prepared.

Nutritional Assessment

Equipment

- Tongue blade
- Penlight
- Scale (weight-bearing or stretcher)
- Tape measure
- Skin fold caliper

Delegation Considerations

The nutritional assessment involves critical thinking and knowledge application. Nutritional assessment is inappropriate to delegate to assistive personnel. Trained assistive personnel can measure and report height and weight values, assist in measuring intake and output (I&O), and estimate solid food intake. Staff should also be informed of clients at risk for eating problems and should be instructed to report to the RN when a client's appetite and dietary intake change.

Client Preparation

- Ideally, client will stand during measurement of height and weight (see Chapter 6).

- Client may sit or lie in bed during remainder of nutritional assessment.
- Client should wear a loose-fitting gown for access to upper extremities.
- Involve a friend, domestic partner, significant other, or family member who helps in preparing food for the client (when applicable).

History

Refer to Chapter 6 for data included within a general diet history.

- Obtain a diet history, including usual intake of foods and liquids, food preferences, snacks, and normal meal times. Giving the client or family member a dietary log to complete for a week to establish food patterns over time may be helpful in determining the client's dietary habits (See Appendixes J, K, and L for food guide pyramids).
- Determine how foods are normally prepared (for example, fried, baked).
- Determine if client is on a prescribed diet or independently follows a weight-loss or special diet. How long has the client followed the diet?
- Ask if client has noticed a recent weight loss or gain and over what time period.

- Does client have any physical limitations affecting the ability to feed self (for example, weak grasp, reduced hand-eye coordination)?
- Does client have current physical status such as burns, sepsis, major skeletal trauma, or fever, that increases metabolic demands?
- Does client have a physical intolerance, such as nausea, vomiting, anorexia, abdominal cramping, or diarrhea, to foods or fluids?
- Is client taking any medications that might influence appetite (for example, captopril, chemotherapy, steroids, antibiotics, insulin, lithium)?

- Is client taking any medications that may interact with nutrients to decrease medication function (for example, vitamin K-rich foods such as dark green vegetables that can change the effectiveness of anticoagulants such as coumadin or warfarin)?
- Does the client follow any cultural, ethnic, or religious traditions that influence the type and intake of food?
- Ask if client has any difficulties in being able to purchase food, travel to grocery store, or maintain utilities to prepare food.
- Determine if client ingests alcohol; determine frequency and amount.

ASSESSMENT TECHNIQUES—NUTRITION

Assessment	Normal Findings	Deviations From Normal
• Review findings from physical examination and note clinical signs of client's nutritional status (for example, condition of skin, nails, and mucous membranes; GI function; condition of muscles; ability to chew and swallow) (Table 21-1).	• Review of systems reveals good condition of integument and musculoskeletal systems.	• See abnormalities listed in Table 21-1.
	• GI function is normal with no palpable masses.	
	• Client has own teeth or properly fitting dentures.	
	• Client is energetic, sleeps well, and has good attention span.	
• Obtain client's height and weight (see Chapter 6).		
If client is unable to stand, the arm span or distance from fingertip to fingertip with arms fully outstretched at shoulder level approximates height for the mature adult.		
• Convert weight to kilograms (2.2 lb = 1 kg).		

Table 21-1 Clinical Signs of Nutritional Status

Body Area	Signs of Good Nutrition	Signs of Poor Nutrition
General appearance	Alert, responsive	Listless, apathetic, cachectic
Weight	Normal for height, age, body build	Overweight or underweight (special concern for underweight)
Posture	Erect, arms and legs straight	Sagging shoulders, sunken chest, humped back
Muscles	Well-developed, firm, good tone, some fat under skin	Flaccid, poor tone, underdeveloped, tender, edematous, wasted appearance, cannot walk properly
Nervous control	Good attention span, not irritable or restless, normal reflexes, psychologic stability	Inattentive, irritable, confused, burning and tingling of hands and feet (paresthesia), loss of position and vibratory sense, weakness and tenderness of muscles (may result in inability to walk), decrease or loss of ankle and knee reflexes, absent vibratory sense
Gastrointestinal function	Good appetite and digestion, normal regular elimination, no palpable organs or masses	Anorexia, indigestion, constipation or diarrhea, liver or spleen enlargement
Gums	Good pink color, healthy, red, no swelling or bleeding	Spongy, bleed easily, marginal redness, inflamed, gums receding

Tongue	Good pink color or deep reddish in appearance, not swollen or smooth, surface papillae present, no lesions	Swelling, scarlet and raw, magenta color, beefy (glossitis), hyperemic and hypertrophic papillae, atrophic papillae
Teeth	No cavities, no pain, bright, straight, no crowding, well-shaped jaw, clean, no discoloration	Unfilled caries, absent teeth, worn surfaces, mottled (fluorosis), malpositioned
Eyes	Bright, clear, shiny, no sores at corner of eye-lids, membranes moist and healthy pink color, no prominent blood vessels or mound of tissue or sclera, no fatigue circles beneath	Eye membranes pale (pale conjunctivae), redness of membrane (conjunctival infection), dryness, signs of infection. Biot's spots, redness and fissuring of eyelid corners (angular palpebritis), dryness of eye membrane (conjunctival xerosis), dull appearance of cornea (corneal xerosis), soft cornea (keratomalacia)
Neck (glands)	No enlargement	Thyroid enlargement
Nails	Firm, pink	Spoon shape (koilonychia), brittle, ridged
Legs, feet	No tenderness, weakness, or swelling; good color	Edema, tender calf, tingling, weakness
Skeleton	No malformations	Bowlegs, knock-knees, chest deformity at diaphragm, beaded ribs, prominent scapulae

From Williams SR: Nutritional assessment and guidance in prenatal care. In Worthington-Roberts BS, Williams SR, eds: *Nutrition in pregnancy and lactation*, ed 6, St Louis, 1997, Mosby.

Assessment	Normal Findings	Deviations From Normal
• Calculate ideal body weight (IBW):	• Client ranges 10% above or 10% below IBW.	• Client ranges exceed 10% above or 10% below IBW.
• Males: 47.7 kg (106 lb) for the first 5 feet, then add 2.25 kg/2.5 cm or 6 lb per additional inch in height.		
• Females: 45 kg (100 lb) for the first 5 feet, then add 2.25 kg/2.5 cm or 5 lb per additional inch in height.		
• Determine body mass index (BMI) (See Appendix D).	• Normal BMI for women is 19 to 23. Normal BMI for men is 20 to 25.	• Women with a BMI value of 23 to 29 are classified as being overweight; a value over 30 indicates obesity.
		• Men with a BMI value of 25 to 30 are classified as overweight; a value over 30 indicates obesity.
• Using tape measure, determine smallest portion of wrist distal to styloid process by measuring circumference in centimeters.	**R Values for Body Frame Size:**	
	• Women: small >11; medium 10.1 to 11.0; large <10.1	

- Divide the wrist circumference into the client's height to calculate the *r* value for body frame size:

  - Men: small >10.4; medium 9.6 to 10.4; large <9.6

- With client's nondominant arm relaxed, measure circumference (in centimeters) at midpoint of arm. The midpoint of the arm is between the tip of the acromial process of scapula and olecranon process of ulna.

  - Normal MAC (see Appendix F).

- Record as mid–upper-arm circumference (MAC) to estimate muscle wasting.

- With thumb and forefinger, pinch a double fold of fat lengthwise about 1 cm above midpoint of the MAC.

  - Triceps skin fold (TSF): men 12.5 mm; women 16.5 mm (see Appendix F).

- With other hand, place teeth of calipers on either side of fat fold.

  - TSF greater than 15 mm in men and 25 mm in women indicates obesity.

- Place calipers below fingers so pressure is exerted from calipers and not fingers.

Assessment	Normal Findings	Deviations From Normal
• Record three separate readings in millimeters and then average to obtain a skin-fold measure (estimate of subcutaneous fat).		
• Calculate midarm muscle circumference (MAMC) to estimate skeletal muscle mass.	• Normal MAMC (see Appendix C).	• MAMC = MAC − (TSF × 3.14)
• Review common laboratory tests to evaluate client's nutritional status.	• No single laboratory or biochemical test is diagnostic for malnutrition.	
• Pay special attention to albumin (indicator of chronic malnutrition), transferrin (indicator of protein and calorie malnutrition), prealbumin, retinol-binding protein, total iron-binding capacity, and hemoglobin.	• Most plasma proteins have a >7-day half-life and will not reflect changes in less than a week.	
	• Consider all of the client's clinical symptoms when reviewing laboratory results.	
• Determine client's caloric needs using the Harris-Benedict equation for basal energy expenditure (BEE):	• Client's daily food intake ranges from 1600 to 1800 kcal/day.	• Client's food intake is less than 1500 kcal or exceeds 2500 kcal/day.

- Dietary fat intake averages 30% or less of total calories, with saturated fat less than 10%.

- Dietary fat intake is 36% or more of total calories, with saturated fat 13% or more.

- Male: BEE = 66 + 13.7W (weight in kilograms) + 5H (height in centimeters) − 6.8A (age of client)

- Female: BEE = 65.5 + .6W + 1.7H − 4.7A

Pediatric Considerations

- Growth is most rapid during an infant's first year of life.
- Some aspects of the assessment could produce anxiety in children. Potential concerns, such as how calipers will be used, should be explained.
- Refer to adjusted height and weight tables based on a child's developmental age and sex (see Appendix E).
- TSF thickness is not routinely measured unless child is at a weight greater than the 90th percentile. TSF thickness often makes it difficult to differentiate fat folds from lean muscle tissue in children (Seidel et al, 1999).

- Toddlers need fewer calories but an increased amount of protein in relation to body weight. Calcium and phosphorus are needed for bone growth. Recommend a daily minimum of two servings from the milk group, four servings from the fruit and vegetable group, four servings from the bread and cereal group, 1 to 3 oz from the meat group, and 1 to 2 tsp of margarine or butter.

- For school-age children, recommend two servings daily from the milk group, 2 to 3 oz from the meat group, four or more servings from the fruit and vegetable group, three to four servings from the bread group, and 1 to 2 tsp of margarine or butter.

- For adolescents, recommend three or more servings daily from the milk group, two or more servings from the meat group, four or more servings from the vegetable and fruit group, four to six or more servings from the bread group, and 1 to 2 tbsp of margarine or butter.

 Gerontologic Considerations

- Older adults have a decreased need for calories as the metabolic rate slows.
- Older adults are particularly prone to fluid imbalance and inadequate intake of fiber nutrients (Lueckenotte, 2000).
- A reduction in the number of taste buds can reduce an older adult's sense of taste and thus reduce appetite.
- Basic tips for older adults in following dietary guidelines include eating a variety of foods; maintaining ideal weight; avoiding excess fat, saturated fat, and cholesterol; eating foods with adequate starch and fiber; avoiding excess sugar, sodium, and salt; and drinking alcohol in moderation.
- Review the following factors with an older adult to determine the risk for poor nutritional health.
  - Illness or condition that makes client change the kind and/or amount of food eaten.
  - Fewer than two meals per day.
  - Eats few fruits/vegetables/milk products.
  - Three or more drinks of beer/liquor/wine almost daily.
  - Tooth or mouth problems.
  - Does not have enough money to buy food needed.
  - Eats alone most of the time.
  - Takes three or more different prescribed over-the-counter drugs.
  - Lost or gained 10 pounds in the last 6 months.
  - Not physically able to shop/cook/feed self.

Cultural Considerations

- Prevalence of being overweight increases with age, for both men and women, but to a greater degree in women. African Americans and Hispanics have a greater prevalence of being overweight than do whites.
- Japanese Americans frequently prepare their food using soy sauce as a seasoning; it is high in sodium.
- There is a growing incidence of childhood obesity among Mexican Americans, which may be related to mothers believing that a fat baby is a healthy baby (Giger, 1999).

- Lactose intolerance is found in over 66% of Mexican Americans and is very common in African Americans, some American Indian tribes, and Orientals (Giger, 1999).
- G6PD is an enzyme constituent of the red blood cells and is involved in the hexose monophosphate pathway, which accounts for 10% of glucose metabolism of the red blood cells. Deficiency of the enzyme causes red blood cells to hemolyze. G6PD deficiency occurs in different forms. The A variety is found in 35% of African Americans. The B variety is found in 65% of African Americans who have the deficiency and in nearly all non–African Americans who have the deficiency. A Chinese and Mediterranean variety of the G6PD deficiency exists (Giger, 1999).
- Elderly Russian women often have a problem with obesity because of the lack of fresh fruits and vegetables in their country. Many culturally prepared foods are high in fat and salts (Giger, 1999).

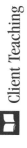 Client Teaching

- Instruct adolescents that vigorous exercise increases needs for kilocalories, fluid, and iron. Stress the need for fluid during exercise. Discuss common myths about nutrition in sports (for example, steak and eggs before competition, sport drinks, carbohydrate loading, high-fat meals).
- Have client develop a 1-week menu to learn how to integrate recommended food groups into daily diet.
- Instruct older clients on the effects certain medications might have on appetite.
- Explain to clients how to read daily reference values (DRVs), which are found on nutritional labeling. DRVs are based on the percentages of 2000 kcal or the highest amount that is recommended (Potter and Perry, 2001).

References

American Academy of Family Physicians (AAFP): *AAFP summary of policy recommendations for periodic health examination*, 1999-2000, AAFP Reference Manual-Clinical Policies.

American Cancer Society: *Breast cancer facts and figures*, Atlanta, 2001, The Society.

American Cancer Society: *2001 cancer facts and figures*, Atlanta, 2000, The Society.

American Heart Association (AHA): 2001 heart and stroke statistical update.

American Heart Association, www.americanheart.org/statistics, 2001.

American Heart Association: About cholesterol. *American Heart Association*, www.americanheart.org/cholesterol, 2000.

American Nurses Association: *Nursing and social policy statement*, Kansas City, MO, 1980, The Association.

American Thoracic Society: Diagnostic standards and classification of tuberculosis in adults and children, *Am J Respir Crit Care Med*, 161, 1376-1395, 2000.

American Thoracic Society: Diagnostic standards and classification of tuberculosis in adults and children, *Am Rev Resp Dis* 161(6): 1376, 2000.

Barkauskas VH et al: *Health and physical assessment*, ed 2, St Louis, 1998, Mosby.

Bates B: *A guide to physical examination*, ed 5, Philadelphia, 1990, JB Lippincott.

Bowers AC, Thompson JM: *Clinical manual of health assessment*, ed 4, St Louis, 1992, Mosby.

Boychuk Duchscher JE: Catching the wave: understanding the concept of critical thinking, *J Adv Nurs* 29(3):577, 1999.

Center for Disease Control and Prevention: Prevention and control of influenza: recommendations of the Advisory Committee on Immunization Practices (ACIP), *MMWR* 1999:48(4).

Center for Disease Control and Prevention: Prevention of pneumococcal disease: recommendations of the Advisory Committee on Immunization Practices (ACIP), *MMWR* 1997:46(8).

Center for Disease Control/National Center for Health Services: *Behavioral risk factor surveillance system*, CDC/NCHS, 1997.

Ebersole P, Hess P: *Toward healthy aging*, ed 5, St Louis, 1998, Mosby.

Folstein MF, Folstein S, McHugh PR: Mini-n-Mental State: a practical method for grading the cognitive state of patients for the clinician, *J Psychiatr Res* 12:189, 1975.

Forgacs P: The functional basis of pulmonary sounds, *Chest* 73:399, 1978.

Giger JN, Davidhizar RE: *Transcultural nursing: assessment and intervention*, ed 3, St Louis, 1999, Mosby.

Gordon M: *Nursing diagnosis, process and application*, ed 3, St Louis, 1994, Mosby.

Hazinski MF: *Manual of pediatric critical care nursing*, St Louis, 1999, Mosby.

Institute for Clinical System Improvement (ICSI), Adult low back pain, ICSI health care guidelines, No. GMSO1, 1999. www.guidelines.gov.

King KB, Mosca L: Prevention of heart disease in women: recommendations for management of risk factors, *Prog Cardiovasc Nurs* 15(2):36-42, 2000.

Kinney MR et al: *AACN's clinical reference for critical care nursing*, ed 4, St Louis, 1998, Mosby.

Kosary CL et al: *SEER cancer statistics review, 1973-1992: tables and graphs*, NIH Pub No 95-2789, Bethesda, Md, 1995, National Cancer Institute.

Lewis SM et al: *Medical-surgical nursing: assessment and management of clinical problems*, ed 5, St Louis, 2000, Mosby.

Lueckenotte A: *Gerontologic nursing*, St Louis, ed 2, 2000, Mosby.

Lueckenotte A: *Pocket guide to gerontologic assessment*, ed 3, St Louis, 1999, Mosby.

McKenry LM, Salerno E: *Mosby's pharmacology in nursing*, ed 21, St Louis, 2000, Mosby.

Morbidity and Mortality Weekly Report (MMWR): Committee on immunization practices (AICP), 48(43), 1999.

National Cancer Institute: What you need to know about oral cancer. *US Department of Health and Human Services, Public Health Service, National Institutes of Health*, NIH Publication No. 97-1574, Bethesda, MD, 1996a.

National Cancer Institute: What you need to know about kidney cancer. National Cancer Institute: What you need to know about oral cancer. *U.S. Department of Health and Human Services, Public Health Service, National Institute of Health*, NIH Publication No. 97-1569, Bethesda, MD, 1996b.

National Cancer Institute: What you need to know about cancer of the colon and rectum. *U.S. Department of Health and Human Services, Public Health Service, National Institutes of Health, National Cancer Institute*, NIH Publication No. 97-1552, Bethesda, MD, 1999.

National Heart, Lung, and Blood Institute (NHLBI): Expert panel on detection, evaluation and treatment of high blood cholesterol in adults. Third report of the national cholesterol education program (NCEP) expert panel on detection, evaluation and treatment of high blood cholesterol in adults (Adult Treatment Panel III), *JAMA* 285:2486, 2001.

Office on Smoking and Health, Division of Adolescent and Health Promotion, Centers for Disease Control and Prevention: Tobacco use among high school students-United States, 1997, *MMWR*, 47(12):229-233, 1998.

Office on Smoking and Health, National Center for Chronic Disease Prevention and Health Promotion, Centers for Disease Control: Cigarette smoking among adults-United States, 1997, *MMWR*, 48:993-996, 1999.

Perry AG, Potter PA: *Clinical nursing skills and techniques*, ed 5, St Louis, 2002, Mosby.

Potter PA, Perry AG: *Fundamentals of nursing: concepts, process, and practice*, ed 5, St Louis, 2001, Mosby.

Ries LAG et al, eds: *SEER cancer statistics review, 1973-1997*, National Cancer Institute, Bethesda, MD, 2000.

Scheffer BK, Rubenfeld MG: A consensus statement on critical thinking in nursing, *Nurs Educ* 39(8):352, 2000.

Seidel HM et al: *Mosby's guide to physical examination*, ed 4, St Louis, 1999, Mosby.

Thibodeau GA, Patton K: *Structure and function of the body*, ed 11, St Louis, 2000, Mosby.

Thompson JM et al: *Mosby's clinical nursing*, ed 5, St Louis, 2001, Mosby.

U.S. Department of Health and Human Services: The initiative to eliminate racial and ethnic disparities in health, *Public Health Services, National Institutes of Health, National Heart, Lung and Blood Institute*, Bethesda, MD, 2001, *www.raceandhealth.gov*.

U.S. Department of Health and Human Services: Sixth report of the joint national committee on prevention, detection, evaluation, and treatment of high blood pressure, *Public Health Service, National Institutes of Health, National Heart, Lung and Blood Institute*, Bethesda, MD, 1997.

Williams SR: *Basic nutrition and diet therapy*, ed 11, St Louis, 2000, Mosby.

Wong DL: *Nursing care of infants and children*, ed 6, St Louis, 1999, Mosby.

APPENDIXES

Potential Nursing Diagnosis by Body System

Skin

- Impaired skin integrity
- Risk for impaired skin integrity
- Deficient fluid volume
- Risk for infection
- Disturbed body image
- Bathing/hygiene self-care deficit

Head and Neck

- Impaired physical mobility
- Fatigue
- Risk for infection

Eye

- Risk for injury
- Disturbed sensory perception: visual
- Pain
- Deficient knowledge: eye care

A

587

- Self-care deficit
- Impaired physical mobility

Ears

- Disturbed sensory perceptions (auditory)
- Deficient knowledge: ear care
- Risk for injury
- Pain

Nose and Sinuses

- Deficient knowledge: use of over-the-counter nasal sprays
- Pain
- Risk for infection

Mouth and Pharynx

- Impaired oral mucous membrane
- Pain
- Deficient knowledge: oral hygiene
- Risk for infection
- Impaired swallowing
- Imbalanced nutrition: less than body requirements
- Ineffective health maintenance

Thorax and Lungs

- Ineffective airway clearance
- Ineffective breathing pattern
- Impaired gas exchange
- Pain
- Impaired mobility
- Deficient knowledge: risks for lung disease

Heart and Vascular System

- Decreased cardiac output
- Anxiety
- Activity intolerance
- Fatigue
- Pain
- Deficient knowledge: risks for heart or vascular disease and/or medical regimen
- Risk for peripheral neurovascular dysfunction

Breasts

- Anxiety
- Deficient knowledge: self-examination of breast

- Impaired skin integrity
- Acute pain
- Disturbed body image
- Ineffective sexuality pattern

Abdomen

- Constipation
- Diarrhea
- Pain
- Imbalanced nutrition: less or more than body requirements
- Deficient knowledge: risks for colon cancer, use of laxatives, and/or diet management

Female and Male Genitalia

- Pain
- Sexual dysfunction
- Deficient knowledge: testicular self-examination and risks of STD
- Impaired urinary elimination
- Impaired tissue integrity

Rectum and Anus

- Deficient knowledge: risk for colorectal cancer
- Deficient knowledge: risk for prostate cancer
- Impaired tissue integrity
- Pain
- Constipation
- Diarrhea
- Anxiety

Musculoskeletal System

- Pain
- Impaired physical mobility
- Bathing/hygiene self-care deficit
- Dressing/grooming self-care deficit
- Feeding self-care deficit
- Toileting self-care deficit
- Risk for injury

Neurological System

- Impaired verbal communication
- Disturbed thought processes

- Ineffective cerebral tissue perfusion
- Risk for injury
- Disturbed sensory perceptions (auditory, gustatory, tactile, olfactory)
- Risk for aspiration related to absent gag reflex
- Impaired swallowing
- Impaired physical mobility

Nutrition

- Imbalanced nutrition: less than body requirements
- Imbalanced nutrition: more than body requirements
- Risk for imbalanced nutrition: more than body requirements
- Risk for infection
- Impaired oral mucous membranes
- Risk for impaired skin integrity
- Impaired swallowing
- Diarrhea
- Feeding self-care deficit

B

Giger and Davidhizar's Transcultural Assessment Model

Culturally Unique Individual

1. Place of birth
2. Cultural definition
   What is . . .
3. Race
   What is . . .
4. Length of time in country (if appropriate)

Communication

1. Voice quality
   a. Strong, resonant
   b. Soft
   c. Average
   d. Shrill
2. Pronunciation and enunciation
   a. Clear

From Giger JN, Davidhizar RE: *Transcultural nursing: assessment and intervention*, ed 3, St Louis, 1999, Mosby.

Continued

Communication—*cont'd*

  b. Slurred

  c. Dialect (geographical)

3. Use of silence

  a. Infrequent

  b. Often

  c. Length

    (1) Brief

    (2) Moderate

    (3) Long

    (4) Not observed

4. Use of nonverbal

  a. Hand movement

  b. Eye movement

  c. Entire body movement

  d. Kinesics (gestures, expression, or stances)

5. Touch

  a. Startles or withdraws when touched

  b. Accepts touch without difficulty

  c. Touches others without difficulty

6. Ask these and similar questions:

  a. How do you get your point across to others?

  b. Do you like communicating with friends, family, and acquaintances?

  c. When asked a question, do you usually respond (in words or body movement, or both)?

  d. If you have something important to discuss with your family, how would you approach them?

Space

1. Degree of comfort

  a. Moves when space invaded

  b. Does not move when space invaded

2. Distance in conversations

  a. 0 to 18 inches

  b. 18 inches to 3 feet

  c. 3 feet or more

3. Definition of space

  a. Describe degree of comfort with closeness when talking with or standing near others.

  b. How do objects (e.g., furniture) in the environment affect your sense of space?

4. Ask these and similar questions:
   a. When you talk with family members, how close do you stand?
   b. When you communicate with co-workers and other acquaintances, how close do you stand?
   c. If a stranger touches you, how do you react or feel?
   d. If a loved one touches you, how do you react or feel?
   e. Are you comfortable with the distance between us now?

Social Organization

1. Normal state of health
   a. Poor
   b. Fair
   c. Good
   d. Excellent
2. Marital status
3. Number of children
4. Parents living or deceased?

5. Ask these and similar questions:
   a. How do you define social activities?
   b. What are some activities that you enjoy?
   c. What are your hobbies, or what do you do when you have free time?
   d. Do you believe in a Supreme Being?
   e. How do you worship that Supreme Being?
   f. What is your function (what do you do) in your family unit/system?
   g. What is your role in your family unit/system (father, mother, child, advisor)?
   h. When you were a child, what or who influenced you most?
   i. What is/was your relationship with your siblings and parents?
   j. What does work mean to you?
   k. Describe your past, present, and future jobs.
   l. What are your political views?
   m. How have your political views influenced your attitude toward health and illness?

Continued

From Giger JN, Davidhizar RE: *Transcultural nursing: assessment and intervention*, ed 3, St Louis, 1999, Mosby.

Giger and Davidhizar's Transcultural Assessment Model **593**

Time

1. Orientation to time
   a. Past-oriented
   b. Present-oriented
   c. Future-oriented
2. View of time
   a. Social time
   b. Clock-oriented
3. Physiochemical reaction to time
   a. Sleeps at least 8 hours a night
   b. Goes to sleep and wakes on a consistent schedule
   c. Understands the importance of taking medication and other treatments on schedule
4. Ask these and similar questions:
   a. What kind of timepiece do you wear daily?
   b. If you have an appointment at 2 PM, what time is acceptable to arrive?
   c. If a nurse tells you that you will receive a medication in "about a half hour," realistically, how much time will you allow before calling the nurses' station?

Environmental Control

1. Locus-of-control
   a. Internal locus-of-control (believes that the power to affect change lies within)
   b. External locus-of-control (believes that fate, luck, and chance have a great deal to do with how things turn out)
2. Value orientation
   a. Believes in supernatural forces
   b. Relies on magic, witchcraft, and prayer to affect change
   c. Does not believe in supernatural forces
   d. Does not rely on magic, witchcraft, or prayer to affect change
3. Ask these and similar questions:
   a. How often do you have visitors at your home?
   b. Is it acceptable to you for visitors to drop in unexpectedly?
   c. Name some ways your parents or other persons treated your illnesses when you were a child.

d. Have you or someone else in your immediate surroundings ever used a home remedy that made you sick?
e. What home remedies have you used that worked? Will you use them in the future?
f. What is your definition of "good health"?
g. What is your definition of illness or "poor health"?

Biologic Variations

1. Conduct a complete physical assessment noting:
   a. Body structure (small, medium, or large frame)
   b. Skin color
   c. Unusual skin discolorations
   d. Hair color and distribution
   e. Other visible physical characteristics (e.g., keloids, chloasma)
   f. Weight
   g. Height
   h. Check lab work for variances in hemoglobin, hematocrit, and sickle phenomena if Black or Mediterranean

2. Ask these and similar questions:
   a. What diseases or illnesses are common in your family?
   b. Describe your family's typical behavior when a family member is ill.
   c. How do you respond when you are angry?
   d. Who (or what) usually helps you to cope during a difficult time?
   e. What foods do you and your family like to eat?
   f. Have you ever had any unusual cravings for:
      (1) White or red clay dirt?
      (2) Laundry starch?
   g. When you were a child what types of foods did you eat?
   h. What foods are family favorites or are considered traditional?

Nursing Assessment

1. Note whether the client has become culturally assimilated or observes own cultural practices.

Continued

From Giger JN, Davidhizar RE: *Transcultural nursing: assessment and intervention*, ed 3, St Louis, 1999, Mosby.

Giger and Davidhizar's Transcultural Assessment Model **595**

Nursing Assessment—*cont'd*

2. Incorporate data into plan of nursing care:
   a. Encourage the client to discuss cultural differences; people from diverse cultures who hold different world views can enlighten nurses.
   b. Make efforts to accept and understand methods of communication.
   c. Respect the individual's personal need for space.
   d. Respect the rights of clients to honor and worship the Supreme Being of their choice.
   e. Identify a clerical or spiritual person to contact.
   f. Determine whether spiritual practices have implications for health, life, and well-being (e.g., Jehovah's Witnesses may refuse blood and blood derivatives; an Orthodox Jew may eat only kosher food high in sodium and may not drink milk when meat is served).
   g. Identify hobbies, especially when devising interventions for a short or extended convalescence or for rehabilitation.
   h. Honor time and value orientations and differences in these areas. Allay anxiety and apprehension if adherence to time is necessary.
   i. Provide privacy according to personal need and health status of the client (NOTE: The perception and reaction to pain may be culturally related.)
   j. Note cultural health practices
      (1) Identify and encourage efficacious practices.
      (2) Identify and discourage dysfunctional practices.
      (3) Identify and determine whether neutral practices will have a long-term ill effect.
   k. Note food preferences
      (1) Make as many adjustments in diet as health status and long-term benefits will allow and that dietary department can provide.
      (2) Note dietary practices that may have serious implications for the client.

From Giger JN, Davidhizar RE: *Transcultural nursing: assessment and intervention*, ed 3, St Louis, 1999, Mosby.

Adult Height and Weight Tables

Adult Height and Weight Table: Weights for Persons 25 to 59 Years According to Build*				
		Men		
Height		Small Frame	Medium Frame	Large Frame
Feet	Inches			
5	2	128-134	131-141	138-150
5	3	130-136	133-143	140-153
5	4	132-138	135-145	142-156

		Women		
Height†		Small Frame	Medium Frame	Large Frame
Feet	Inches			
4	10	102-111	109-121	118-131
4	11	103-113	111-123	120-134
5	0	104-115	113-126	122-137

Courtesy Metropolitan Life Insurance Company, Statistical Bulletin, 2000. This information is not intended to be a substitute for professional medical advice and should not be regarded as an endorsement or approval of any product or service.
*Indoor clothing weighing 5 pounds for men and 3 pounds for women.
†Shoes with 1-inch heels.

Adult Height and Weight Table: Weights for Persons 25 to 59 Years According to Build*—cont'd

Men

Height		Small Frame	Medium Frame	Large Frame
Feet	Inches			
5	5	134-140	137-148	144-160
5	6	136-142	139-151	146-164
5	7	138-145	142-154	149-168
5	8	140-148	145-157	152-172
5	9	142-151	148-160	155-176
5	10	144-154	151-163	158-180
5	11	146-157	154-166	161-184
6	0	149-160	157-170	164-188
6	1	152-164	160-174	168-192
6	2	155-168	164-178	172-197
6	3	158-172	167-182	176-202
6	4	162-176	171-187	181-207

Women

Height†		Small Frame	Medium Frame	Large Frame
Feet	Inches			
5	1	106-118	115-129	125-140
5	2	108-121	118-132	128-143
5	3	111-124	121-135	131-147
5	4	114-127	124-138	134-151
5	5	117-130	127-141	137-155
5	6	120-133	130-144	140-159
5	7	123-136	133-147	143-163
5	8	126-139	136-150	146-167
5	9	129-142	139-153	149-170
5	10	132-145	142-156	152-173
5	11	135-148	145-159	155-176
6	0	138-151	148-162	158-179

Courtesy Metropolitan Life Insurance Company, Statistical Bulletin, 2000. This information is not intended to be a substitute for professional medical advice and should not be regarded as an endorsement or approval of any product or service.
*Indoor clothing weighing 5 pounds for men and 3 pounds for women.
†Shoes with 1-inch heels.

Body Mass Index

Height	120	130	140	150	160	170	180	190	200	210	220	230	240	250	260	270	280	290	300	310	320	330
												Weight										
4'5"	30	33	35	38	40	43	45	48	50	53	55	58	60	63	65	68	70	73	75	78	80	83
4'6"	29	31	34	36	39	41	43	46	48	51	53	56	58	60	63	65	68	70	72	75	77	80
4'7"	28	30	33	35	37	40	42	44	47	49	51	54	56	58	61	63	65	68	70	72	75	77
4'8"	27	29	31	34	36	38	40	43	45	47	49	52	54	56	58	61	63	65	67	70	72	74
4'9"	26	28	30	33	35	37	39	41	43	46	48	50	52	54	56	59	61	63	65	67	69	72
4'10"	25	27	29	31	34	36	38	40	42	44	46	48	50	52	54	57	59	61	63	65	67	69
4'11"	24	26	28	30	32	34	36	38	40	43	45	47	49	51	53	55	57	59	61	63	65	67
5'0"	23	25	27	29	31	33	35	37	39	41	43	45	47	49	51	53	55	57	59	61	63	65
5'1"	22	25	27	28	30	32	34	36	38	40	42	44	46	47	49	51	53	55	57	59	61	62

Adapted from Roche Pharmaceuticals Body Mass Index and Risks of Overweight, 2001.

Height		Weight																				
	21	24	26	27	29	31	33	35	37	38	40	42	44	46	48	49	51	53	55	57	59	60
5'2"	21	24	26	27	29	31	33	35	37	38	40	42	44	46	48	49	51	53	55	57	59	60
5'3"	21	23	25	27	28	30	32	34	36	37	39	41	43	44	46	48	50	51	53	55	57	59
5'4"	20	22	24	26	28	29	31	33	34	36	38	40	41	43	45	46	48	50	52	53	55	57
5'5"	19	22	23	25	27	28	30	32	33	35	37	38	40	42	43	45	47	48	50	52	53	55
5'6"	19	21	22	24	26	27	29	31	32	34	36	37	39	40	42	44	45	47	49	50	52	53
5'7"	18	20	21	24	25	27	28	30	31	33	35	36	38	39	41	42	44	46	47	49	50	52
5'8"	18	20	21	23	24	26	27	29	30	32	34	35	37	38	40	41	43	44	46	47	49	50
5'9"	18	19	21	22	24	25	27	28	30	31	33	34	36	37	38	40	41	43	44	46	47	49
5'10"	17	19	20	22	23	24	26	27	29	30	32	33	35	36	37	39	40	42	43	45	46	47
5'11"	16	18	20	21	22	24	25	27	28	29	31	32	34	35	36	38	39	41	42	43	45	46
6'0"	16	18	19	21	22	23	24	26	27	29	30	31	33	34	35	37	38	39	41	42	43	45
6'1"	15	17	19	20	21	22	24	25	26	28	29	30	32	33	34	36	37	38	40	41	42	44
6'2"	15	17	18	20	21	22	23	24	26	27	28	30	31	32	33	35	36	37	39	40	41	42
6'3"	15	16	18	19	20	21	23	24	25	26	28	29	30	31	33	34	35	36	38	39	40	41
6'4"	14	16	17	19	20	21	22	23	24	26	27	28	29	30	32	33	34	35	37	38	39	40
6'5"	14	15	17	18	19	20	21	23	24	25	26	27	29	30	31	32	33	34	36	37	38	39
6'6"	14	15	16	18	19	20	21	22	23	24	25	27	28	29	30	31	32	33	35	36	37	38
6'7"	13	15	16	17	18	19	20	21	23	24	25	26	27	28	29	30	32	33	34	35	36	37
6'8"	13	14	16	17	18	19	20	21	22	24	24	25	26	28	29	30	31	32	33	34	35	36
6'9"	13	14	15	17	18	18	19	21	21	23	24	25	26	27	28	29	30	31	32	33	34	35
6'10"	13	14	15	16	17	18	19	20	21	22	23	24	25	26	27	28	29	30	31	32	34	35

Adapted from Roche Pharmaceuticals Body Mass Index and Risks of Overweight, 2001.

E

Physical Growth
Curves for Children

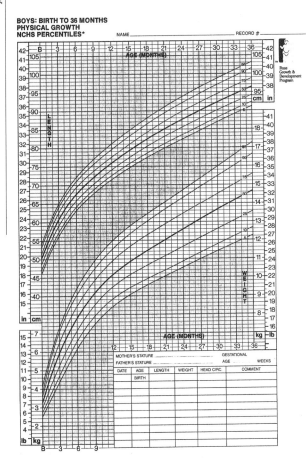

BOYS: BIRTH TO 36 MONTHS
PHYSICAL GROWTH
NCHS PERCENTILES*

Courtesy Ross Laboratories, Columbus, Ohio.

BOYS: BIRTH TO 36 MONTHS
PHYSICAL GROWTH
NCHS PERCENTILES*

NAME _____ RECORD # _____

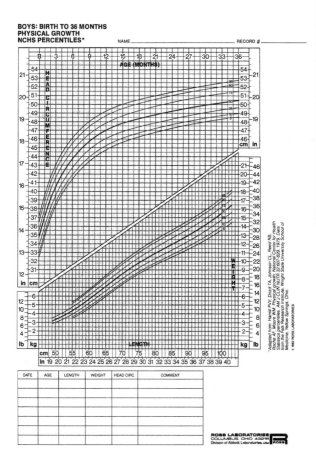

DATE	AGE	LENGTH	WEIGHT	HEAD CIRC	COMMENT

*Adapted from: Hamill PVV, Drizd TA, Johnson CL, Reed RB, Roche AF, Moore WM. Physical growth: National Center for Health Statistics percentiles. AM J CLIN NUTR 32:607-629 1979. Data from the Fels Research Institute, Wright State University School of Medicine, Yellow Springs, Ohio.

© 1982 ROSS LABORATORIES

ROSS LABORATORIES
COLUMBUS, OHIO 43216
Division of Abbott Laboratories, USA

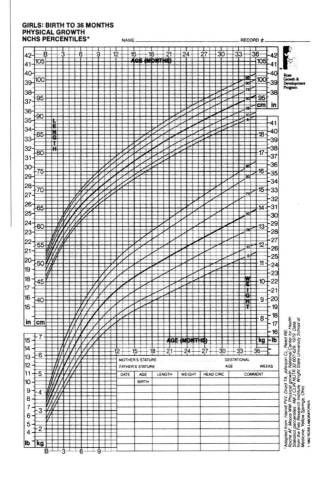

GIRLS: BIRTH TO 36 MONTHS
PHYSICAL GROWTH
NCHS PERCENTILES*

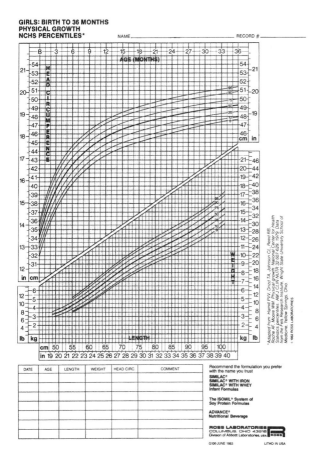

GIRLS: BIRTH TO 36 MONTHS
PHYSICAL GROWTH
NCHS PERCENTILES*

Mid–Upper-Arm Muscle Circumference and Triceps Skin Fold Percentiles

F

Mid–Upper-Arm Muscle Circumference Percentiles (cm)

Age (yr)	Female Percentiles					Male Percentiles				
	5th	25th	50th	75th	95th	5th	25th	50th	75th	95th
1	10.5	11.7	12.4	13.9	14.3	11.0	11.9	12.7	13.5	14.7
2	11.1	11.9	12.6	13.3	14.7	11.1	12.2	13.0	14.0	15.0
3	11.3	12.4	13.2	14.0	15.2	11.7	13.1	13.7	14.3	15.3
4	11.5	12.8	13.8	14.4	15.7	12.3	13.3	14.1	14.8	15.9
5	12.5	13.4	14.2	15.1	16.5	12.8	14.0	14.7	15.4	16.9

Age										
6	13.0	13.8	14.5	15.4	17.1	13.1	14.2	15.1	16.1	17.7
7	12.9	14.2	15.1	16.0	17.6	13.7	15.1	16.0	16.8	19.0
8	13.8	15.1	16.0	17.1	19.4	14.0	15.4	16.2	17.0	18.7
9	14.7	15.8	16.7	18.0	19.8	15.1	16.1	17.0	18.3	20.2
10	14.8	15.9	17.0	18.0	19.7	15.6	16.6	18.0	19.1	22.1
11	15.0	17.1	18.1	19.6	22.3	15.9	17.3	18.3	19.5	23.0
12	16.2	18.0	19.1	20.1	22.0	16.7	18.2	19.5	21.0	24.1
13	16.9	18.3	19.8	21.1	24.0	17.2	19.6	21.1	22.6	24.5
14	17.4	19.0	20.1	21.6	24.7	18.9	21.2	22.3	24.0	26.4
15	17.5	18.9	20.2	21.5	24.4	19.9	21.8	23.7	25.4	27.2
16	17.0	19.0	20.2	21.6	24.9	21.3	23.4	24.9	26.9	29.6
17	17.5	19.4	20.5	22.1	25.7	22.4	24.5	25.8	27.3	31.2
18	17.4	19.1	20.2	21.5	24.5	22.6	25.2	26.4	28.3	32.4
19-25	17.9	19.5	20.7	22.1	24.9	23.8	25.7	27.3	28.9	32.1
25-35	18.3	19.9	21.2	22.8	26.4	24.3	26.4	27.9	29.8	32.6
35-45	18.6	20.5	21.8	23.6	27.2	24.7	26.9	28.6	30.2	32.7
45-55	18.7	20.6	22.0	23.8	27.4	23.9	26.5	28.1	30.0	32.6
55-65	18.7	20.9	22.5	24.4	28.0	23.6	26.0	27.8	29.5	32.0
65-75	18.5	20.8	22.5	24.4	27.9	22.3	25.1	26.8	28.4	30.6

Values derived by formula calculation. Data derived from the Health and Nutrition Examination Survey data of 1971-1974, using same population samples as those of the National Center for Health Statistics (NCHS) growth percentiles for children. Adapted from Frisancho AR: New norms of upper limb fat and muscle areas for assessment of nutritional status, *Am J Clin Nutr* 34:2540, 1981.

Mid–Upper-Arm Muscle Circumference and Triceps Skin Fold Percentiles

Triceps Skin Fold Percentiles (mm)

Age (yr)	Female Percentiles					Male Percentiles				
	5th	25th	50th	75th	95th	5th	25th	50th	75th	95th
1	6	8	10	12	16	6	8	10	12	16
2	6	9	10	12	16	6	8	10	12	15
3	7	9	11	12	15	6	8	10	11	15
4	7	8	10	12	16	6	8	9	11	14
5	6	8	10	12	18	6	8	9	11	15
6	6	8	10	12	16	5	7	8	10	16
7	6	9	11	13	18	5	7	9	12	17
8	6	9	12	15	24	5	7	8	10	16
9	8	10	13	16	22	6	7	10	13	18
10	7	10	12	17	27	6	8	10	14	21
11	7	10	13	18	28	6	8	11	16	24

12	8	11	14	18	27	6	8	11	14	28
13	8	12	15	21	30	5	7	10	14	26
14	9	13	16	21	28	4	7	9	14	24
15	8	12	17	21	32	4	6	8	11	24
16	10	15	18	22	31	4	6	8	12	22
17	10	13	19	24	37	5	6	8	12	19
18	10	15	18	22	30	4	6	9	13	24
19-25	10	14	18	24	34	4	7	10	15	22
25-35	10	16	21	27	37	5	8	12	16	24
35-45	12	18	23	29	38	5	8	12	16	23
45-55	12	20	25	30	40	6	8	12	15	25
55-65	12	20	25	31	38	5	8	11	14	22
65-75	12	18	24	29	36	4	8	11	15	22

Data derived from the Health and Nutrition Examination Survey data of 1971-1974, using same population samples as those of the National Center for Health Statistics (NCHS) growth percentiles for children. Adapted from Frisancho AR: New norms of upper limb fat and muscle areas for assessment of nutritional status. *Am J Clin Nutr* 34:2540, 1981.

G

Recommended Schedule for Immunization of Healthy Infants and Children in the United States

Recommended Age[b]	Immunization(s)[c]	Comments
Birth	HBV[d]	
1-2 months	HBV[d]	
2 months	DTP, Hib, IPV	DTP and IPV can be initiated as early as 4 weeks after birth in areas of high endemicity or during outbreaks
4 months	DTP, Hib, IPV	2-month interval (minimum of 6 weeks) recommended for IPV
6 months	DTP, (Hib[e])	

Age	Vaccines	Notes
6-18 months	HBV[a], IPV	
12-15 months	Hib, MMR Varicella	MMR should be given at 12 months of age in high-risk areas; if indicated, tuberculin testing may be done at the same visit
15-18 months	DTaP or DTP Varicella	The fourth dose of diphtheria-tetanus-pertussis vaccine should be given 6 to 12 months after the third dose of DTP and may be given as early as 12 months of age, provided that the interval between doses 3 and 4 is at least 6 months and DTP is given; DTaP is not currently licensed for use in children younger than 15 months
24 months-11 years	Hep A in selected areas	
4-6 years	DTaP or DTP, IPV	DTaP or DTP and OPV should be given at or before school entry; DTP or DTaP should not be given at or after the seventh birthday
11-12 years	MMR	MMR should be given at entry to middle school or junior high school unless 2 doses were given after the first birthday
14-16 years	Td	Repeat every 10 years throughout life

From MMWR: 48(43)1999 Committee on Immunization Practices (AICP).

Recommended Schedule for Immunization of Healthy Infants and Children in the United States **611**

Routine Primary Immunization Schedule for Infants and Children in Canada

	Immunization Against			
Age				
2 months	Diphtheria	Pertussis	Tetanus	Poliomyelitis IPV/OPV	Haemophilus influenzae b[1]
4 months	Diphtheria	Pertussis	Tetanus	Poliomyelitis IPV/OPV	Haemophilus influenzae b
6 months	Diphtheria	Pertussis	Tetanus	Poliomyelitis IPV/OPV	Haemophilus influenzae b
12 months	Measles	Mumps	Rubella		
18 months	Diphtheria	Pertussis	Tetanus	Poliomyelitis IPV/OPV	Haemophilus influenzae b
4-6 years	Diphtheria	Pertussis	Tetanus	Poliomyelitis OPV	
	Measles	Mumps	Rubella		
14-16 years	Diphtheria[3]		Tetanus[3]	Poliomyelitis[2]	

From The Canadian guide to clinical preventive healthcare: Chapter 33. Childhood immunizations, Sept 1994 (Reviewed: 1998, Canadian Task Force on the Periodic Health Examination.)

[1]Hib schedule shown is for HbOC or PRP-T vaccine. If PRP-OMP is used, give at 2, 4, and 12 months of age.

[2]Omit this dose if OPV is used exclusively.

[3]Td (tetanus and diphtheria toxoid), a combined absorbed "adult-type" preparation for use in persons ≥7 years of age, contains less diptheria toxoid than preparations given to younger children and is less likely to cause reactions in older persons. Repeat every 10 years throughout life.

Snellen and E Eye Charts

E

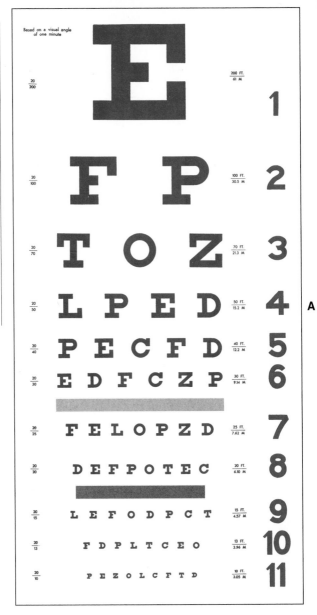

Fig. E-1 **A,** Snellen chart for testing distant vision.
(From Seidel et al: *Mosby's guide to physical examination*, ed 4, St Louis, 1999, Mosby.)

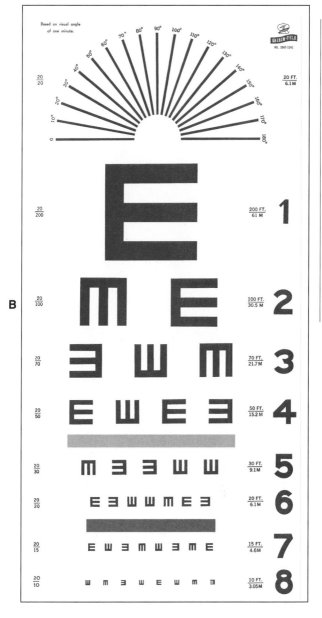

Fig. E-1, cont'd **B,** E chart for testing distant vision.
(From Seidel et al: *Mosby's guide to physical examination,* ed 4, St Louis, 1999, Mosby.)

U.S. Food Guide Pyramid

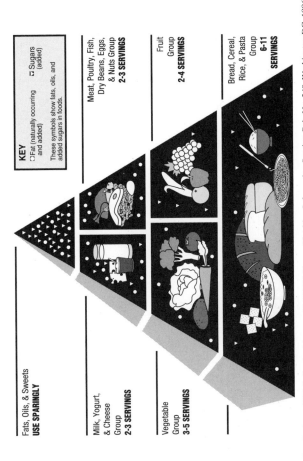

Fats, Oils, & Sweets
USE SPARINGLY

KEY
□ Fat (naturally occurring and added)   ▽ Sugars (added)

These symbols show fats, oils, and added sugars in foods.

Milk, Yogurt, & Cheese Group
2-3 SERVINGS

Meat, Poultry, Fish, Dry Beans, Eggs, & Nuts Group
2-3 SERVINGS

Vegetable Group
3-5 SERVINGS

Fruit Group
2-4 SERVINGS

Bread, Cereal, Rice, & Pasta Group
6-11 SERVINGS

From U.S. Department of Agriculture: USDA's food guide pyramid, USDA Human Nutrition Information Service, Pub. No. 249, Washington DC, 1996, U.S. Government Printing Office.

K

Canada's Food Guide to Healthy Eating

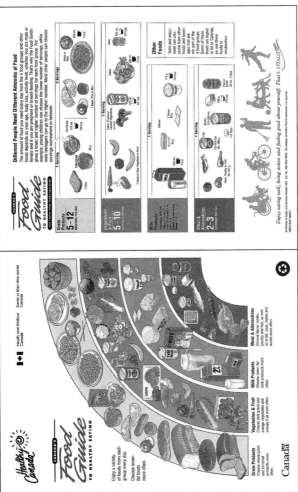

Canada's Food Guide to Healthy Eating 619

The Vegetarian Food Pyramid

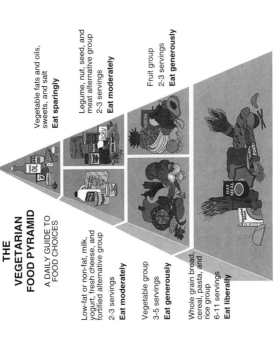

THE VEGETARIAN FOOD PYRAMID

A DAILY GUIDE TO FOOD CHOICES

Vegetable fats and oils, sweets, and salt
Eat sparingly

Legume, nut, seed, and meat alternative group
2-3 servings
Eat moderately

Fruit group
2-3 servings
Eat generously

Low-fat or non-fat, milk, yogurt, fresh cheese, and fortified alternative group
2-3 servings
Eat moderately

Vegetable group
3-5 servings
Eat generously

Whole grain bread, cereal, pasta, and rice group
6-11 servings
Eat liberally

Courtesy The Health Connection (Illustration by Merle Poirier).

The Vegetarian Food Pyramid **621**

M

Normal Reference Laboratory Values

Blood, Plasma, or Serum Values

Test	Reference Range	
	Conventional Values	SI Units*
Acetoacetate plus acetone	0.30-2.0 mg/dl	3-20 mg/l
Acetone	Negative	Negative
Acid phosphatase	Adults:	28-175 nmol/s/L
	0.10-0.63 U/ml (Bessey-Lowry)	
	0.5-2.0 U/ml (Bodansky)	
	1.0-4.0 U/ml (King-Armstrong)	
	Children: 6.4-15.2 U/L	

Test	Conventional Values	SI Units
Activated partial thromboplastin time (APTT)	30-40 sec	30-40 sec
Adrenocorticotropic hormone (ACTH)	6 AM 15-100 pg/ml 6 PM <50 pg/ml	10-80 ng/L <50 ng/L
Alanine aminotransferase (ALT)	5-35 IU/L	5-35 U/L
Albumin	3.2-4.5 g/dl	35-55 g/L
Alcohol	Negative	Negative
Aldolase	Adults: 3.0-8.2 Sibley-Lehninger units/dl Children: approximately 2 × adult values Newborns: approximately 4 × adult values	22-59 mU/L at 37° C
Aldosterone	Peripheral blood: Supine: 7.4 ± 4.2 ng/dl Upright: 1-21 ng/dl Adrenal vein: 200-800 ng/dl	0.08-0.3 nmol/L 0.14-0.8 nmol/L
Alkaline phosphatase	Adults: 30-85 ImU/ml Children and adolescents: <2 years: 85-235 ImU/ml 2-8 years: 65-210 ImU/ml 9-15 years: 60-300 ImU/ml (active bone growth) 16-21 years: 30-200 ImU/ml	

*The use of the System of International Units (SI) was recommended at the 30th World Health Assembly in 1977 to implement an international language of measurement. Because this system is being adopted by numerous laboratories, many of the common values are expressed in both conventional and SI units. SI units are calculated by multiplying the conventional unit by a number factor. The SI measurement system uses *moles* as the basic unit for the amount of a substance, *kilograms* for its mass, and *meter* for its length.

Continued

Blood, Plasma, or Serum Values—cont'd

Test	Reference Range		
	Conventional Values	SI Units*	
Alpha-aminonitrogen	3-6 mg/dl	2.1-3.9 mmol/L	
Alpha-1-antitrypsin	>250 mg/dl		
Alpha fetoprotein (AFP)	<25 ng/ml		
Ammonia	Adults: 15-110 μg/dl	47-65 μmol/L	
	Children: 40-80 μg/dl		
	Newborns: 90-150 μg/dl		
Amylase	56-190 IU/L	25-125 U/L	
	80-150 Somogyi units/ml		
Angiotensin-converting enzyme (ACE)	23-57 U/ml		
Antinuclear antibodies (ANA)	Negative		
Antistreptolysin O (ASO)	Adults: ≤160 Todd units/ml		
	Children:		
	Newborns: similar to mother's value		
	6 months-2 years: ≤50 Todd units/ml		
	2-4 years: ≤160 Todd units/ml		
	5-12 years: ≤200 Todd units/ml		
Antithyroid microsomal antibody	Titer <1:100		
Antithyroglobulin antibody	Titer <1:100		

Ascorbic acid (vitamin C)	0.6-1.6 mg/dl	23-57 μmol/L
Aspartate aminotransferase (AST, SGOT)	12-36 U/ml	0.10-0.30 μmol/s/L
	5-40 IU/L	5-40 U/L
Australian antigen (hepatitis-associated antigen, HAA)	Negative	Negative
Barbiturates	Negative	Negative
Base excess	Men: −3.3 to +1.2	0 ± 2 mmol/L
	Women: −2.4 to +2.3	0 ± 2 mmol/L
Bicarbonate (HCO$_3^-$)	22-26 mEq/L	22-26 mmol/L
Bilirubin		
Direct (conjugated)	0.1-0.3 mg/dl	1.7-5.1 μmol/L
Indirect (unconjugated)	0.2-0.8 mg/dl	3.4-12.0 μmol/L
Total	Adults and children: 0.1-1.0 mg/dl	5.1-17.0 μmol/L
	Newborns: 1-12 mg/dl	
Bleeding time (Ivy method)	1-9 min	
Blood count (see Complete blood count)		
Blood gases (arterial)		
pH	7.35-7.45	
PCO$_2$	35-45 mm Hg	4.7-6.0 kPa
HCO$_3^-$	22-26 mEq/L	21-28 nmol/L
PO$_2$	80-100 mm Hg	11-13 kPa
O$_2$ saturation	95%-100%	

*The use of the System of International Units (SI) was recommended at the 30th World Health Assembly in 1977 to implement an international language of measurement. Because this system is being adopted by numerous laboratories, many of the common values are expressed in both conventional and SI units. SI units are calculated by multiplying the conventional unit by a number factor. The SI measurement system uses *moles* as the basic unit for the amount of a substance, *kilograms* for its mass, and *meter* for its length.
Continued

Blood, Plasma, or Serum Values—cont'd

Test	Reference Range	
	Conventional Values	SI Units*
Blood urea nitrogen (BUN)	5-20 mg/dl	3.6-7.1 mmol/L
Bromide	Up to 5 mg/dl	0-63 mmol/L
Bromsulphalein (BSP)	<5% retention after 45 min	
CA 15-3	<22 U/ml	
CA-125	0-35 U/ml	
CA 19-9	<37 U/ml	
C-reactive protein (CRP)	<6 μg/ml	
Calcitonin	<50 pg/ml	<50 pmol/L
Calcium (Ca)	9.0-10.5 mg/dl (total)	2.25-2.75 mmol/L
	3.9-4.6 mg/dl (ionized)	1.05-1.30 mmol/L
Carbon dioxide (CO_2) content	23-30 mEq/L	21-30 mmol/L
Carboxyhemoglobin (COHb)	3% of total hemoglobin	
Carcinoembryonic antigen (CEA)	<2 ng/ml	
Carotene	50-200 μg/dl	0.2-5 μg/L
Chloride (Cl)	90-110 mEq/L	0.74-3.72 μmol/L
Cholesterol	150-250 mg/dl	98-106 mmol/L
Clot retraction	50%-100% clot retraction in 1-2 hours, complete retraction within 24 hours	3.90-6.50 mmol/L

Complement	C_3: 70-176 mg/dl	0.55-1.20 g/L
	C_4: 16-45 mg/dl	0.20-0.50 g/L
Complete blood count (CBC)		
Red blood cell (RBC) count	Men: 4.7-6.1 million/mm³	
	Women: 4.2-5.4 million/mm³	
	Infants and children: 3.8-5.5 million/mm³	
	Newborns: 4.8-7.1 million/mm³	
Hemoglobin (Hgb)	Men: 14-18 g/dl	8.7-11.2 mmol/L
	Women: 12-16 g/dl (pregnancy: >11 g/dl)	7.4-9.9 mmol/L
	Children: 11-16 g/dl	1.74-2.56 mmol/L
	Infants: 10-15 g/dl	
	Newborns: 14-24 g/dl	2.56-3.02 mmol/L
Hematocrit (Hct)	Men: 42%-52%	
	Women: 37%-47% (pregnancy: >33%)	
	Children: 31%-43%	
	Infants: 30%-40%	
	Newborns: 44%-64%	
Mean corpuscular volume (MCV)	Adults and children: 80-95 µ³	80-95 fl
	Newborns: 96-108 µ³	
Mean corpuscular hemoglobin (MCH)	Adults and children: 27-31 pg	0.42-0.48 fmol
	Newborns: 32-34 pg	

Continued

*The use of the System of International Units (SI) was recommended at the 30th World Health Assembly in 1977 to implement an international language of measurement. Because this system is being adopted by numerous laboratories, many of the common values are expressed in both conventional and SI units. SI units are calculated by multiplying the conventional unit by a number factor. The SI measurement system uses *moles* as the basic unit for the amount of a substance, *kilograms* for its mass, and *meter* for its length.

Blood, Plasma, or Serum Values—cont'd

Test	Reference Range	
	Conventional Values	SI Units*
Mean corpuscular hemoglobin concentration (MCHC)	Adults and children: 32-36 g/dl	0.32-0.36
	Newborns: 32-33 g/dl	
White blood cell (WBC) count	Adults and children >2 years: 5,000-10,000/mm³	
	Children ≤2 years; 6,200-17,000/mm³	
	Newborns: 9,000-30,000/mm³	
Differential count		
Neutrophils	55%-70%	
Lymphocytes	20%-40%	
Monocytes	2%-8%	
Eosinophils	1%-4%	
Basophils	0.5%-1%	
Platelet count	150,000-400,000/mm³	
Coombs' test		
Direct	Negative	Negative
Indirect	Negative	Negative
Copper (Cu)	70-140 µg/dl	11.0-24.3 µmol/L

Cortisol	6-28 μg/dl (AM)	170-635 nmol/L
	2-12 μg/dl (PM)	82-413 nmol/L
CPK isoenzyme (MB)	<5% total	
Creatinine	0.7-1.5 mg/dl	<133 μmol/L
Creatinine clearance	Men: 95-104 ml/min	<133 μmol/L
	Women: 95-125 ml/min	
Creatinine phosphokinase (CPK)	5-75 mU/ml	12-80 units/L
Cryoglobulin	Negative	Negative
Differential (WBC) count (see Complete blood count)		
Digoxin	Therapeutic level: 0.5-2.0 ng/ml	40-79 μmol/L
	Toxic level: >2.4 ng/ml	>119 μmol/L
Erythrocyte count (see Complete blood count)		
Erythrocyte sedimentation rate (ESR)	Men: up to 15 mm/hour	
	Women: up to 20 mm/hour	
	Children: up to 10 mm/hour	
Ethanol	80-200 mg/dl (mild to moderate intoxication)	17-43 mmol/L
	250-400 mg/dl (marked intoxication)	54-87 mmol/L
	>400 mg/dl (severe intoxication)	>87 mmol/L
Euglobulin lysis test	90 min-6 hours	
Fats	Up to 200 mg/dl	

*The use of the System of International Units (SI) was recommended at the 30th World Health Assembly in 1977 to implement an international language of measurement. Because this system is being adopted by numerous laboratories, many of the common values are expressed in both conventional and SI units. SI units are calculated by multiplying the conventional unit by a number factor. The SI measurement system uses *moles* as the basic unit for the amount of a substance, *kilograms* for its mass, and *meter* for its length.

Continued

Blood, Plasma, or Serum Values—cont'd

Test	Reference Range	
	Conventional Values	SI Units*
Ferritin	15-200 ng/dl	15-200 µg/L
Fibrin degradation products (FDP)	<10 µg/ml	
Fibrinogen (factor I)	200-400 mg/dl	5.9-11.7 µmol/L
Fibrinolysis/euglobulin lysis test	90 min-6 hours	
Fluorescent treponemal antibody (FTA)	Negative	Negative
Fluoride	<0.05 mg/dl	<0.027 mmol/L
Folic acid (Folate)	5-20 µg/ml	14-34 mmol/L
Follicle-stimulating hormone (FSH)	Men: 0.1-15.0 ImU/ml	
	Women: 6-30 ImU/ml	
	Children: 0.1-12.0 ImU/ml	
	Castrate and postmenopausal: 30-200 ImU/ml	
Free thyroxine index (FTI)	0.9-2.3 ng/dl	
Galactose-1-phosphate uridyl transferase	18.5-28.5 U/g hemoglobin	
Gammaglobulin	0.5-1.6 g/dl	
Gamma-glutamyl transpeptidase (GGTP)	Men: 8-38 U/L	5-40 U/L at 37° C
	Women: <45 years: 5-27 U/L	
Gastrin	40-150 pg/ml	40-150 ng/L
Glucagon	50-200 pg/ml	14-56 pmol/L

Test	Value	SI Units
Glucose, fasting (FBS)	Adults: 70-115 mg/dl Children: 60-100 mg/dl Newborns: 30-80 mg/dl	3.89-6.38 mmol/L
Glucose, 2-hour postprandial (2-hour PPG)	<140 mg/dl	
Glucose-6-phosphate dehydrogenase (G-6-PD)	8.6-18.6 IU/g of hemoglobin	
Glucose tolerance test (GTT)	Fasting: 70-115 mg/dl 30 min: <200 mg/dl 1 hour: <200 mg/dl 2 hours: <140 mg/dl 3 hours: 70-115 mg/dl 4 hours: 70-115 mg/dl	
Glycosylated hemoglobin	Adults: 2.2%-4.8% Children: 1.8%-4.0% Good diabetic control: 2.5%-6% Fair diabetic control: 6.1%-8% Poor diabetic control: >8%	
Growth hormone	<10 ng/ml	<10 µg/L
Haptoglobin	100-150 mg/dl	16-31 µmol/L

*The use of the System of International Units (SI) was recommended at the 30th World Health Assembly in 1977 to implement an international language of measurement. Because this system is being adopted by numerous laboratories, many of the common values are expressed in both conventional and SI units. SI units are calculated by multiplying the conventional unit by a number factor. The SI measurement system uses *moles* as the basic unit for the amount of a substance, *kilograms* for its mass, and *meter* for its length.

Continued

Blood, Plasma, or Serum Values—cont'd

Test	Reference Range	
	Conventional Values	SI Units*
Hematocrit (Hct)	Men: 42%-52%	
	Women: 37%-47% (pregnancy: >33%)	
	Children: 31%-43%	
	Infants: 30%-40%	
	Newborns: 44%-64%	
Hemoglobin (HgB)	Men: 14-18 g/dl	8.7-11.2 mmol/L
	Women: 12-16 g/dl (pregnancy: >11 g/dl)	7.4-9.9 mmol/L
	Children: 11-16 g/dl	
	Infants: 10-15 g/dl	
	Newborns: 14-24 g/dl	
Hemoglobin electrophoresis	Hgb A₁: 95%-98%	
	Hgb A₂: 2%-3%	
	Hgb F: 0.8%-2%	
	Hgb S: 0	
	Hgb C: 0	
Hepatitis B surface antigen (HB$_s$AG)	Nonreactive	Nonreactive
Heterophil antibody	Negative	Negative
HLA-B27	None	None

Test	Conventional	SI Units
Human chorionic gonadotropin (HCG)	Negative	Negative
Human placental lactogen (HPL)	Rise during pregnancy	
5-Hydroxyindoleacetic acid (5-HIAA)	2.8–8.0 mg/24 hours	
Immunoglobulin quantification	IgG: 550–1900 mg/dl	5.5–19.0 g/L
	IgA: 60–333 mg/dl	0.6–3.3 g/L
	IgM: 45–145 mg/dl	0.45–1.5 g/L
Insulin	4–20 μU/ml	36–179 pmol/L
Iron (Fe)	60–190 μg/dl	13–31 μmol/L
Iron-binding capacity, total (TIBC)	250–420 μg/dl	45–73 μmol/L
Iron (transferrin) saturation	30%–40%	
Ketone bodies	Negative	Negative
Lactic acid	0.6–1.8 mEq/L	0.4–1.7 μmol/s/L
Lactic dehydrogenase (LDH) isoenzymes	90–200 ImU/ml	
	LDH-1: 17%–27%	
	LDH-2: 28%–38%	
	LDH-3: 19%–27%	
	LDH-4: 5%–16%	
	LDH-5: 6%–16%	
Lead	120 μg/dl or less	<1.0 μmol/L
Leucine aminopeptidase (LAP)	Men: 80–200 U/ml	
	Women: 75–185 U/ml	

*The use of the System of International Units (SI) was recommended at the 30th World Health Assembly in 1977 to implement an international language of measurement. Because this system is being adopted by numerous laboratories, many of the common values are expressed in both conventional and SI units. SI units are calculated by multiplying the conventional unit by a number factor. The SI measurement system uses *moles* as the basic unit for the amount of a substance, *kilograms* for its mass, and *meter* for its length.

Continued

Blood, Plasma, or Serum Values—cont'd

Test	Reference Range		
	Conventional Values		SI Units*
Leukocyte count (see Complete blood count)			
Lipase	Up to 1.5 units/ml		0-417 U/L
Lipids			
Total	400-1000 mg/dl		4-8 g/L
Cholesterol	150-250 mg/dl		3.9-6.5 mmol/L
Triglycerides	40-150 mg/dl		0.4-1.5 g/L
Phospholipids	150-380 mg/dl		1.9-3.9 mmol/L
Lithium			
Long-acting thyroid-stimulating hormone (LATS)	Negative		Negative
Magnesium (Mg)	1.6-3.0 mEq/L		0.8-1.3 mm/L
Methanol	Negative		Negative
Mononucleosis spot test	Negative		Negative
Nitrogen, nonprotein	15-35 mg/dl		10.7-25.0 mmol/L
Nuclear antibody (ANA)	Negative		Negative
5'-Nucleotidase	Up to 1.6 units		27-233 nmol/s/L
Osmolality	275-300 mOsm/kg		

Oxygen saturation (arterial)	95%-100%	0.95-1.00 of capacity
Parathormone (PTH)	<2000 pg/ml	
Partial thromboplastin time, activated (APTT)	30-40 sec	
PCO_2	35-45 mm Hg	7.35-7.45
pH	7.35-7.45	
Phenylalanine	Up to 2 mg/dl	<0.18 mmol/L
Phenylketonuria (PKU)	Negative	Negative
Phenytoin (Dilantin)	Therapeutic level: 10-20 µg/ml	
Phosphatase (acid)	0.10-0.63 U/ml (Bessey-Lowry)	0.11-0.60 U/L
	0.5-2.0 U/ml (Bodansky)	
	1.0-4.0 U/ml (King-Armstrong)	
Phosphatase (alkaline)	Adults: 30-85 ImU/ml	20-90 units/L
	Children and adolescents:	
	<2 years: 85-235 ImU/ml	
	2-8 years: 65-210 ImU/ml	
	9-15 years: 60-300 ImU/ml (active bone growth)	
	16-21 years: 30-200 ImU/ml	
Phospholipids (see Lipids)		

*The use of the System of International Units (SI) was recommended at the 30th World Health Assembly in 1977 to implement an international language of measurement. Because this system is being adopted by numerous laboratories, many of the common values are expressed in both conventional and SI units. SI units are calculated by multiplying the conventional unit by a number factor. The SI measurement system uses *moles* as the basic unit for the amount of a substance, *kilograms* for its mass, and *meter* for its length.

Continued

Blood, Plasma, or Serum Values—cont'd

Test	Reference Range		SI Units*
	Conventional Values		
Phosphorus (P, PO₄)	Adults: 2.5-4.5 mg/dl		0.78-1.52 mmol/L
	Children: 3.5-5.8 mg/dl		1.29-2.26 mmol/L
Platelet count	150,000-400,000/mm³		
PO₂	80-100 mm Hg		
Potassium (K)	3.5-5.0 mEq/L		3.5-5.0 mmol/L
Progesterone	Men, prepubertal girls, and postmenopausal women: <2 ng/ml		6 nmol/L
	Women, luteal: peak >5 ng/ml		>16 nmol/L
Prolactin	2-15 ng/ml		2-15 µg/L
Prostate-specific antigen (PSA)	<4 ng/ml		
Protein (total)	6-8 g/dl		55-80 g/L
Albumin	3.2-4.5 g/dl		35-55 g/L
Globulin	2.3-3.4 g/dl		20-35 g/L
Prothrombin time (PT)	11.0-12.5 sec		11.0-12.5 sec
Pyruvate	0.3-0.9 mg/dl		34-103 µmol/L
Red blood cell count (see Complete blood count)			
Red blood cell indexes (see Complete blood count)			
Renin			

Reticulocyte count	Adults and children: 0.5%–2% of total erythrocytes	
	Infants: 0.5%–3.1% of total erythrocytes	
	Newborns: 2.5%–6.5% of total erythrocytes	
Rheumatoid factor	Negative	Negative
Rubella antibody test		
Salicylates	Negative	
	Therapeutic: 20–25 mg/dl (to age 10: 25–30 mg/dl)	1.4–1.8 mmol/L
	Toxic: >30 mg/dl (after age 60: >20 mg/dl)	>2.2 mmol/L
Schilling test (vitamin B_{12} absorption)	8%–40% excretion/24 hours	
Serologic test for syphilis (STS)	Negative (nonreactive)	
Serum glutamic oxaloacetic transaminase (SGOT, AST)	12–36 U/ml	
	5–40 IU/L	0.10–0.30 μmol/s/L
Serum glutamic-pyruvic transaminase (SGPT, ALT)	5–35 IU/L	0.5–0.43 μmol/s/L
Sickle cell	Negative	
Sodium (Na^+)	136–145 mEq/L	136–145 mmol/L
Sugar (see Glucose)		
Syphilis (see Serologic tests for syphilis, Fluorescent treponemal antibody, Venereal Disease Research Laboratory)		

*The use of the System of International Units (SI) was recommended at the 30th World Health Assembly in 1977 to implement an international language of measurement. Because this system is being adopted by numerous laboratories, many of the common values are expressed in both conventional and SI units. SI units are calculated by multiplying the conventional unit by a number factor. The SI measurement system uses *moles* as the basic unit for the amount of a substance, *kilograms* for its mass, and *meter* for its length.

Continued

Blood, Plasma, or Serum Values—cont'd

Test	Reference Range	
	Conventional Values	SI Units*
Testosterone	Men: 300-1200 ng/dl	10-42 nmol/L
	Women: 30-95 ng/dl	1.1-3.3 nmol/L
	Prepubertal boys and girls: 5-20 ng/dl	0.165-0.70 nmol/L
Thymol flocculation	Up to 5 units	
Thyroglobulin antibody (see Antithyroglobulin antibody)		
Thyroid-stimulating hormone (TSH)	1-4 µIU/ml	5 mU/L
	Neonates: <25 µIU/ml by 3 days	
Thyroxine (T₄)	Murphy-Pattee:	50-154 nmol/L
	Neonates: 10.1-20.1 µg/dl	
	1-6 years: 5.6-12.6 µg/dl	
	6-10 years: 4.9-11.7 µg/dl	
	>10 years: 4-11 µg/dl	
	Radioimmunoassay: 5-10 µg/dl	
Thyroxine-binding globulin (TBG)	12-28 µg/ml	129-335 nmol/L
Toxoplasmosis antibody titer		

Transaminase (see Serum glutamic-oxaloacetic transaminase, Serum glutamic pyruvic transaminase)	
Triglycerides	40-150 mg/dl	0.4-1.5 g/L
Triiodothyronine (T_3)	110-230 ng/dl	1.2-1.5 nmol/L
Triiodothyronine (T_3) resin uptake	25%-35%	
Tubular phosphate reabsorption (TPR)	80%-90%	
Urea nitrogen (see Blood urea nitrogen)	
Uric acid	Men: 2.1-8.5 mg/dl	0.15-0.48 mmol/L
	Women: 2.0-6.6 mg/dl	0.09-0.36 mmol/L
	Children: 2.5-5.5 mg/dl	
Venereal Disease Research Laboratory (VDRL)	Negative	Negative
Vitamin A	20-100 g/dl	0.7-3.5 μmol/L
Vitamin B_{12}	200-600 pg/ml	148-443 pmol/L
Vitamin C	0.6-1.6 mg/dl	23-57 μmol/L
Whole blood clot retraction (see Clot retraction)	
Zinc	50-150 μg/dl	

*The use of the System of International Units (SI) was recommended at the 30th World Health Assembly in 1977 to implement an international language of measurement. Because this system is being adopted by numerous laboratories, many of the common values are expressed in both conventional and SI units. SI units are calculated by multiplying the conventional unit by a number factor. The SI measurement system uses *moles* as the basic unit for the amount of a substance, *kilograms* for its mass, and *meter* for its length.

Continued

Urine Values

Test	Reference Range		SI Units*
	Conventional Values		
Acetone plus acetoacetate (ketone bodies)	Negative		Negative
Addis count (12-hour)	Adults:		Negative
	WBCs and epithelial cells: 1.8 million/12 hours		
	RBCs: 500,000/12 hours		
	Hyaline casts: Up to 5000/12 hours		
	Children:		
	WBCs: <1 million/12 hours		
	RBCs: <250,000/12 hours		
	Casts: >5000/12 hours		
	Protein: <20 mg/12 hours		
Albumin	Random: ≦8 mg/dl		Negative
	24-hour: 10-100 mg/24 hours		10-100 mg/24 hr
Aldosterone	2-16 µg/24 hours		5.5-72 nmol/24 hours
Alpha-aminonitrogen	0.4-1.0 g/24 hours		28-71 nmol/24 hours
Amino acid	50-200 mg/24 hours		
Ammonia (24-hour)	30-50 mEq/24 hours		30-50 nmol/24 hours
	500-1200 mg/24 hours		
Amylase	≦5000 Somogyi units/24 hours		6.5-48.1 U/hr
	3-35 IU/hour		

Arsenic (24-hour)	<50 µg/L	<0.65 mol/L
Ascorbic acid (vitamin C)	Random: 1-7 ng/dl	0.06-0.40 mmol/L
	24-hour: >50 mg/24 hours	>0.29 mmol/24 hours
Bacteria	None	None
Bence Jones protein	Negative	Negative
Bilirubin	Negative	Negative
Blood or hemoglobin	Negative	Negative
Borate (24-hour)	<2 mg/L	<32 µmol/L
Calcium	Random: 1 + turbidity	1 + turbidity
	24-hour: 1-300 mg (diet dependent)	
Catecholamines (24-hour)	Epinephrine: 5-40 µg/24 hours	<55 nmol/24 hours
	Norepinephrine: 10-80 µg/24 hours	
	Metanephrine: 24-96 µg/24 hours	<590 nmol/24 hours
	Normetanephrine: 75-375 µg/24 hours	0.5-8.1 µmol/24 hours
Chloride (24-hour)	140-250 mEq/24 hours	140-250 mmol/24 hours
Color	Amber-yellow	Amber-yellow
Concentration test (Fishberg test)	Specific gravity: >1.025	>1.025
	Osmolality: 850 mOsm/L	>850 mOsm/L

*The use of the System of International Units (SI) was recommended at the 30th World Health Assembly in 1977 to implement an international language of measurement. Because this system is being adopted by numerous laboratories, many of the common values are expressed in both conventional and SI units. SI units are calculated by multiplying the conventional unit by a number factor. The SI measurement system uses *moles* as the basic unit for the amount of a substance, *kilograms* for its mass, and *meter* for its length.

Continued

Urine Values—cont'd

Test	Reference Range	
	Conventional Values	SI Units*
Copper (CU) (24-hour)	Up to 25 µg/24 hours	0-0.4 µmol/24/hours
Coproporphyrin (24-hour)	100-300 µg/24 hours	150-460 nmol/24 hours
Creatine	Adults: <100 mg/24 hours or <6% creatinine	
	Pregnant women: ≦12%	
	Infants <1 year: equal to creatinine	
	Older children: ≦30% of creatinine	
Creatinine (24-hour)	15-25 mg/kg body wt/24 hours	0.13-0.22 nmol/kg⁻¹ body wt/24 hours
Creatinine clearance (24-hour)	Men: 90-140 ml/min	90-140 ml/min
	Women: 85-125 ml/min	85-125 ml/min
Crystals	Negative	Negative
Cystine or cysteine	Negative	Negative
Delta-aminolevulinic acid (ΔALA)	1-7 mg/24 hours	10-53 µmol/24 hours
Epinephrine (24-hour)	5-40 µg/24 hours	
Epithelial cells and casts	Occasional	Occasional
Estriol (24-hour)	>12 mg/24 hours	
Fat	Negative	Negative
Fluoride (24-hour)	<1 mg/24 hours	0.053 mmol/24 hours

Follicle-stimulating hormone (FSH) (24-hour)	Men: 2-12 IU/24 hours
	Women:
	   During menses: 8-60 IU/24 hours
	   During ovulation: 30-60 IU/24 hours
	   During menopause: >50 IU/24 hours	

Glucose	Negative	Negative
Granular casts	Occasional	Occasional
Hemoglobin and myoglobin	Negative	Negative
Homogentisic acid	Negative	Negative
Human chorionic gonadotropin (HCG)	Negative	Negative
Human placental lactogen (HPL)	Negative	Negative
Hyaline casts	Occasional	Occasional
17-Hydroxycorticosteroids (17-OCHS) (24-hour)	Men: 5.5-15.0 mg/24 hours Women: 5.0-13.5 mg/24 hours Children: lower than adult values	8.3-25 μmol/24 hours 5.5-22 μmol/24 hours
5-Hydroxyindoleacetic acid (5-HIAA, serotonin) (24-hour)	Men: 2-9 mg/24 hours Women: lower than men	10-47 μmol/24 hours
Ketones (see Acetone plus acetoacetate)		
17-Ketosteroids (17-KS) (24-hour)	Men: 8-15 mg/24 hours Women: 6-12 mg/24 hours	21-62 μmol/24 hours 14-45 μmol/24 hours

*The use of the System of International Units (SI) was recommended at the 30th World Health Assembly in 1977 to implement an international language of measurement. Because this system is being adopted by numerous laboratories, many of the common values are expressed in both conventional and SI units. SI units are calculated by multiplying the conventional unit by a number factor. The SI measurement system uses *moles* as the basic unit for the amount of a substance, *kilograms* for its mass, and *meter* for its length.
Continued

Urine Values—cont'd

Test	Reference Range		
	Conventional Values	SI Units*
17-Ketosteroids (17-KS) (24-hour)—cont'd	Children:		
	12-15 yr: 5-12 mg/24 hours		
	<12 yr: <5 mg/24 hours		
Lactose (24-hour)	14-40 mg/24 hours	41-116 μm	
Lead	<0.08 g/ml or <120 g/24 hours	0.39 μmol/L	
Leucine aminopeptidase (LAP)	2-18 U/24 hours		
Magnesium (24-hour)	6.8-8.5 mEq/24 hours	3.0-4.3 mmol/24 hours	
Melanin	Negative	Negative	
Odor	Aromatic	Aromatic	
Osmolality	500-800 mOsm/L	38-1400 mmol/kg water	
pH	4.6-8.0	4.6-8.0	
Phenolsulfonphthalein (PSP)	15 min: at least 25%	At least 0.25	
	30 min: at least 40%	At least 0.40	
	120 min: at least 60%	At least 0.60	
Phenylketonuria (PKU)	Negative	Negative	
Phenylpyruvic acid	Negative	Negative	
Phosphorus (24-hour)	0.9-1.3 g/24 hours	29-42 mmol/24 hours	
Porphobilinogen	Random: negative	Negative	
	24-hour: up to 2 mg/24 hours		

Test	Conventional	SI
Porphyrin (24-hour)	50-300 mg/24 hours	25-100 nmol/24 hours
Potassium (K+) (24-hour)	25-100 mEq/24 hours	
Pregnancy test	Positive in normal pregnancy or with tumors producing HCG	Positive in normal pregnancy or with tumors producing HCG
Pregnanediol	After ovulation: >1 mg/24 hours	>0.05 g/24 hours
Protein (albumin)	Random: ≤8 mg/dl	
	10-100 mg/24 hours	100-260 nmol/24 hours
Sodium (Na+) (24-hour)	100-260 mEq/24 hours	1.010-1.025
Specific gravity	1.010-1.025	
Steroids (see 17-Hydroxycorticosteroids, 17-Ketosteroids)		
Sugar (see Glucose)		
Titratable acidity (24-hour)	20-50 mEq/24 hours	20-50 mmol/24 hours
Turbidity	Clear	Clear
Urea nitrogen (24-hour)	6-17 g/24 hours	0.21-0.60 mol/24 hours
Uric acid (24-hour)	250-750 mg/24 hours	1.48-4.43 mmol/24 hours
Urobilinogen	0.1-1.0 Ehrlich U/dl	0.1-1.0 Ehrlich U/dl
Uroporphyrin	Negative	Negative
Vanillylmandelic acid (VMA) (24-hour)	1-9 mg/24 hours	
Zinc (24-hour)	0.20-0.75 mg/24 hours	<40 µmol/day

*The use of the System of International Units (SI) was recommended at the 30th World Health Assembly in 1977 to implement an international language of measurement. Because this system is being adopted by numerous laboratories, many of the common values are expressed in both conventional and SI units. SI units are calculated by multiplying the conventional unit by a number factor. The SI measurement system uses *moles* as the basic unit for the amount of a substance, *kilograms* for its mass, and *meter* for its length.

Index

Overview of CDC Hand Hygiene Guidelines

The Centers for Disease Control and Prevention recently released new recommendations for hand hygiene in health care settings. Hand hygiene is a term that applies to either handwashing, use of an antiseptic hand rub, or surgical hand antisepsis. Evidence suggests that hand antisepsis, the cleansing of hands with an antiseptic hand rub is more effective in reducing nosocomial infections than plain handwashing.

Follow these guidelines in the care of all patients

- Continue to wash hands with either a non-antimicrobial or an antimicrobial soap and water whenever the hands are visibly soiled.
- Use an alcohol-based hand rub to routinely decontaminate the hands in the following clinical situations: (Note: if alcohol-based hand rubs are not available, the alternative is hand washing)
  - Before and after client contact.
  - Before donning sterile gloves when inserting central intravascular catheters.
  - Before performing non-surgical invasive procedures (e.g., urinary catheter insertion, nasotracheal suctioning).
  - After contact with body fluids or excretions, mucous membranes, nonintact skin, and wound dressings.
  - If moving from a contaminated-body site (rectal area or mouth) to a clean-body site (surgical wound, urinary meatus) during client care.
  - After contact with inanimate objects (including medical equipment) in the immediate vicinity of the client.
  - After removing gloves.
- Before eating and after using a restroom, wash hands with a non-antimicrobial or an antimicrobial soap and water.
- Antimicrobial-impregnated wipes (i.e., towelettes) are not a substitute for using an alcohol-based hand rub or antimicrobial soap.
- If exposure to Bacillus anthracis is suspected or proven, wash hands with a non-antimicrobial or an antimicrobial soap and water. The physical action of washing and rinsing hands is recommended because alcohols, chlorhexidine, iodophors, and other antiseptic agents have poor activity against spores.

Method for decontaminating hands

When using an alcohol-based hand rub, apply product to palm of one hand and rub hands together, covering all surfaces of hands and fingers, until hands are dry. Follow the manufacturer's recommendations regarding the volume of product to use.

Follow these guidelines for surgical hand antisepsis

- Surgical hand antisepsis reduces the resident microbial count on the hands to a minimum.
  - The CDC recommends using an antimicrobial soap, and to scrub hands and forearms for the length of time recommended by the manufacturer, usually 2–6 minutes. The Association of Operating Room Nurses recommends 5 to 10 minutes. Refer to agency policy for time required.
  - When using an alcohol-based surgical hand-scrub product with persistent activity, follow the manufacturer's instructions. Before applying the alcohol solution, prewash hands and forearms with a non-antimicrobial soap and dry hands and forearms completely. After application of

the alcohol-based product as recommended, allow hands and forearms to dry thoroughly before donning sterile gloves.

General Recommendations for Hand Hygiene

- Use hand lotions or creams to minimize the occurrence of irritant contact dermatitis associated with hand antisepsis or handwashing.
- Do not wear artificial fingernails or extenders when having direct contact with clients at high risk (e.g., those in intensive-care units or operating rooms).
- Keep natural nails tips less than 1/4-inch long.
- Wear gloves when contact with blood or other potentially infectious materials, mucous membranes, and nonintact skin could occur.
- Remove gloves after caring for a client. Do not wear the same pair of gloves for the care of more than one client, and do not wash gloves between uses with different clients.
- Change gloves during client care if moving from a contaminated body site to a clean body site.

(From Centers for Disease Control and Prevention (Morbidity and Mortality Weekly Report [MMWR], October 25, 2002 51 (RR16): 1-44 www.cdc.gov/handhygiene)